Newborn Screening for Diseases and Disorders

Newborn Screening for Diseases and Disorders

Newborn Screening for Diseases and Disorders

Editor: Elizabeth Curling

AMERICAN
MEDICAL PUBLISHERS
www.americanmedicalpublishers.com

AMERICAN
MEDICAL PUBLISHERS
www.americanmedicalpublishers.com

Cataloging-in-Publication Data

Newborn screening for diseases and disorders / edited by Elizabeth Curling.
p. cm.
Includes bibliographical references and index.
ISBN 978-1-63927-754-4
1. Newborn screening. 2. Newborn infants--Diseases--Diagnosis. 3. Newborn infants--Medical examinations.
4. Newborn infants—Diseases--Treatment. 5. Child health services. I. Curling, Elizabeth.
RJ255.5 .N48 2023
618.920 1--dc23

American Medical Publishers,
41 Flatbush Avenue,
1st Floor, New York,
NY 11217, USA

ISBN 978-1-63927-754-4 (Hardback)

Contents

Preface

Newborn screening refers to tests that aim to find out the risk of developing uncommon but severe medical conditions that could affect the growth in infants. It seeks to identify metabolic, genetic and developmental disorders as early as possible. Newborn screening allows for rapid diagnosis of the conditions of newborns and then initiating treatment, at the earliest possible time. The forms of newborn screening tests include hearing test, blood tests and critical congenital heart disease screen. Infants undergo a simple blood test, as soon as they are born to look for conditions that do not manifest directly after birth. Galactosemia, biotinidase deficiency, maple syrup urine disease, congenital hypothyroidism, sickle cell disease, homocystinuria, hearing loss and congenital adrenal hyperplasia are a few of the conditions that may be detected during newborn screening tests. This book explores all the important aspects of newborn screening in the modern day. It provides comprehensive insights on newborn screening and its significance in the diagnosis of diseases and disorders. This book will prove to be immensely beneficial to students and researchers in the field of pediatrics.

The researches compiled throughout the book are authentic and of high quality, combining several disciplines and from very diverse regions from around the world. Drawing on the contributions of many researchers from diverse countries, the book's objective is to provide the readers with the latest achievements in the area of research. This book will surely be a source of knowledge to all interested and researching the field.

In the end, I would like to express my deep sense of gratitude to all the authors for meeting the set deadlines in completing and submitting their research chapters. I would also like to thank the publisher for the support offered to us throughout the course of the book. Finally, I extend my sincere thanks to my family for being a constant source of inspiration and encouragement.

Editor

Preface

Newborn screening refers to tests that aim to find out the risk of developing uncommon but severe medical conditions that could affect the growth in infants. It seeks to identify metabolic, genetic and developmental disorders as early as possible. Newborn screening allows for rapid diagnosis of the conditions of newborns and then initiating treatment, at the earliest possible time. The forms of newborn screening tests include hearing test, blood tests and critical congenital heart disease screen. Infants undergo a simple blood test, as soon as they are born to look for conditions that do not manifest directly after birth. Galactosemia, biotinidase deficiency, maple syrup urine disease, congenital hypothyroidism, sickle cell disease, homocystinuria, hearing loss and congenital adrenal hyperplasia are a few of the conditions that may be detected during newborn screening tests. This book explores all the important aspects of newborn screening in the modern day. It provides comprehensive insights on newborn screening and its significance in the diagnosis of diseases and disorders. This book will prove to be immensely beneficial to students and researchers in the field of pediatrics.

The researches compiled throughout the book are authentic and of high quality, combining several disciplines and from very diverse regions from around the world. Drawing on the contributions of many researchers from diverse countries, the book's objective is to provide the readers with the latest achievements in the area of research. This book will surely be a source of knowledge to all interested and researching the field.

In the end, I would like to express my deep sense of gratitude to all the authors for meeting the set deadlines in completing and submitting their research chapters. I would also like to thank the publisher for the support offered to us throughout the course of the book. Finally, I extend my sincere thanks to my family for being a constant source of inspiration and encouragement.

Editor

Next Generation Sequencing in Newborn Screening in the United Kingdom National Health Service

Julia C. van Campen [1,*,†,‡], Elizabeth S. A. Sollars [1,†], Rebecca C. Thomas [1,†], Clare M. Bartlett [1], Antonio Milano [1,§], Matthew D. Parker [1,||], Jennifer Dawe [1], Peter R. Winship [1], Gerrard Peck [1], Darren Grafham [1], Richard J. Kirk [1], James R. Bonham [2], Anne C. Goodeve [1,3] and Ann Dalton [1,*]

1 Sheffield Diagnostic Genetics Service (SDGS), Sheffield Children's NHS Foundation Trust, Western Bank, Sheffield S10 2TH, UK; elizabeth.sollars@nhs.net (E.S.A.S.); rebecca.thomas@sch.nhs.uk (R.C.T.); clare_gladding@yahoo.co.uk (C.M.B.); amilano@sidra.org (A.M.); matthew.parker@sheffield.ac.uk (M.D.P.); Jennifer.Dawe@sch.nhs.uk (J.D.); Peter.Winship@sch.nhs.uk (P.R.W.); Gerrard.Peck@lwh.nhs.uk (G.P.); darrengrafham@gmail.com (D.G.); Richard.Kirk@sch.nhs.uk (R.J.K.); a.goodeve@sheffield.ac.uk (A.C.G.)

2 Division of Pharmacy, Diagnostics and Genetics, Sheffield Children's NHS Foundation Trust, Western Bank, Sheffield S10 2TH, UK; Jim.Bonham@sch.nhs.uk

3 Department of Infection, Immunity & Cardiovascular Disease, Faculty of Medicine, Dentistry & Health, University of Sheffield Medical School, Beech Hill Road, Sheffield S10 2RX, UK

* Correspondence: julia.vancampen@gstt.nhs.uk (J.C.v.C.); anndalton2015@gmail.com (A.D.)

† These authors contributed equally to this work.

‡ Present address: Genetics Centre, Guy's Hospital, Great Maze Pond, London SE1 9RT, UK.

§ Present address: Pathology Department, Sidra Medicine, Main Hospital, H2M-24091, PO Box 26999, Doha, Qatar.

|| Present address: Sheffield Bioinformatics Core, Sheffield Biomedical Research Centre, The University of Sheffield, Western Bank, Sheffield S10 2TN, UK.

Abstract: Next generation DNA sequencing (NGS) has the potential to improve the diagnostic and prognostic utility of newborn screening programmes. This study assesses the feasibility of automating NGS on dried blood spot (DBS) DNA in a United Kingdom National Health Service (UK NHS) laboratory. An NGS panel targeting the entire coding sequence of five genes relevant to disorders currently screened for in newborns in the UK was validated on DBS DNA. An automated process for DNA extraction, NGS and bioinformatics analysis was developed. The process was tested on DBS to determine feasibility, turnaround time and cost. The analytical sensitivity of the assay was 100% and analytical specificity was 99.96%, with a mean 99.5% concordance of variant calls between DBS and venous blood samples in regions with ≥30× coverage (96.8% across all regions; all variant calls were single nucleotide variants (SNVs), with indel performance not assessed). The pipeline enabled processing of up to 1000 samples a week with a turnaround time of four days from receipt of sample to reporting. This study concluded that it is feasible to automate targeted NGS on routine DBS samples in a UK NHS laboratory setting, but it may not currently be cost effective as a first line test.

Keywords: newborn screening; next generation sequencing; automation

---

1. Introduction

Newborn screening (NBS) programmes worldwide provide early diagnosis and intervention for infants affected with rare disorders which, if untreated, are associated with progressive deterioration, disability and potentially fatal outcomes [1]. In the UK, NBS is carried out through measurement of biomarkers in a dried blood spot (DBS) taken 5–8 days after birth [2–8]. Currently, DNA testing is only undertaken as a second line test in the NBS protocol for cystic fibrosis, as part of the follow-up diagnostic protocol for suspected cases of medium-chain acyl-coenzyme A dehydrogenase deficiency (MCADD), isovaleric acidaemia (IVA) and glutaric aciduria type 1 (GA1) and for further characterisation of a subset of suspected haemoglobinopathy cases [3,6,9]. However, the advent of next generation sequencing (NGS) has resulted in attempts to expand the use of DNA sequencing in NBS to improve diagnostic and prognostic utility [10–13]. Several key features of NGS make it a potentially powerful technology in NBS. A single assay can be used for a range of disorders regardless of whether a biochemical marker is available; simultaneous analysis of large numbers of genetic loci and samples can drive down costs; and laboratory processes can largely be automated. The increasing trend toward provision of genetic laboratory services in larger centralised units in the UK has the potential to enable greater access to high throughput NGS technology. Thus, it is timely and relevant to investigate the potential of NGS in NBS in a UK NHS context.

1.1. Next Generation Sequencing in Newborn Screening: Genome Wide or Targeted Assays?

Routine NGS in healthy newborns has predominantly gained attention through studies proposing whole exome sequencing (WES) or whole genome sequencing (WGS) as a first line screening test [12,13]. These studies have shown that WES and WGS from DBS samples are technically feasible; that WGS can identify a wider range of disorders than current NBS methods and may, in some cases, yield fewer false positives and that, although ethical concerns exist, there is considerable interest in it from parents of healthy newborns in the postpartum period [12–14].

However, using a targeted NGS panel, where only a subset of genetic loci is analysed rather than a WGS approach, has advantages over WGS. Compared to WGS/WES, targeted approaches minimize the amount of sequence to be covered, reducing data processing time and data storage cost, thus reducing the cost per sample and turnaround time. The inclusion of loci relevant to additional screening disorders could likely be achieved rapidly through NGS panel expansion where necessary.

Two possible targeted approaches can be defined: the entire coding sequence of a selected set of genes can be analysed or analysis can be limited to a panel of known pathogenic variants. The key trade-off in defining how targeted to make any NGS-based NBS assay is that of ease of interpretation versus diagnostic sensitivity. Targeted NGS, especially if only a panel of known variants is analysed, has the benefit of limiting the number of variants of uncertain significance found and the time required for interpretation. However, clinical sensitivity may be unacceptably reduced by only targeting a known panel of variants. Given these considerations, this study took a semi-targeted approach, with the entire coding sequence of a selected set of genes analysed.

1.2. Applications of NGS in NBS as an Adjunct Test or Primary Screening Test

Next generation sequencing has the potential to benefit NBS in two modalities, namely, a) as an adjunct test to enhance the utility of current NBS protocols or b) as a primary (first line) screening test used to detect disorders deemed suitable for NBS, but with no existing biochemical marker. The approach described in this study could be used in either modality.

As an adjunct test, DNA sequencing can aid clarification of ambiguous or borderline biochemical screening results. Adjunct genetic testing may also improve the prognostic utility of NBS results, particularly for inborn errors of metabolism, in which variable presentation is a key feature [15–26]. Currently, the correct treatment option can be difficult to determine in asymptomatic screen-positive infants [16,22,23]. This can lead to less effective treatment or to unnecessary medicalisation of healthy infants. Adjunct DNA sequencing can pinpoint those screen positive cases which have a mild variant of the disorder and may not require any clinical intervention, such as IVA cases with the benign c.941C>T variant or MCADD cases with the mild c.199T>C variant [25,26]. It also enables precision medicine, for example, in selecting optimal treatment for cystic fibrosis patients [27–29].

Alternatively, DNA sequencing may be used as a first line NBS test, particularly for disorders not amenable to biochemical analysis. A timely rare disease diagnosis can prevent the cost and distress associated with an extensive diagnostic odyssey [30–33]. In addition to the impact on the health and wellbeing of the affected newborn, many rare diseases are heritable, and rapid diagnosis of an infant proband can thus have an impact on relatives' reproductive decisions [33]. The number of candidate NBS disorders may increase in the future as therapeutic progress opens up new avenues for treatment of rare disorders currently deemed untreatable [34–38].

1.3. Development of a Rapid Targeted NGS Assay Utilising DBS DNA

As the collection and analysis of the DBS is at the core of the UK NBS programme, any novel NBS assay must work robustly on this sample [2–6]. Liquid capillary heel prick sampling alternatives are available and would potentially yield better quality DNA than DBS. However, their introduction would require a major change to the UK NBS process, which is not currently anticipated. Targeted NGS from DBS samples has been previously described, but no targeted automated assay is currently available at scale, at a cost, and in a sufficiently fast turnaround time to be appropriate for NBS in a UK National Health Service context [10,11,39–41]. Previous work has described manual DNA extraction and library preparation from DBS, automated DNA extraction from DBS followed by manual NGS library preparation or protocols only suitable for the processing of relatively small numbers of samples at once [11,41]. However, DNA in DBS is stable and analytical validity is independent of the baby's age, condition, feeding or gestation. As such, DBS samples are highly suitable for NBS using targeted NGS. The current study evaluated the technical feasibility and cost of automated, high throughput, fast turnaround, targeted NGS on DBS samples in the UK using a targeted AmpliSeq NGS panel assay and Ion Torrent (semiconductor) sequencing [42].

2. Materials and Methods

2.1. Sample Collection

The DBS samples were taken by an experienced midwife from fingertips of adult healthy volunteers who were not affected by any of the disorders analysed and did not have a family history of these disorders. All subjects gave their informed consent for the sharing of anonymised data outside the study. The study was conducted in accordance with the Declaration of Helsinki, and the protocol was approved by the London-Brent Research Ethics Committee (REC reference 14/LO/1715) and the UK Health Research Authority (IRAS ID 159179). The DBS samples were stored at room temperature for up to two weeks prior to extraction and sequencing. Six-millimetre disks were punched from Guthrie cards (Perkin Elmer 226) using the Panthera DBS Puncher (Perkin Elmer) into 0.8 mL 96 well plates (Thermo Fisher Scientific, Altrincham, UK). The DNA contamination of the punch head through repeated punching of DBS disks was found not to be an issue (Figure S1).

2.2. DNA Extraction

For extraction of DNA from venous blood, Qiagen DSP DNA kits were used with the Qiasymphony liquid handling platform (Qiagen, Manchester, UK). For extraction of DNA from DBS, the United States Centers for Disease Control and Prevention (CDC) DBS DNA extraction method [43] was modified and automated using a custom program on the Biomek FXp liquid handling platform (Beckmann Coulter, Brea, CA, USA) (Figure S2). Single 6 mm DBS punches in a 0.8 mL 96 well plate covered with a pierceable adhesive plastic seal were used as the input material. Following the addition of the final 60 uL of Qiagen Elution Solution, plates were covered with a non-pierceable adhesive plastic seal and incubated at 99 °C for 15 min. The eluate was then transferred into a new 96 well plate using the Biomek FXp liquid handling platform.

2.3. Panel Design and Validation

A custom targeted Ion AmpliSeq panel (WG_IAD48658, hereafter referred to as the "NBS2" panel) was designed to cover all coding regions of the following genes associated with disorders screened for in the UK: *ACADM* (Medium Chain Acyl Co-A Dehydrogenase Deficiency), *PAH* (phenylketonuria), *TSHR* (congenital hypothyroidism), *CFTR* (cystic fibrosis) and *HBB* (sickle cell disease). The panel also covers 3′ untranslated regions (UTRs) of these genes and extends 5 bp either side of each exon. The total size of the panel was 50.054 kb (see Supplementary Materials Data S2, NBS2 panel. BED file for genomic coordinates).

Validation of the panel was carried out according to the American College of Medical Genetics (ACMG) Guidelines for Targeted Sequencing [44], with library preparation carried out manually according to the standard Ion AmpliSeq protocol (Thermo Fisher Scientific; [45]). Sequencing of two high-confidence cell line DNA truth sets was undertaken on the Ion S5 sequencer (Thermo Fisher Scientific), namely, "Genome in a Bottle" (GIAB, sample NA12878, Corriell), with truth set of variants generated by Zook et al. 2014 [46], and the Human Reference Genome (HuRef; sample GM25430, Corriell), with truth set of variants generated by Mu et al. 2015 [47]. Thirty-two DBS samples from healthy controls were also sequenced on the Ion S5 sequencer. In addition, 66 paired venous blood and DBS samples from 33 healthy controls were sequenced on the Ion PGM sequencer (Thermo Fischer Scientific, Altrincham, UK) to assess concordance of variant calling (defined as the percentage of variants matching) between DBS and venous blood DNA samples.

2.4. Semi-Automated Library Preparation

Semi-automated library preparation was carried out using the AmpliSeq library preparation protocol (Thermo Fischer Scientific) modified for automation using the Biomek FXp and Biomek NXp liquid handling platforms (Beckmann Coulter) (Figure S3). Three microlitres of undiluted DBS DNA extracted using the automated CDC DBS DNA extraction method was used immediately after extraction in the initial AmpliSeq reaction, and 2 uL HiFi Mastermix and 5 uL primer pool were added to this in 96 well plates using the Biomek Fxp liquid handling platform. The "NBS2" AmpliSeq panel used is made up of two primer pools; as such, two reactions were set-up per sample. After amplification (two minutes at 99 °C, followed by 22 cycles of 15 s at 99 °C and four minutes at 60 °C), the two pools were combined manually and 2 µL FuPa was added manually. Samples were incubated at 50 °C for 10 min, 55 °C for 10 min, and 60 °C for 20 min. Within an hour of the end of this incubation, 4 µL Switch solution, 2 µL DNA Ligase and 1.5 µL of a unique molecular barcode were added to each sample using the Biomek NXp automated liquid handling platform. This reaction was incubated at 22 °C for 30 min, followed by heat inactivation at 72 °C for 10 min. At this stage, library quality and molarity were assessed (TapeStation 2200, Agilent). Library products with sizes between 150 bp and 450 bp were included in molarity determination. Equimolar library pooling was carried out using a custom spreadsheet application and the Biomek NXp liquid handling platform. Assessment of the concentration of input DBS DNA samples or the molarity of each initial AmpliSeq library pool (after the first amplification step) were not found to improve performance during routine high throughput processing; therefore, these steps were omitted from the final process.

2.5. Chip Loading and Sequencing

Chip loading was carried out using the Ion Chef liquid handling platform (Thermo Fisher Scientific), with 96 NBS2 panel libraries loaded per Ion 540 chip. Seven high throughput sequencing runs were carried out: four on the Ion S5 sequencer and three on the Ion S5 Prime sequencer (Thermo Fisher Scientific). The run plan had the following parameters: analysis parameters: default; reference library: hg19; target regions: NBS2 panel BED file; hotspot regions: none; read length: 200 bp; flows: 500; base calibration mode: default. The plugins used were coverageAnalysis, DataExport and variantCaller.

2.6. Data Analysis

Read mapping was performed automatically in TorrentSuite (v5.2 for S5 runs and v5.8 for S5 Prime runs). Indel re-alignment was carried out using the command-line version of TMAP (ThermoFisher) using v5.2 for S5 runs and v5.4 for S5 Prime runs. Variant calling was then performed using the command-line version of TVC (ThermoFisher) using v5.2 for S5 runs and v5.4 for S5 Prime runs, and v.5.8 for the DBS versus VB comparison. The following parameters were changed from default to improve variant calling sensitivity: Minimum variant score (quality) = 10, minimum allele frequency = 0.1, minimum coverage = 10, min coverage each strand = 0, maximum strand bias = 1 and strand bias *p*-value = 0, homopolymer maximum length = 9 bp. Variant calling was performed on the designed panel regions (WG_IAD48658), decomposed and normalised using vt (v0.5772), and then restricted down to the NBS2 panel regions (exon ± 5 bp) using the Bedtools (v2.25.0) "intersect" command [48,49]. Base-by-base coverage across the NBS2 panel was ascertained using the Sambamba (v0.6.7) "depth base" command [50].

Sequencing quality of the NBS2 panel regions was evaluated using "% bases with 50x coverage" cut-offs of 90% (samples below this were deemed to have failed), 97% (samples in this range may have gaps) and 99.5% (samples above this are unlikely to have substantial gaps). Comparison of variant calls from cell lines to their respective truth sets was performed using the Bcftools (v1.3.1) "isec" command [50,51].

3. Results

3.1. Validation of the Custom Targeted Ion AmpliSeq Panel for Use on DBS DNA

The genes targeted by our custom NGS panel were selected for proof of principle following discussion with the National Screening Committee and alignment with the existing UK screening programmes; development of alternative screening programmes by NGS was not a project aim. The designed panel covered 3′ UTRs of these genes and extended 5 bp either side of each exon. No additional intronic regions were targeted to maximise coverage of exonic regions and to facilitate rapid and unambiguous interpretation in the context of NBS. We used the Ion Torrent S5 XL platform, as the rapid amplicon-based library preparation enables a fast turnaround time; it has the potential for good cost effectiveness and it affords a high degree of sample multiplexing and, thus, throughput.

The NBS2 panel was validated using cell line truth sets as well as DNA from both venous blood (VB) and DBS (Figure S4 and S5). The overall analytical sensitivity of the panel across both cell line truth sets (GIAB and HuRef) was 100%, specificity was 99.96% and Matthew's correlation coefficient was 0.963, with 85 unique variants matching the truth sets sequenced. There were 130 correctly called true positive variants, 49,905 true negative reference calls and no false negative (missed) calls. Out of a total of ten false positive calls across the GIAB and HuRef samples, eight were in the same intronic short tandem repeat (STR) region upstream of exon 8 of the *TSHR* gene, which would be excluded in a targeted analysis in which only exons ± 5 bp would be analysed. All true variants in these cell line samples were SNVs; no data on analytical sensitivity or specificity for indels are available. Low coverage areas were limited in number. There was one small exonic region that had an average coverage below 30× (part of *TSHR* exon 10) and another that had an average coverage between 30 and 50× (*CFTR* exon 1), with all other regions having an average coverage of ≥50× (Figure S4).

Mean concordance of variant calling between sequencing from VB DNA and DBS DNA was 96.8% (99.5% in regions of >30× read depth, based on 3166 variant calls in 33 paired samples), with a total of 215 unique variants displaying concordance between venous blood and DBS samples (Figure 1; Table S1). Discordant variants were not correctly called for a variety of reasons including low allele frequency causing false positives and STR regions causing misalignments. Out of a total of 3166 variant calls, four false positive SNVs were called in DBS (of which three were in areas with a coverage ≤30×), two false positive SNVs were called in VB (both in areas with a coverage ≤30×), 29 SNVs were missed in DBS (DBS false negatives; of which 26 in areas with a coverage ≤30×), and 38 SNVs were missed in VB (VB false negatives; of which 36 in areas with a coverage ≤30×). There were five false positive indel calls in DBS (one of which was in an area with a coverage ≤30×; the other four calls were all at the same position in a poly-T tract) and no false positive indel calls in VB. There was one indel present in two individuals for whom paired DBS and VB samples were analysed (Phe508del, the common pathogenic variant in the *CFTR* gene). This indel was correctly called from both VB and DBS samples for both individuals. The panel met the ACGS acceptance criteria for NGS panels (Supplementary Materials Section S4, Figure S4, and Table S1; [44]) and was validated as suitable for sequencing from DBS DNA as well as from VB DNA.

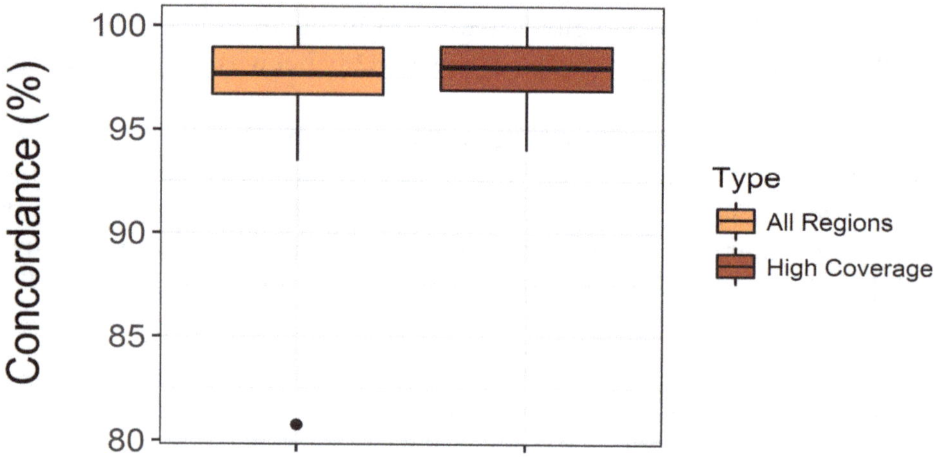

Figure 1. Concordance of variant calls, dried blood spot (DBS) versus venous blood. Variant calls were compared in both the whole panel ("All Regions") or in regions with coverage over 50× only ("High Coverage"). $n = 33$.

3.2. Performance of Semi-Automated Next Generation Sequencing from DBS

Libraries were prepared from healthy control venous blood (VB) samples manually and using a semi-automated process. This semi-automated process was found to result in improved uniformity and an improved percentage of reads on target compared to manual library preparation (Figure S6).

Libraries were also prepared from DBS using semi-automated processes for DNA extraction and library preparation. Four runs of 96 samples were carried out on the Ion S5 sequencer (Figure S7) and three runs of 96 samples were carried out on the Ion S5 Prime sequencer (Figure 2). Automated DNA extraction yielded DNA of a satisfactory concentration (0.79–1.77 ng/µL) in 96/96 samples in run 1 and 95/96 samples in run 2 (S5 runs). Across the three S5 Prime runs, 78% of samples (225/288) had 50× coverage for ≥99.5% of bases, 92% of samples (264/288) had 50× coverage for ≥97% of bases and 98% of samples (281/288) had 50× coverage for ≥90% of bases.

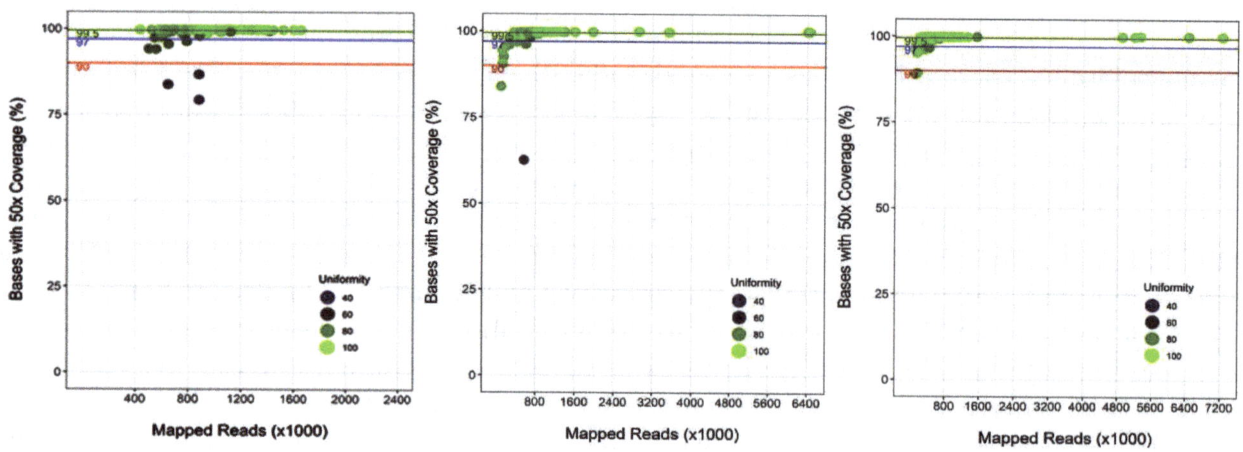

Figure 2. Quality of three high throughput sequencing runs (96 samples per run) from dried blood spots (Ion S5 Prime). Libraries were prepared using the semi-automated AmpliSeq library preparation process.

3.3. *Timeline for High Throughput Sequencing from DBS*

Using this semi-automated sequencing pipeline, up to 192 (2 × 96) libraries can be prepared from DBS DNA in one day, with the entire process from booking on of samples to reporting of results fitting into a four-day turnaround time (Figure 3; Figure S8). Booking on of Guthrie cards, DBS punching, DNA extraction and the initial step of AmpliSeq library preparation were carried out on day 1; FuPa digestion, barcode ligation, library quality control, equimolar library pooling and chip loading on day 2; sequencing and data processing on day 3; and data analysis and reporting on day 4. Repeated daily in the context of a seven-day service, this pipeline was capable of processing over 1000 samples per week. The cost of this semi-automated process including punching of samples, DNA extraction, library preparation and sequencing was calculated at approximately £62.41/sample (including labour) or £60.58/sample (excluding labour), based on a full run of 96 samples per sequencer chip (with a repeat rate of 3/96 samples).

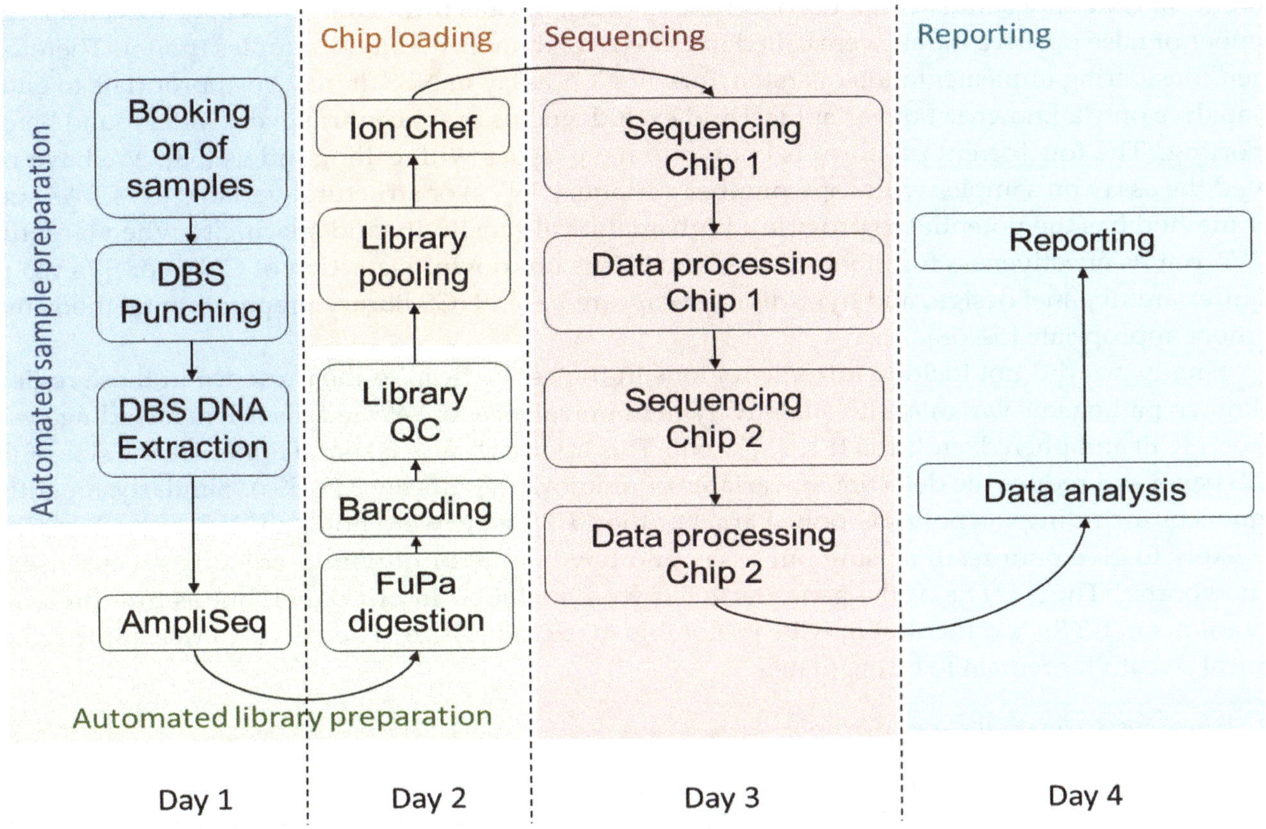

Figure 3. Timeline for automated fast turnaround time NGS from DBS. Booking on of samples and DNA extraction were carried out on Day 1. Automated AmpliSeq library preparation was initiated on Day 1 and PCR was run overnight. FuPa digestion (manual pooling and FuPa enzyme addition), automated barcoding, automated library QC, and automated library pooling were carried out on Day 2. The Ion Chef was used for automated loading of libraries onto sequencing chips overnight on Day 2. Sequencing and data processing were carried out on Day 3, with data analysis (assuming all samples were run in parallel) and reporting on Day 4.

4. Discussion

We set out to explore the feasibility of targeted NGS from DBS as a high throughput NBS assay using a semi-automated protocol. The only step of NGS library preparation that was not automated was the addition of the FuPa enzyme, which is highly viscous and, in our hands, not amenable to automated liquid handling. A fully automated library preparation process would be preferable for assay robustness and avoidance of operator error, although the difference in time required would be negligible. Alternative rapid, potentially fully automatable amplicon-based library preparation methods are now also available for other NGS platforms [52]. Our assay was developed in a UK NHS diagnostic genetics laboratory, and this study provides proof of principle that targeted NGS can be carried out in this setting on a scale and in a timeframe compatible with the demands of routine NBS. However, the cost of the assay is not currently comparable to that of existing biochemical assays used in first line screening.

4.1. Assay Performance

The assay has an analytical sensitivity of 100% and analytical specificity of 99.96% (figures are for SNVs only; the number of indels called was too low to estimate figures for this variant class). When comparing VB and DBS sequencing, we found good concordance between sample types (96.8% in all areas or 99.5% excluding areas with ≤30× coverage). The vast majority of the discrepancies between VB and DBS samples were false negative SNV calls (in both DBS and VB) due to the low coverage; there were generally similar numbers of erroneous variant calls from DBS and VB; however, a larger number of false positive indels were called in DBS (five) than in VB blood samples (none). Therefore, when considering implementation of an Ion Torrent NGS assay in NBS, it may be appropriate to either (a) analyse only a known set of variant loci and exclude indels or (b) confirm every indel found before reporting. The Ion Torrent platform is known to have issues with calling indels [53]. We have not tested the assay on samples with copy number variants (CNVs) or structural variants (SVs). As such, our method has the potential to provide a high analytical sensitivity and specificity when targeting SNVs, but its effectiveness for indels, CNVs and SVs is unknown. Detection of CNVs or SVs would require careful panel design, and hybridisation capture-based NGS library preparation methods may be more appropriate [54–58].

Finally, we did not include intronic regions in the assay, despite the presence in these regions of known pathogenic variants with a relatively high prevalence for selected disorders including cystic fibrosis (CF) and phenylketonuria (PKU) [59,60]. This approach was taken to minimise the size of the NGS panel and reduce the detection of variants of unknown significance (VUSs). Similarly, repetitive sequences including the poly-TG poly-T tract of the *CFTR* gene were not included, as such regions are likely to give poor results using our assay and have limited utility in predicting severe disease in newborns. The 3′UTRs of the genes targeted were included in our panel, but as interpretation of variants in UTRs is difficult it may be preferable to exclude them. The effects of this approach on clinical sensitivity remain to be evaluated.

4.2. Turnaround Time of the Assay

A robust fast turnaround time is essential for any NBS assay. In total across the three runs, we estimated that 92% (with ≥97% of bases having 50× coverage) to 98% (with ≥90% of bases having 50× coverage) of samples had sequencing data of sufficient quality for clinical interpretation within a four-day turnaround time, without the need for repeat testing or Sanger sequencing confirmation of variants found. Any samples requiring repeat testing would have a turnaround time of at least eight days.

For adjunct genetic testing, the NGS assay described here could be carried out within a turnaround time compatible with current UK requirements [61]. However, a faster turnaround time would be required if the assay were to be used as a first line test. Currently, in the UK, the target time of the first clinical appointment for screen positive babies is by 17 days of age (metabolic disorders), with longer times to first clinical appointment acceptable for CF (28 days of age) and for screen negative results (issued within six weeks) [61]. This is particularly challenging in the light of the fact that the DBS sample is not taken until 5–8 days of age. If the DBS sample were taken at birth, this would allow for earlier initiation of the laboratory assay, enabling current target times to the first appointment to be met.

This study provides a proof of principle that a targeted NGS assay on DBS samples can be automated such that over 1000 samples a week can be processed. This throughput would require a seven-day lab service, with two 96 sample runs set-up daily and overlapping four-day periods of sample processing. A doubling of the capacity to 2000 samples per week is feasible with duplicate key equipment (Ion Chef and S5 Prime sequencer). In the UK, the average newborn screening laboratory tests around 50,000 babies tested per year, an achievable throughput using our setup [61].

4.3. Cost of High throughput NGS for NBS

The cost of this assay was approximately £71.14/sample. This included booking on samples, DBS punching, DNA extraction, the NGS assay, equipment and labour. Variant interpretation and reporting costs are excluded as an automated process is likely required (not developed in this study). Our cost estimate was based on a full run of 96 samples per sequencer chip, required for economies of scale. Given the current cost per sample (approximately £25 per baby including equipment, staffing, biochemical assays and reporting, Jim Bonham, personal communication), the NGS assay developed here is unlikely to be deemed cost effective as a first line NBS test in the UK in its current form.

However, sampling at birth could result in a major cost saving compared to current practice. This would avoid the community midwife visit at day 5–8, the costliest element of UK NBS, in all hospital births (97.7% of births, 2013 [62]). Secondly, NGS may offer a cost saving by the avoidance of carrier status reporting in recessive disorders. In NBS cases in which only a single pathogenic variant is found in a gene with an autosomal recessive inheritance pattern, this variant could be filtered out before raw data are reported on by the analyst. In cystic fibrosis screening in a UK context, where the laboratory guide to NBS for cystic fibrosis states: "The UK protocol is intended to minimise detection of unaffected heterozygotes", such filtering may be considered desirable [5]. This could lead to a reduced requirement for second bloodspots at day 21 (~84% of which currently result in a "cystic fibrosis not suspected" report [61]) and a reduction in requests for genetic counselling in unaffected carriers. This would improve the cost effectiveness of the screening pathway. In other screening contexts or populations with high consanguinity, reporting carrier status may be considered beneficial, and a reporting pipeline appropriate to the screening context should be designed.

4.4. Expansion of Newborn Screening through Targeted NGS as a First Line Test

As the cost of targeted NGS falls, it has the potential to allow for expansion of NBS to disorders for which a suitable screening technology is currently not available. Targeted sequencing rather than a genome- or exome-wide approach enables addition of screening programmes to continue on a disorder-by-disorder basis, as is currently preferred by the UK National Screening Committee, rather than in response to any technological imperative [63–67]. A targeted analysis also reduces the risk of incidental findings [68–71]. Targeted rather than genome scale sequencing may also help prevent any drop in screening uptake due to the fact of parental fears of inappropriate use of genetic data [72,73].

The degree to which any NBS-based NGS assay should be targeted requires careful thought. Analysing the entire coding sequence of selected genes has the advantage of increasing sensitivity, as all coding variants are likely to be detected, including rare or previously unseen variants. However, variant interpretation is time consuming and the return of VUSs is undesirable. Reporting of VUSs carries a risk of unnecessary medicalisation of false positive or ambiguous screening cases, the avoidance of which is key to UK screening policy [7,61]. This is especially relevant for disorders with a high degree of genetic or allelic variation or with variable penetrance [74–76]. Variant interpretation in NBS would be complicated by the absence of phenotype information or family segregation studies. It may be possible to ameliorate these issues by developing adjunct biochemical or RNA testing on either DBS or liquid blood samples and by developing a thorough understanding of genotype–phenotype correlations in candidate NBS disorders [77–84].

An alternative way of using NGS in NBS is to target specific genetic variants, rather than analysing the entire coding sequence of genes [11,81,82]. A major advantage of this approach is that the number of newborns in whom a VUS is detected can be reduced to zero. However, this approach may limit clinical sensitivity, as rare or previously unseen variants would go undetected. As new treatment options for rare diseases become available, studies of genotype–treatment response correlations may inform which subset of pathogenic/likely pathogenic variants are considered actionable and, therefore, which variants to include in any targeted panel [27,85–88].

The analytical platform studied here could be used for the analysis of either the entire coding sequence of a set of genes, or of only a selected set of variants. Further studies on the two approaches would be needed to assess the optimal balance of clinical sensitivity and ease of interpretation.

5. Summary

Here, we have demonstrated that it is technically feasible to perform targeted NGS on DBS DNA with a sufficiently high throughput and fast turnaround time that the assay could be used in a UK NBS pathway. To assess clinical sensitivity and specificity, the implementation of any targeted NGS assay for NBS should be carefully evaluated through pilot studies in the population to be screened [82,83]. This assessment was not an aim of our study. Further work would be required using samples from both affected patients (with as wide a range of variant types as is relevant to the disorder to be screened for) and a cohort representative of the population to be screened. Although the aim of this study was to assess the potential of targeted NGS in routine NBS, targeted NGS from DBS may also be applicable in a range of other clinical pathways [89–91]. This assay thus provides a basis for further work to develop cost effective, fast, high throughput targeted NGS from DBS.

Supplementary Materials:
Figure S1: Absence of DNA contamination on punch head; Figure S2: Automated DNA extraction protocol for dried blood spots; Figure S3: Semi-automated protocol for AmpliSeq library preparation; Figure S4: Average coverage for 30 dried blood spot samples across exons in the NBS2 panel; Figure S5: Percentage of amplicons with 100× coverage, reads on target and uniformity in dried blood spot (DBS) versus venous blood (VB) samples; Figure S6: Sequencing quality metrics, manual versus automated library preparation; Figure S7: Quality of high throughput sequencing from dried blood spots on Ion S5 sequencer; Figure S8: Detailed timings for automated dried blood spot DNA extraction, AmpliSeq library preparation, Ion Chef chip loading and sequencing; Table S1: Comparison of variant calls from venous blood (VB) and blood spot (DBS) extraction methods for 33 samples, Supplementary Materials 2, NBS2 panel .BED file.

Author Contributions: Conceptualization, J.R.B. and A.D.; Funding acquisition, D.G., J.R.B., A.C.G. and A.D.; Project administration, C.M.B.; Supervision, C.M.B., M.D.P., R.J.K., J.R.B. and A.D.; Methodology, A.M., J.D. and D.G.; Validation, J.C.v.C., R.C.T., P.R.W. and G.P.; Formal analysis, J.C.v.C., E.S.A.S. and M.D.P.; Writing—Original draft, J.C.v.C. and E.S.A.S.; Writing—Review and editing, J.C.v.C., E.S.A.S., R.C.T., D.G., R.J.K., J.R.B. and A.D.

Acknowledgments: The authors would like to thank Sian Richards for technical assistance; Carole Chambers for taking dried blood spot samples from healthy volunteers; Joyce Baston for help with the Panthera dried blood spot puncher; Lindsay Weaver and Metabolic Support UK for guidance during the project; and all subjects who donated dried blood spot samples for assay development.

References

1. Almannai, M.; Marom, R.; Sutton, V.R. Newborn screening: A review of history, recent advancements, and future perspectives in the era of next generation sequencing. *Curr. Opin. Pediatr.* **2016**, *28*, 694–699. [CrossRef] [PubMed]
2. Guthrie, R.; Susi, A. A Simple Phenylalanine Method for Detecting Phenylketonuria in Large Populations of Newborn Infants. *Pediatrics* **1963**, *32*, 338–343. [PubMed]
3. Public Health England. *A Laboratory Guide to Newborn Blood Spot Screening for Inherited Metabolic Diseases*; PHE Publications: London, UK, 2017.
4. Public Health England. *A Laboratory Guide to Newborn Screening in the UK for Congenital Hypothyroidism*; PHE Publications: London, UK, 2014.
5. Public Health England. *A Laboratory Guide to Newborn Screening in the UK for Cystic Fibrosis*; PHE Publications: London, UK, 2014.

6. Public Health England. *NHS Sickle Cell and Thalassaemia Screening Programme, Handbook for Laboratories*, 4th ed.; PHE Publications: London, UK, 2017.
7. Bonham, J.R. Expanded newborn screening—Progress into practice. *Clin. Biochem.* **2014**, *47*, 697–698. [CrossRef] [PubMed]
8. Chilcott, J.; Bessey, A.; Pandor, A.; Paisley, S. Expanded Newborn Screening for Inborn Errors of Metabolism. *Health Econ.* **2013**, *111*, 1399–1406.
9. Barrett, A.N.; Saminathan, R.; Choolani, M. Thalassaemia screening and confirmation of carriers in parents. *Best Pract. Res. Clin. Obstet. Gynaecol.* **2017**, *39*, 27–40. [CrossRef]
10. Smon, A.; Repic Lampret, B.; Groselj, U.; Zerjav Tansek, M.; Kovac, J.; Perko, D.; Bertok, S.; Battelino, T.; Trebusak Podkrajsek, K. Next generation sequencing as a follow-up test in an expanded newborn screening programme. *Clin. Biochem.* **2017**, *52*, 48–55. [CrossRef]
11. Bhattacharjee, A.; Sokolsky, T.; Wyman, S.K.; Reese, M.G.; Puffenberger, E.; Strauss, K.; Morton, H.; Parad, R.B.; Naylor, E.W. Development of DNA confirmatory and high-risk diagnostic testing for newborns using targeted next-generation DNA sequencing. *Genet. Med.* **2015**, *17*, 337–347. [CrossRef]
12. Hollegaard, M.V.; Grauholm, J.; Nielsen, R.; Grove, J.; Mandrup, S.; Hougaard, D.M. Archived neonatal dried blood spot samples can be used for accurate whole genome and exome-targeted next-generation sequencing. *Mol. Genet. Metab.* **2013**, *110*, 65–72. [CrossRef]
13. Bodian, D.L.; Klein, E.; Iyer, R.K.; Wong, W.S.; Kothiyal, P.; Stauffer, D.; Huddleston, K.C.; Gaither, A.D.; Remsburg, I.; Khromykh, A.; et al. Utility of whole-genome sequencing for detection of newborn screening disorders in a population cohort of 1696 neonates. *Genet. Med.* **2016**, *18*, 221–230. [CrossRef]
14. Waisbren, S.E.; Back, D.K.; Liu, C.; Kalia, S.S.; Ringer, S.A.; Holm, I.A.; Green, R.C. Parents are interested in newborn genomic testing during the early postpartum period. *Genet. Med.* **2015**, *17*, 501–504. [CrossRef]
15. Dercksen, M.; Duran, M.; Ijlst, L.; Mienie, L.J.; Reinecke, C.J.; Ruiter, J.P.; Waterham, H.R.; Wanders, R.J. Clinical variability of isovaleric acidemia in a genetically homogeneous population. *J. Inherit. Metab. Dis.* **2012**, *35*, 1021–1029. [CrossRef] [PubMed]
16. Barends, M.; Pitt, J.; Morrissy, S.; Tzanakos, N.; Boneh, A.; Newborn Screening Laboratory Staff. Biochemical and molecular characteristics of patients with organic acidaemias and urea cycle disorders identified through newborn screening. *Mol. Genet. Metab.* **2014**, *113*, 46–52. [CrossRef] [PubMed]
17. Grunert, S.C.; Wendel, U.; Lindner, M.; Leichsenring, M.; Schwab, K.O.; Vockley, J.; Lehnert, W.; Ensenauer, R. Clinical and neurocognitive outcome in symptomatic isovaleric acidemia. *Orphanet J. Rare Dis.* **2012**, *7*, 9. [CrossRef] [PubMed]
18. Kolker, S.; Valayannopoulos, V.; Burlina, A.B.; Sykut-Cegielska, J.; Wijburg, F.A.; Teles, E.L.; Zeman, J.; Dionisi-Vici, C.; Baric, I.; Karall, D.; et al. The phenotypic spectrum of organic acidurias and urea cycle disorders. Part 2: The evolving clinical phenotype. *J. Inherit. Metab. Dis.* **2015**, *38*, 1059–1074. [CrossRef] [PubMed]
19. Jacob, M.; Lopata, A.L.; Dasouki, M.; Abdel Rahman, A.M. Metabolomics toward personalized medicine. *Mass Spectrom. Rev.* **2019**, *38*, 221–238. [CrossRef]
20. Olpin, S.E. Pathophysiology of fatty acid oxidation disorders and resultant phenotypic variability. *J. Inherit. Metab. Dis.* **2013**, *36*, 645–658. [CrossRef] [PubMed]
21. Grunert, S.C. Clinical and genetical heterogeneity of late-onset multiple acyl-coenzyme A dehydrogenase deficiency. *Orphanet J. Rare Dis.* **2014**, *9*, 117. [CrossRef] [PubMed]
22. Almannai, M.; Marom, R.; Divin, K.; Scaglia, F.; Sutton, V.R.; Craigen, W.J.; Lee, B.; Burrage, L.C.; Graham, B.H. Milder clinical and biochemical phenotypes associated with the c.482G > A(p.Arg161Gln) pathogenic variant in cobalamin C disease: Implications for management and screening. *Mol. Genet. Metab.* **2017**, *122*, 60–66. [CrossRef]
23. Kang, E.; Kim, Y.M.; Kang, M.; Heo, S.H.; Kim, G.H.; Choi, I.H.; Choi, J.H.; Yoo, H.W.; Lee, B.H. Clinical and genetic characteristics of patients with fatty acid oxidation disorders identified by newborn screening. *BMC Pediatr.* **2018**, *18*, 103. [CrossRef]
24. Landau, Y.E.; Waisbren, S.E.; Chan, L.M.; Levy, H.L. Long-term outcome of expanded newborn screening at Boston children's hospital: Benefits and challenges in defining true disease. *J. Inherit. Metab. Dis.* **2017**, *40*, 209–218. [CrossRef]

25. Ensenauer, R. A Common Mutation is Associated with a Mild, Potentially Asymptomatic Phenotype in Patients with Isovaleric Acidemia Diagnosed by Newborn Screening. *Am. J. Hum. Genet.* **2004**, *75*, 1136–1142. [CrossRef] [PubMed]
26. Andresen, B.S.; Dobrowolski, S.F.; O'Reilly, L.; Muenzer, J.; McCandless, S.E.; Frazier, D.M.; Udvari, S.; Bross, P.; Knudsen, I.; Banas, R.; et al. Medium-chain acyl-CoA dehydrogenase (MCAD) mutations identified by MS/MS-based prospective screening of newborns differ from those observed in patients with clinical symptoms: Identification and characterization of a new, prevalent mutation that results in mild MCAD deficiency. *Am. J. Hum. Genet.* **2001**, *68*, 1408–1418. [CrossRef] [PubMed]
27. Harutyunyan, M.; Huang, Y.; Mun, K.S.; Yang, F.; Arora, K.; Naren, A.P. Personalized Medicine in CF: From Modulator Development to Therapy for Cystic Fibrosis Patients with Rare CFTR Mutations. *Am. J. Physiol. -Lung Cell. Mol. Physiol.* **2017**. [CrossRef] [PubMed]
28. Lucarelli, M.; Bruno, S.M.; Pierandrei, S.; Ferraguti, G.; Testino, G.; Truglio, G.; Strom, R.; Quattrucci, S. The Impact on Genetic Testing of Mutational Patterns of CFTR Gene in Different Clinical Macrocategories of Cystic Fibrosis. *J. Mol. Diagn.* **2016**, *18*, 554–565. [CrossRef]
29. Lucarelli, M.; Bruno, S.M.; Pierandrei, S.; Ferraguti, G.; Stamato, A.; Narzi, F.; Amato, A.; Cimino, G.; Bertasi, S.; Quattrucci, S.; et al. A Genotypic-Oriented View of CFTR Genetics Highlights Specific Mutational Patterns Underlying Clinical Macrocategories of Cystic Fibrosis. *Mol. Med.* **2015**, *21*, 257–275. [CrossRef]
30. UK Department of Health. *The UK Strategy for Rare Diseases*; UK Department of Health: London, UK, 2013.
31. Bouwman, M.G.; De Ru, M.H.; Linthorst, G.E.; Hollak, C.E.; Wijburg, F.A.; Van Zwieten, M.C. Fabry patients' experiences with the timing of diagnosis relevant for the discussion on newborn screening. *Mol. Genet. Metab.* **2013**, *109*, 201–207. [CrossRef]
32. De Ru, M.H.; Bouwman, M.G.; Wijburg, F.A.; Van Zwieten, M.C. Experiences of parents and patients with the timing of Mucopolysaccharidosis type I (MPS I) diagnoses and its relevance to the ethical debate on newborn screening. *Mol. Genet. Metab.* **2012**, *107*, 501–507. [CrossRef]
33. Boycott, K.M.; Vanstone, M.R.; Bulman, D.E.; MacKenzie, A.E. Rare-disease genetics in the era of next-generation sequencing: Discovery to translation. *Nat. Rev. Genet.* **2013**, *14*, 681–691. [CrossRef]
34. Schneller, J.L.; Lee, C.M.; Bao, G.; Venditti, C.P. Genome editing for inborn errors of metabolism: Advancing towards the clinic. *BMC Med.* **2017**, *15*, 43. [CrossRef]
35. Schiroli, G.; Ferrari, S.; Conway, A.; Jacob, A.; Capo, V.; Albano, L.; Plati, T.; Castiello, M.C.; Sanvito, F.; Gennery, A.R.; et al. Preclinical modeling highlights the therapeutic potential of hematopoietic stem cell gene editing for correction of SCID-X1. *Sci. Transl. Med.* **2017**, *9*. [CrossRef]
36. Diez, B.; Genovese, P.; Roman-Rodriguez, F.J.; Alvarez, L.; Schiroli, G.; Ugalde, L.; Rodriguez-Perales, S.; Sevilla, J.; Diaz de Heredia, C.; Holmes, M.C.; et al. Therapeutic gene editing in CD34(+) hematopoietic progenitors from Fanconi anemia patients. *EMBO Mol. Med.* **2017**, *9*, 1574–1588. [CrossRef] [PubMed]
37. Naldini, L. Gene therapy returns to centre stage. *Nature* **2015**, *526*, 351–360. [CrossRef] [PubMed]
38. Aartsma-Rus, A.; Straub, V.; Hemmings, R.; Haas, M.; Schlosser-Weber, G.; Stoyanova-Beninska, V.; Mercuri, E.; Muntoni, F.; Sepodes, B.; Vroom, E.; et al. Development of Exon Skipping Therapies for Duchenne Muscular Dystrophy: A Critical Review and a Perspective on the Outstanding Issues. *Nucleic Acid Ther.* **2017**, *27*, 251–259. [CrossRef] [PubMed]
39. Bassaganyas, L.; Freedman, G.; Vaka, D.; Wan, E.; Lao, R.; Chen, F.; Kvale, M.; Currier, R.J.; Puck, J.M.; Kwok, P.Y. Whole exome and whole genome sequencing with dried blood spot DNA without whole genome amplification. *Hum. Mutat.* **2018**, *39*, 167–171. [CrossRef]
40. Baudhuin, L.M.; Leduc, C.; Train, L.J.; Avula, R.; Kluge, M.L.; Kotzer, K.E.; Lin, P.T.; Ackerman, M.J.; Maleszewski, J.J. Technical Advances for the Clinical Genomic Evaluation of Sudden Cardiac Death: Verification of Next-Generation Sequencing Panels for Hereditary Cardiovascular Conditions Using Formalin-Fixed Paraffin-Embedded Tissues and Dried Blood Spots. *Circ. Cardiovasc. Genet.* **2017**, *10*, e001844. [CrossRef]
41. Baker, M.W.; Atkins, A.E.; Cordovado, S.K.; Hendrix, M.; Earley, M.C.; Farrell, P.M. Improving newborn screening for cystic fibrosis using next-generation sequencing technology: A technical feasibility study. *Genet. Med.* **2016**, *18*, 231–238. [CrossRef]
42. Rothberg, J.M.; Hinz, W.; Rearick, T.M.; Schultz, J.; Mileski, W.; Davey, M.; Leamon, J.H.; Johnson, K.; Milgrew, M.J.; Edwards, M.; et al. An integrated semiconductor device enabling non-optical genome sequencing. *Nature* **2011**, *475*, 348–352. [CrossRef]

43. Cordovado, S.K. Dried Blood Spot DNA Extraction Guidelines to Ensure Robust Performance in NBS Molecular Assays. In Proceedings of the APHL Newborn Screening Symposium, Atlanta, GA, USA, 2–5 June 2013.
44. Deans, Z.; Watson, C.; Charlton, R.; Ellard, S.; Wallis, Y.; Mattocks, C.; Abbs, S. *Practice guidelines for Targeted Next Generation Sequencing Analysis and Interpretation*; ACGS: London, UK, 2015.
45. Fisher, T. Ion AmpliSeq Library Kit 2.0 User Guide. Available online: https://tools.thermofisher.com/content/sfs/manuals/MAN0006735_AmpliSeq_DNA_RNA_LibPrep_UG.pdf (accessed on 16 September 2019).
46. Zook, J.M.; Chapman, B.; Wang, J.; Mittelman, D.; Hofmann, O.; Hide, W.; Salit, M. Integrating human sequence data sets provides a resource of benchmark SNP and indel genotype calls. *Nat. Biotechnol.* **2014**, *32*, 246–251. [CrossRef]
47. Mu, J.C.; Tootoonchi Afshar, P.; Mohiyuddin, M.; Chen, X.; Li, J.; Bani Asadi, N.; Gerstein, M.B.; Wong, W.H.; Lam, H.Y. Leveraging long read sequencing from a single individual to provide a comprehensive resource for benchmarking variant calling methods. *Sci. Rep.* **2015**, *5*, 14493. [CrossRef]
48. Tan, A.; Abecasis, G.R.; Kang, H.M. Unified representation of genetic variants. *Bioinformatics* **2015**, *31*, 2202–2204. [CrossRef]
49. Quinlan, A.R.; Hall, I.M. BEDTools: A flexible suite of utilities for comparing genomic features. *Bioinformatics* **2010**, *26*, 841–842. [CrossRef] [PubMed]
50. Tarasov, A.; Vilella, A.J.; Cuppen, E.; Nijman, I.J.; Prins, P. Sambamba: Fast processing of NGS alignment formats. *Bioinformatics* **2015**, *31*, 2032–2034. [CrossRef] [PubMed]
51. Li, H.; Handsaker, B.; Wysoker, A.; Fennell, T.; Ruan, J.; Homer, N.; Marth, G.; Abecasis, G.; Durbin, R.; 1000 Genome Project Data Processing Subgroup. The Sequence Alignment/Map format and SAMtools. *Bioinformatics* **2009**, *25*, 2078–2079. [CrossRef] [PubMed]
52. Illumina. AmpliSeq for Illumina Targeted Resequencing Solution Data Sheet 770-2017-022-C. 2018. Available online: https://www.illumina.com/content/dam/illumina-marketing/documents/products/datasheets/ampliseq-for-illumina-targeted-resequencing-solution-data-sheet-770-2017-022.pdf (accessed on 3 October 2019).
53. Tarabeux, J.; Zeitouni, B.; Moncoutier, V.; Tenreiro, H.; Abidallah, K.; Lair, S.; Legoix-Ne, P.; Leroy, Q.; Rouleau, E.; Golmard, L.; et al. Streamlined ion torrent PGM-based diagnostics: BRCA1 and BRCA2 genes as a model. *Eur. J. Hum. Genet.* **2014**. [CrossRef] [PubMed]
54. Belkadi, A.; Bolze, A.; Itan, Y.; Cobat, A.; Vincent, Q.B.; Antipenko, A.; Shang, L.; Boisson, B.; Casanova, J.L.; Abel, L. Whole-genome sequencing is more powerful than whole-exome sequencing for detecting exome variants. *Proc. Natl. Acad. Sci. USA* **2015**, *112*, 5473–5478. [CrossRef] [PubMed]
55. Abel, H.J.; Duncavage, E.J. Detection of structural DNA variation from next generation sequencing data: A review of informatic approaches. *Cancer Genet.* **2013**, *206*, 432–440. [CrossRef]
56. Mu, W.; Li, B.; Wu, S.; Chen, J.; Sain, D.; Xu, D.; Black, M.H.; Karam, R.; Gillespie, K.; Farwell Hagman, K.D.; et al. Detection of structural variation using target captured next-generation sequencing data for genetic diagnostic testing. *Genet. Med.* **2018**. [CrossRef]
57. Kerkhof, J.; Schenkel, L.C.; Reilly, J.; McRobbie, S.; Aref-Eshghi, E.; Stuart, A.; Rupar, C.A.; Adams, P.; Hegele, R.A.; Lin, H.; et al. Clinical Validation of Copy Number Variant Detection from Targeted Next-Generation Sequencing Panels. *J. Mol. Diagn.* **2017**, *19*, 905–920. [CrossRef]
58. Feng, Y.; Ge, X.; Meng, L.; Scull, J.; Li, J.; Tian, X.; Zhang, T.; Jin, W.; Cheng, H.; Wang, X.; et al. The next generation of population-based spinal muscular atrophy carrier screening: Comprehensive pan-ethnic SMN1 copy-number and sequence variant analysis by massively parallel sequencing. *Genet. Med.* **2017**, *19*, 936–944. [CrossRef]
59. Martinez-Pizarro, A.; Dembic, M.; Pérez, B.; Andresen, B.S.; Desviat, L.R. Intronic PAH gene mutations cause a splicing defect by a novel mechanism involving U1snRNP binding downstream of the 5′ splice site. *PLoS Genet.* **2018**. [CrossRef]
60. Bergougnoux, A.; Deletang, K.; Pommier, A.; Varilh, J.; Houriez, F.; Altieri, J.P.; Koenig, M.; Férec, C.; Claustres, M.; Lalau, G.; et al. Functional characterization and phenotypic spectrum of three recurrent disease-causing deep intronic variants of the CFTR gene. *J. Cyst. Fibros.* **2019**, *18*, 468–475. [CrossRef] [PubMed]
61. Public Health England. *Data Collection and Performance Analysis Report, Newborn Bloodspot Screening in the UK, 2016/17*; PHE Publications: London, UK, 2018.

62. Office of National Statistics. *Birth Characteristics in England and Wales*; ONS Publications: London, UK, 2016.
63. Jansen, M.E.; Metternick-Jones, S.C.; Lister, K.J. International differences in the evaluation of conditions for newborn bloodspot screening: A review of scientific literature and policy documents. *Eur. J. Hum. Genet.* **2016**, *25*, 10–16. [CrossRef] [PubMed]
64. Mackie, A. UK National Screening Committee Criteria: Clarification of two misunderstandings. *Eur. J. Hum. Genet.* **2017**, *25*, 791. [CrossRef] [PubMed]
65. Faulkner, A. Resisting the screening imperative: Patienthood, populations and politics in prostate cancer detection technologies for the UK. *Sociol. Health Illn.* **2012**, *34*, 221–233. [CrossRef] [PubMed]
66. Taylor-Phillips, S.; Boardman, F.; Seedat, F.; Hipwell, A.; Gale, N.K.; Clarke, A.; Slowther, A.; Sime, M.; Thomas, S.; Davis, H.; et al. *The Ethical, Social and Legal Issues with Expanding the Newborn Blood Spot Test*; The University of Warwick: Warwick, UK, 2014.
67. Laberge, A.-M.; Burke, W. Avoiding the Technological Imperative: Criteria for Genetic Screening Programs. *OBM Genet.* **2017**, *1*. [CrossRef]
68. Johnston, J.; Lantos, J.D.; Goldenberg, A.; Chen, F.; Parens, E.; Koenig, B.A.; Members of the NSIGHT Ethics and Policy Advisory Board. Sequencing Newborns: A Call for Nuanced Use of Genomic Technologies. *Hastings Cent. Rep.* **2018**, *48*, S2–S6. [CrossRef]
69. Lim, E.C.; Brett, M.; Lai, A.H.; Lee, S.P.; Tan, E.S.; Jamuar, S.S.; Ng, I.S.; Tan, E.C. Next-generation sequencing using a pre-designed gene panel for the molecular diagnosis of congenital disorders in pediatric patients. *Hum. Genom.* **2015**, *9*, 33. [CrossRef]
70. Green, R.C.; Berg, J.S.; Grody, W.W.; Kalia, S.S.; Korf, B.R.; Martin, C.L.; McGuire, A.L.; Nussbaum, R.L.; O'Daniel, J.M.; Ormond, K.E.; et al. ACMG recommendations for reporting of incidental findings in clinical exome and genome sequencing. *Genet. Med.* **2013**, *15*, 565–574. [CrossRef]
71. Abdul-Karim, R.; Berkman, B.E.; Wendler, D.; Rid, A.; Khan, J.; Badgett, T.; Hull, S.C. Disclosure of incidental findings from next-generation sequencing in pediatric genomic research. *Pediatrics* **2013**, *131*, 564–571. [CrossRef]
72. Hasegawa, L.E.; Fergus, K.A.; Ojeda, N.; Au, S.M. Parental attitudes toward ethical and social issues surrounding the expansion of newborn screening using new technologies. *Public Health Genom.* **2011**, *14*, 298–306. [CrossRef]
73. Waisbren, S.E.; Weipert, C.M.; Walsh, R.C.; Petty, C.R.; Green, R.C. Psychosocial Factors Influencing Parental Interest in Genomic Sequencing of Newborns. *Pediatrics* **2016**, *137*, S30–S35. [CrossRef] [PubMed]
74. Ellard, S.; Baple, E.L.; Owens, M.; Eccles, D.M.; Abbs, S.; Deans, Z.C.; Newman, W.G.; McMullan, D.J. *ACGS Best Practice Guidelines for Variant Classification*; ACGS: London, UK, 2017.
75. Yang, S.; Lincoln, S.E.; Kobayashi, Y.; Nykamp, K.; Nussbaum, R.L.; Topper, S. Sources of discordance among germ-line variant classifications in ClinVar. *Genet. Med.* **2017**, *19*, 1118–1126. [CrossRef] [PubMed]
76. Whiffin, N.; Minikel, E.; Walsh, R.; O'Donnell-Luria, A.H.; Karczewski, K.; Ing, A.Y.; Barton, P.J.R.; Funke, B.; Cook, S.A.; MacArthur, D.; et al. Using high-resolution variant frequencies to empower clinical genome interpretation. *Genet. Med.* **2017**, *19*, 1151–1158. [CrossRef] [PubMed]
77. Garbade, S.F.; Shen, N.; Himmelreich, N.; Haas, D.; Trefz, F.K.; Hoffmann, G.F.; Burgard, P.; Blau, N. Allelic phenotype values: A model for genotype-based phenotype prediction in phenylketonuria. *Genet. Med.* **2019**, *21*, 580–590. [CrossRef] [PubMed]
78. Grauholm, J.; Khoo, S.K.; Nickolov, R.Z.; Poulsen, J.B.; Baekvad-Hansen, M.; Hansen, C.S.; Hougaard, D.M.; Hollegaard, M.V. Gene expression profiling of archived dried blood spot samples from the Danish Neonatal Screening Biobank. *Mol. Genet. Metab.* **2015**, *116*, 119–124. [CrossRef] [PubMed]
79. Gonorazky, H.D.; Naumenko, S.; Ramani, A.K.; Nelakuditi, V.; Mashouri, P.; Wang, P.; Kao, D.; Ohri, K.; Viththiyapaskaran, S.; Tarnopolsky, M.A.; et al. Expanding the Boundaries of RNA Sequencing as a Diagnostic Tool for Rare Mendelian Disease. *Am. J. Hum. Genet.* **2019**, *104*, 466–483. [CrossRef] [PubMed]
80. Wai, H.; Douglas, A.G.L.; Baralle, D. RNA splicing analysis in genomic medicine. *Int. J. Biochem. Cell Biol.* **2019**, *108*, 61–71. [CrossRef] [PubMed]
81. Ferraguti, G.; Pierandrei, S.; Bruno, S.M.; Ceci, F.; Strom, R.; Lucarelli, M. A template for mutational data analysis of the CFTR gene. *Clin. Chem. Lab. Med.* **2011**, *49*, 1447–1451. [CrossRef]
82. Cutting, G.R. Cystic fibrosis genetics: From molecular understanding to clinical application. *Nat. Rev. Genet.* **2015**, *16*, 45–56. [CrossRef]

83. Reinstein, E. Challenges of using next generation sequencing in newborn screening. *Genet. Res.* **2015**, *97*, e21. [CrossRef]
84. Brookes, A.J.; Robinson, P.N. Human genotype-phenotype databases: Aims, challenges and opportunities. *Nat. Rev. Genet.* **2015**, *16*, 702–715. [CrossRef] [PubMed]
85. Wilson, J.M.G.; Jungner, G. *Principles and Practice of Screening for Disease*; WHO: Geneva, Switzerland, 1968.
86. Richer, J.; Laberge, A.M. Secondary findings from next-generation sequencing: What does actionable in childhood really mean? *Genet. Med.* **2019**, *21*, 124–132. [CrossRef] [PubMed]
87. Dabrowski, M.; Bukowy-Bieryllo, Z.; Zietkiewicz, E. Advances in therapeutic use of a drug-stimulated translational readthrough of premature termination codons. *Mol. Med.* **2018**, *24*, 25. [CrossRef] [PubMed]
88. Welch, E.M.; Barton, E.R.; Zhuo, J.; Tomizawa, Y.; Friesen, W.J.; Trifillis, P.; Paushkin, S.; Patel, M.; Trotta, C.R.; Hwang, S.; et al. PTC124 targets genetic disorders caused by nonsense mutations. *Nature* **2007**, *447*, 87–91. [CrossRef] [PubMed]
89. Brentnall, A.R.; Evans, D.G.; Cuzick, J. Distribution of breast cancer risk from SNPs and classical risk factors in women of routine screening age in the UK. *Br. J. Cancer* **2014**, *110*, 827–828. [CrossRef]
90. Zhang, L.; Bao, Y.; Riaz, M.; Tiller, J.; Liew, D.; Zhuang, X.; Amor, D.J.; Huq, A.; Petelin, L.; Nelson, M.; et al. Population genomic screening of all young adults in a health-care system: A cost-effectiveness analysis. *Genet. Med.* **2019**. [CrossRef]
91. Schuurmans, J.; Birnie, E.; Van den Heuvel, L.M.; Plantinga, M.; Lucassen, A.; Van der Kolk, D.M.; Abbott, K.M.; Ranchor, A.V.; Diemers, A.D.; Van Langen, I.M. Feasibility of couple-based expanded carrier screening offered by general practitioners. *Eur. J. Hum. Genet.* **2019**. [CrossRef]

2

Pulse Oximetry Screening Adapted to a System with Home Births: The Dutch Experience

Ilona C. Narayen [1,*], Nico A. Blom [2] and Arjan B. te Pas [1]

[1] Department of Paediatrics, Division of Neonatology, Leiden University Medical Center, P.O. Box 9200, 2300 RC Leiden, The Netherlands; a.b.te_pas@lumc.nl

[2] Division of Paediatric Cardiology, Leiden University Medical Center, 2333 ZA Leiden, The Netherlands; N.A.Blom@lumc.nl

* Correspondence: i.c.narayen@lumc.nl

Abstract: Neonatal screening for critical congenital heart defects is proven to be safe, accurate, and cost-effective. The screening has been implemented in many countries across all continents in the world. However, screening for critical congenital heart defects after home births had not been studied widely yet. The Netherlands is known for its unique perinatal care system with a high rate of home births (18%) and early discharge after an uncomplicated delivery in hospital. We report a feasibility, accuracy, and acceptability study performed in the Dutch perinatal care system. Screening newborns for critical congenital heart defects using pulse oximetry is feasible after home births and early discharge, and acceptable to mothers. The accuracy of the test is comparable to other early-screening settings, with a moderate sensitivity and high specificity.

Keywords: neonates; screening; congenital heart defects; home births

---

1. Background

To increase the number of timely diagnoses, several studies on screening newborns for critical congenital heart defects (CCHD) using pulse oximetry (PO) have been performed since 2000 and led to an increasing implementation of PO screening across all continents [1,2]. This non-invasive screening method was proven to be reliable, easy to perform, and easy to implement in hospitals. Although studies only investigated the costs, without the long-term benefits, the screening is likely to be cost-effective and studies using questionnaires have shown that the screening was acceptable for parents and caregivers [2–5].

However, all large studies performed so far were in hospital settings and with a postnatal stay of more than five hours. In contrast, The Netherlands has a different perinatal care setting with the highest rate of home births (18%), which are supervised by community midwives [6]. The midwives stay for approximately three hours after birth and come back for their first follow-up visit at day two or three after birth (day of birth is day one). Also, in The Netherlands, mother and newborn are discharged early (within five hours) after uncomplicated vaginal delivery in hospital. For these reasons, the published protocols used in other countries do not match with the Dutch perinatal logistics and it is not possible to extrapolate the results of other PO screening studies to the Dutch perinatal care setting. We therefore performed studies with an adapted PO screening protocol to fit home births and early discharge in the Dutch unique perinatal care setting.

2. Discussion in The Netherlands

After publication of the meta-analysis on PO screening in the Lancet in 2012 it was stated that in The Netherlands it would be difficult to train all 1850 community midwives in performing PO measurements and to provide them all with PO devices [7]. Although the Dutch Association of Pediatricians (NVK) recommends the use of PO in case of resuscitation of a newborn, PO has not been implemented as standard practice in community midwifery [8,9]. The Netherlands has a history of having a high rate of 'natural' deliveries at home, without medical intervention [10]. Community midwives in The Netherlands are traditionally trained in clinical assessment and intervention with little use of technical devices [9]. However, in the Leiden region there is a well-organized clinical and research collaboration between hospitals and community midwives. The midwives participated in a study with recording PO measurements at birth at home. The midwives were trained in one afternoon session and experienced no problems with the use of PO during the study. The study showed that using the PO at home birth was feasible and almost all midwives were enthusiastic about having a PO available, especially in situations with a suboptimal condition of the newborn [9]. We considered the Leiden region the optimal region to pilot PO screening in the Dutch perinatal care setting.

The screening protocol used in the United States and Scandinavia needed to be adapted and made to fit with the visiting scheme of community midwives in The Netherlands [10,11]. Instead of performing one pre- and post-ductal SpO_2 reading 24–48 h after birth, we decided to perform these measurements at two separate time points: the first measurement at least one hour after birth, and the second measurement on day two or three of the newborn's life (day of birth is day one). The first measurement should be performed in the first hours after birth, since community midwives stay for approximately three hours after a delivery and because of discharge within five hours after in-hospital delivery. We were aware that performing screening early (before 24 h) is accompanied with a higher false positive rate due to transitional circulation [2]. However, studies also demonstrated that when the screening was performed after 24 h of life, some CCHD already presented with severe symptoms before the screening was performed [5,12]. The intention of screening is to detect pathology before symptoms occur, making early screening pivotal. Early screening also enables timely detection of other significant pathology, such as infections and respiratory morbidity. We added the second measurement on day two or three of life using the same protocol, at the first follow-up visit of the community midwife, because it is possible that a widely patent ductus arteriosus can cause normal SpO_2 values in newborns with CCHD in the first hours of life. Midwives and nurses were trained in performing and interpreting the PO measurements in a one-day education session. A web-based entry form with an automatic algorithm interpretation was used for quality assurance, and the research team could be reached 24/7 for questions regarding the screening. Handheld pulse oximeters were used for both studies, supplied by Medtronic (Dublin, Ireland). Reusable sensors were used in order to reduce the costs.

3. Pilot Study

We first piloted the adapted protocol in a feasibility study in the Leiden region, in which one academic hospital, two regional hospitals, and 14 midwifery practices are situated [13]. In this study, the Pulse Oximetry Leiden Screening (POLS) study, screening could only be performed after parental consent. Almost all parents who were approached consented and 99% (3059/3090) of the newborns with parental consent were screened. It was reassuring to observe that during the first screening episode in most of the healthy term newborns the pre- and post-ductal SpO_2 was already above 95% in the first hours after birth (10th percentile was 97% pre-ductally and 96% post-ductally within the first hour after birth, $n = 394$). This implies that newborns with SpO_2 values below 95% should be evaluated when they are measured at least one hour after birth. Indeed, in 50% of the newborns with a false positive screening result other morbidities than CCHD were diagnosed, including infections, wet lungs, PPHN, or non-critical congenital heart defects.

4. Acceptability to Mothers

We then assessed the acceptability of performing PO screening at home amongst 1172 mothers participating in the feasibility study by using questionnaire [14]. In this group, screening measurements were performed at least once at home by their community midwife. The response rate was acceptable (77%) and the vast majority (93%) of mothers considered the screening test important for all babies and would recommend the test to someone else.

We concluded that PO screening for CCHD, using the adapted protocol, was feasible in the Dutch perinatal care setting and that screening at home is acceptable to mothers [13,14].

5. Accuracy Study

In order to assess the accuracy of the adapted PO screening, we performed an implementation study in a larger cohort in a much larger region (Leiden–Amsterdam Region (POLAR) study) [15]. This study was carried out in three academic hospitals, 11 regional hospitals and 75 midwifery practices and included 23,959 newborns. The prenatal detection rate was 73% and the sensitivity was 50%, with a specificity of 99%. Four out of five detected CCHD were identified in the first screening test, in the first hours after birth. The fifth CCHD was diagnosed at 12 h after birth, on the day after the date of birth (day 2 of life). Serious illnesses such as infections and respiratory pathology were detected in 61% of all newborns with false positive screening results (Table 1). This study demonstrated that PO screening adapted to home births and early post-delivery hospital discharge contributes to the detection of CCHD in an early, asymptomatic stage. The early detection of CCHD, but also other significant pathologies, such as infections and respiratory morbidity, could be considered as a safety net when newborns are born at home or early discharged after delivery in hospital. In that view, the PO screening has the potential to decrease morbidity and mortality of newborns in The Netherlands.

Table 1. Overview of screening parameters for pilot and accuracy study

	Pilot Study (*n* = 3059)	**Accuracy Study (*n* = 23,959)**
True positive screens, *n* (%)	0 (0)	5 (0.02)
False negative screens, *n* (%)	0 (0)	5 (0.02)
False positive screens, *n* (%)	32 (1.0)	221 (0.9)
Respiratory pathology	8	88
Infection/sepsis	3	31
Non-critical CHD	3	3
Other pathology	2	12
Healthy	16	87

6. Costs

Before screening programs can be recommended for universal implementation, cost effectiveness should be considered. Cost analyses have shown that the PO screening is likely to be cost effective, but only screening in hospitals was taken into account [3,4,16]. The outcome of children after pediatric cardiac surgery has considerably improved in the last decades, but recent data on gained quality-adjusted life years (QALYs) are lacking. However, it is known that a timely diagnosis of CCHD decreases the risk of mortality and morbidity, and also the length of hospital stay [17,18].

In the way our screening was set up, all community midwives would require a pulse oximeter, and positive screenings at home should be transported and referred to hospital. This is likely to increase the costs when performing the screening in the Dutch perinatal care system as compared to settings with deliveries and screening in hospital. Therefore, we also performed a cost-effectiveness analysis with the results of the implementation study. These results will also be published in another article.

7. Prenatal Detection and Sensitivity of PO Screening

PO screening is not a replacement for other screening methods for CCHD, but should be considered as an addition to prenatal screening and physical examination. An early prenatal diagnosis of CCHD allows the parents to be mentally prepared, and gives them the opportunity to terminate the pregnancy. Furthermore, it allows the medical team to prepare a treatment strategy and the delivery can be planned in a congenital heart disease center with a level 3 NICU facility to enable acute surgical or catheter interventions. Prenatal detection varies between countries, and regions within countries, and can be improved with training and logistic interventions [19]. The sensitivity of PO screening is correlated with the prenatal detection rate of CCHD, which ranged from 0 to 82% within performed accuracy studies [20]. Fetal screening, which includes structural anomaly scans, is well organized and highly accessible in The Netherlands; there are strict nationwide requirements regarding the performance of the fetal ultrasounds. Intensive training and audit programs are regionally organized. The prenatal detection rate of CCHD was high in the region where the implementation study was performed [15], but the prenatal detection rate in the other regions of The Netherlands is currently unknown.

Although the overall prenatal detection of CCHD is high, specific defects remain difficult to detect prenatally, such as transposition of the great arteries (TGA), total anomalous pulmonary venous return (TAPVR), pulmonary valve stenosis, aortic valve stenosis, and coarctation of the aorta (CoA) [19,21]. PO screening is efficient at detecting low SpO_2 caused by TGA, TAPVR, and pulmonary valve stenosis, but left-sided obstructive lesions—such as CoA—are frequently missed with PO screening [2,22,23]. It remains challenging to detect CoA in an early stage even in combination with antenatal screening, PO screening and neonatal physical examination. In conclusion, PO is an effective screening method for identifying CCHD, but results of PO screening are correlated with the prenatal detection rate of CCHD. When considering the implementation of PO screening in The Netherlands and anticipating a variable prenatal detection rate in the Dutch regions, the sensitivity is likely to be somewhere between 50% and 70% [15].

8. Comparison with Other Studies

Several studies on PO screening in hospitals were performed which led to implementation in many countries. We performed the first studies, including a feasibility study and a large implementation study, with an adapted protocol for PO screening in a perinatal care system with home births and early postnatal discharge from hospital. Smaller pilot studies on PO screening out-of-hospital settings were performed in the United Kingdom (n = 90) and in the plain community in Wisconsin (n = 440) [24,25]. In The Netherlands, only women with low-risk pregnancies can choose to have a home birth, while in the Plain community in Wisconsin place of birth is not selected based on a risk profile. Instead it is culturally, religiously or financially based and many pregnant women in the Plain community do not receive prenatal screening. The detection of CCHD in this group will probably be higher when compared to our population of home birth deliveries.

This was the first screening set up where two separate screening episodes were used. Also, the first screening moment was earlier when compared to other early screening studies (8, 30). In general, it is not recommended to perform PO screening in the first hours after birth, because of the probability of having a higher false positive rate due to transitional circulation. In our Leiden pilot study, however, we demonstrated that SpO_2 values in healthy newborns were above 95% within the first hour of life [13].

9. Current Status

After finalizing the studies, a large number of caregivers did not want to await a governmental decision regarding top-down universal implementation, which can take several years. Bottom-up implementation has already begun in the studied region using the logistics that was set up for the study; the screening is continued in all participating hospitals in the POLAR study, as well as by 36% of all participating community midwifery practices, and this rate is still increasing. The perinatal caregivers in these hospitals and practices were convinced of the usefulness of PO screening.

10. Conclusions

PO screening for CCHD is feasible to perform and acceptable to mothers in the Dutch perinatal care setting with an adapted protocol for home births and early postnatal discharge from hospital. The screening detects CCHD at an early symptomatic stage with the extra benefit of detecting other significant and potentially life-threatening morbidities, such as infections and respiratory pathology. Implementation of PO screening for CCHD and other morbidities has the potential to decrease infant morbidity and mortality and increase the safety of newborns born at home or discharged from hospital in the first hours of life.

Author Contributions: Ilona C. Narayen performed literature review and analysis, wrote the first draft of the article, and gave final approval for publication of the report. Nico A. Blom supervised the writing of the report, reviewed and edited the manuscript, and gave final approval for publication of the report. Arjan B. te Pas supervised the analysis and writing of the article, reviewed and edited the manuscript, and gave final approval for publication of the report.

References

1. Hom, L.A.; Martin, G.R. U.S. international efforts on critical congenital heart disease screening: Can we have a uniform recommendation for Europe? *Early Hum. Dev.* **2014**, *90*, S11–S14. [CrossRef]
2. Thangaratinam, S.; Brown, K.; Zamora, J.; Khan, K.S.; Ewer, A.K. Pulse oximetry screening for critical congenital heart defects in asymptomatic newborn babies: A systematic review and meta-analysis. *Lancet* **2012**, *379*, 2459–2464. [CrossRef]
3. Peterson, C.; Grosse, S.D.; Oster, M.E.; Olney, R.S.; Cassell, C.H. Cost-effectiveness of routine screening for critical congenital heart disease in US newborns. *Pediatrics* **2013**, *132*, e595–e603. [CrossRef] [PubMed]
4. Roberts, T.E.; Barton, P.M.; Auguste, P.E.; Middleton, L.J.; Furmston, A.T.; Ewer, A.K. Pulse oximetry as a screening test for congenital heart defects in newborn infants: A cost-effectiveness analysis. *Arch. Dis. Child.* **2012**, *97*, 221–226. [CrossRef] [PubMed]
5. Ewer, A.K.; Furmston, A.T.; Middleton, L.J.; Deeks, J.J.; Daniels, J.P.; Pattison, H.M.; Powell, R.; Roberts, T.E.; Barton, P.; Auguste, P.; et al. Pulse oximetry as a screening test for congenital heart defects in newborn infants: A test accuracy study with evaluation of acceptability and cost-effectiveness. *Health Technol. Assess.* **2012**, *16*, 1–184. [CrossRef] [PubMed]
6. Netherlands Statistics; CBS Statline. Delivery and Birth: 1989–2015; Netherlands Statistics: The Hague, The Netherlands. Available online: http://statline.cbs.nl/Statweb/publication/?DM=SLNL&PA=81628NED&D1=0-22&D2=a&VW=T (accessed on 7 April 2017).
7. De Visser, E. Hartonderzoek BIJ Baby's Effectief. *Volkskrant*, 2 May 2012.
8. Nederlandse Vereniging voor Kindergeneesunde. Richtlijn Reanimatie van Het Kind BIJ de Geboorte. 2014. Available online: http://www.nvk.nl/Portals/0/richtlijnen/reanimatie/Reanimatie%20van%20het%20kind%20bij%20de%20geboorte_%20NVK%20richtlijn%202014_revisie%2011%20dec%202014.pdf (accessed on 7 April 2017).
9. Smit, M.; Ganzeboom, A.; Dawson, J.A.; Walther, F.J.; Bustraan, J.; van Roosmalen, J.J.; te Pas, A.B. Feasibility of pulse oximetry for assessment of infants born in community based midwifery care. *Midwifery* **2014**, *30*, 539–543. [CrossRef] [PubMed]
10. Kemper, A.R.; Mahle, W.T.; Martin, G.R.; Cooley, W.C.; Kumar, P.; Morrow, W.R.; Kelm, K.; Pearson, G.D.; Glidewell, J.; Grosse, S.D.; et al. Strategies for implementing screening for critical congenital heart disease. *Pediatrics* **2011**, *128*, e1259–e1267. [CrossRef] [PubMed]
11. Narayen, I.C.; Blom, N.A.; Verhart, M.S.; Smit, M.; Posthumus, F.; van den Broek, A.J.; Havers, H.; Haak, M.C.; te Pas, A.B. Adapted protocol for pulse oximetry screening for congenital heart defects in a country with homebirths. *Eur. J. Pediatr.* **2015**, *174*, 129–132. [CrossRef] [PubMed]
12. De-Wahl Granelli, A.; Wennergren, M.; Sandberg, K.; Mellander, M.; Bejlum, C.; Inganas, L.; Eriksson, M.; Segerdahl, N.; Agren, A.; Ekman-Joelsson, B.M.; et al. Impact of pulse oximetry screening on the detection of duct dependent congenital heart disease: A Swedish prospective screening study in 39,821 newborns. *BMJ* **2009**, *338*, a3037. [CrossRef] [PubMed]

13. Narayen, I.C.; Blom, N.A.; Bourgonje, M.S.; Haak, M.C.; Smit, M.; Posthumus, F.; van den Broek, A.J.; Havers, H.M.; te Pas, A.B. Pulse Oximetry Screening for Critical Congenital Heart Disease after Home Birth and Early Discharge. *J. Pediatr.* **2016**, *170*, 188–192. [CrossRef] [PubMed]
14. Narayen, I.C.; Kaptein, A.A.; Hogewoning, J.A.; Blom, N.A.; te Pas, A.B. Maternal acceptability of pulse oximetry screening at home after home birth or very early discharge. *Eur. J. Pediatr.* **2017**, *176*, 669–672. [CrossRef] [PubMed]
15. Narayen, I.C.; Blom, N.A.; van Geloven, N.; Blankman, E.I.; van den Broek, A.J.M.; Bruijn, M.; Clur, S.B.; van den Dungen, F.A.; Havers, H.M.; van Laerhoven, H.; et al. Accuracy of pulse oximetry screening for critical congenital heart defects after home birth and early postnatal discharge. *J. Pediatr.* **2018**. [CrossRef] [PubMed]
16. Griebsch, I.; Knowles, R.L.; Brown, J.; Bull, C.; Wren, C.; Dezateux, C.A. Comparing the clinical and economic effects of clinical examination, pulse oximetry, and echocardiography in newborn screening for congenital heart defects: A probabilistic cost-effectiveness model and value of information analysis. *Int. J. Technol. Assess. Health Care* **2007**, *23*, 192–204. [CrossRef] [PubMed]
17. Brown, K.L.; Ridout, D.A.; Hoskote, A.; Verhulst, L.; Ricci, M.; Bull, C. Delayed diagnosis of congenital heart disease worsens preoperative condition and outcome of surgery in neonates. *Heart* **2006**, *92*, 1298–1302. [CrossRef] [PubMed]
18. Peterson, C.; Dawson, A.; Grosse, S.D.; Riehle-Colarusso, T.; Olney, R.S.; Tanner, J.P.; Kirby, R.S.; Correia, J.A.; Watkins, S.M.; Cassell, C.H. Hospitalizations, costs, and mortality among infants with critical congenital heart disease: How important is timely detection? *Birth Defects Res. A Clin. Mol. Teratol.* **2013**, *97*, 664–672. [CrossRef] [PubMed]
19. Van Velzen, C.L.; Clur, S.A.; Rijlaarsdam, M.E.; Bax, C.J.; Pajkrt, E.; Heymans, M.W.; Bekker, M.N.; Hruda, J.; de Groot, C.J.; Blom, N.A.; et al. Prenatal detection of congenital heart disease—Results of a national screening programme. *BJOG* **2016**, *123*, 400–407. [CrossRef] [PubMed]
20. Narayen, I.C.; Blom, N.A.; Ewer, A.K.; Vento, M.; Manzoni, P.; te Pas, A.B. Aspects of pulse oximetry screening for critical congenital heart defects: When, how and why? *Arch. Dis. Child. Fetal Neonatal Ed.* **2016**, *101*, F162–F167. [CrossRef] [PubMed]
21. Van Velzen, C.L.; Clur, S.A.; Rijlaarsdam, M.E.; Pajkrt, E.; Bax, C.J.; Hruda, J.; de Groot, C.J.; Blom, N.A.; Haak, M.C. Prenatal diagnosis of congenital heart defects: Accuracy and discrepancies in a multicenter cohort. *Ultrasound Obstet Gynecol.* **2016**, *47*, 616–622. [CrossRef] [PubMed]
22. Ewer, A.K. Evidence for CCHD screening and its practical application using pulse oximetry. *Early Hum. Dev.* **2014**, *90*, S19–S21. [CrossRef]
23. Riede, F.T.; Schneider, P. Most wanted, least found: Coarctation. *Neonatology* **2012**, *101*, 13. [CrossRef] [PubMed]
24. Cawsey, M.J.; Noble, S.; Cross-Sudworth, F.; Ewer, A.K. Feasibility of pulse oximetry screening for critical congenital heart defects in homebirths. *Arch. Dis. Child. Fetal Neonatal Ed.* **2016**, *101*, F349–F351. [CrossRef] [PubMed]
25. Lhost, J.J.; Goetz, E.M.; Belling, J.D.; van Roojen, W.M.; Spicer, G.; Hokanson, J.S. Pulse oximetry screening for critical congenital heart disease in planned out-of-hospital births. *J. Pediatr.* **2014**, *165*, 485–489. [CrossRef] [PubMed]

3

Pulse Oximetry Values in Newborns with Critical Congenital Heart Disease upon ICU Admission at Altitude

John S. Kim [1,*], Merlin W. Ariefdjohan [2], Marci K. Sontag [2,3] and Christopher M. Rausch [1]

1 Department of Pediatrics, Heart Institute, Children's Hospital Colorado, University of Colorado School of Medicine, Aurora, CO 80045, USA; Christopher.Rausch@childrenscolorado.org

2 Department of Epidemiology, Colorado School of Public Health, University of Colorado Anschutz Medical Campus, Aurora, CO 80045, USA; Merlin.Ariefdjohan@ucdenver.edu (M.W.A.); msontag@ciinternational.com (M.K.S.)

3 Center for Public Health Innovation at CI International, Littleton, CO 80120, USA

* Correspondence: john.kim@childrenscolorado.org;

Abstract: Pulse oximetry screening for critical congenital heart disease (CCHD) has been recommended by the American Academy of Pediatrics (AAP). The objectives of this study are to describe saturation data, and to evaluate the effectiveness of AAP-recommended pulse oximetry screening guidelines applied retrospectively to a cohort of newborns with known CCHD at moderate altitude (5557 feet, Aurora, Colorado). Data related to seven critical congenital heart disease diagnoses were extracted from electronic health records (pulse oximetry, prostaglandin administration, and oxygen supplementation). Descriptive epidemiologic data were calculated. 158 subjects were included in this analysis; the AAP pulse oximetry screening protocol was applied to 149 subjects. Mean pre-ductal and post-ductal pulse oximetry values of the infants known to have CCHD at 24 h of life were 87.1% $\pm$ 7.2 and 87.8% $\pm$ 6.3, respectively. Infants treated with prostaglandins and oxygen had lower oximetry readings. The screening algorithm would have identified 80.5% of infants with known CCHDs (120/149 subjects). Additionally, sequential pulse oximetry screening based on the AAP-recommended protocol was able to identify a true positive screen capture rate of 80.5% at moderate altitude.

Keywords: critical congenital heart disease; pulse oximetry; newborn screening; altitude

1. Introduction

Congenital heart disease is among the most common birth defects, with an incidence of approximately 1 per 100 live births. Critical congenital heart disease (CCHD) is defined as a structural heart defect with significant risk for mortality without intensive intervention. CCHD occurs in approximately 4 per 1000 live births, and it is estimated that 13–55% of newborns with CCHD are discharged from hospital undiagnosed [1–3].

Screening with pulse oximetry has been identified as a low-cost non-invasive test that improves the ability to diagnose CCHD when compared to physical examination alone [4,5]. Several CCHD lesions are particularly amenable to identification via pulse oximetry screening, including truncus arteriosus (TA), transposition of the great arteries (TGA), tricuspid valve atresia (TVA), tetralogy of Fallot (TOF), total anomalous pulmonary venous return (TAPVR), hypoplastic left heart syndrome (HLHS), and pulmonary valve atresia with intact ventricular septum (PA/IVS) [6–8]. The most widely utilized pulse oximetry screening guidelines recommend initiation at or beyond 24 h of life with measurement of pre- and post-ductal saturations (right hand and foot, respectively) [8]. Pulse oximetry screening in the first 24–48 h after birth has been found to be highly specific (99.9% specificity; 95% confidence interval (CI) 99.7, 99.9), but with a lower sensitivity of 76.3% (95% CI 69.5, 82.0) in one meta-analysis [9].

The performance of pulse oximetry screening has been evaluated in many studies performed at sea level [10], however, studies at altitude are limited [3,11]. Evaluation of the effectiveness of pulse oximetry screening guidelines is complicated due to the small number of infants likely to be identified through newborn screening as many infants with CCHD are diagnosed prenatally or in the first 24 h of life, thereby reducing the potential number of infants with undiagnosed CCHD eligible for screening with pulse oximetry. Furthermore, studies of newborn oxygen saturations have suggested a wider range and lower average saturations for infants born at higher altitude, further complicating evaluation of the utility of pulse oximetry in this population [12–15]. We retrospectively reviewed pulse oximetry values for a population of newborns between 24 and 48 h of life who were known to have CCHD to provide an epidemiologic description of saturation data in newborns with CCHD at altitude.

2. Materials and Methods

We performed a retrospective cohort study at a regional tertiary children's hospital at moderate altitude (5557 feet, Aurora, CO, USA). We queried the electronic health record (EHR) for newborns presenting within the first 24–48 h of life with one of the 7 CCHD diagnoses using International Classification of Disease (ICD) codes in the years 2006–2013 (i2b2; Informatics for Integrating Biology and the Bedside, Version 1.7, Partners HealthCare System, Boston, MA, USA). Subjects included both prenatally and postnatally diagnosed CCHD. We reviewed the EHR for confirmation of diagnosis, pulse oximetry readings, prostaglandin (PGE) administration, and oxygen supplementation data at 24, 28, 36, and 48 h ($\pm$2 h) of life. These time points were within the American Academy of Pediatrics (AAP)-recommended window of screening between 24 and 48 h [8]. Pulse oximetry was measured continuously in all subjects with simultaneous pre- and post-ductal saturation values recorded in the EHR. Pulse oximetry values were recorded hourly in the EHR via standard clinical practice upon bedside nurse confirmation of the plethysmograph waveform during the patient's usual calm physiologic state.

In a secondary analysis of the pulse oximetry data, we applied a simulated pulse oximetry screening protocol modeled after the recommended AAP algorithm [8]. Pulse oximetry values were categorized based on the AAP screening protocol: (1) passed screen (no concern for CCHD, false negative): saturation $\geq$95% and $\leq$3% difference between pre- and post-ductal readings; (2) borderline reading (to be repeated at next time point): saturation 90–94% and/or >3% difference between pre- and post-ductal readings; (3) failed screen (concern for CCHD, true positive): saturation <90% in either pre- or post-ductal reading. Up to 3 total hypothetical screens were applied to the retrospective data collected at times closest to 28, 36, and 48 h of life. Data that resulted in a positive or negative screen for CCHD (based on the AAP protocol) were not evaluated in subsequent time points. Subjects with borderline pulse oximetry values at 3 consecutive readings were considered to meet screening criteria for concern for CCHD. Since all participating subjects had a CCHD diagnosis, subjects in whom pulse oximetry readings raised no concern for CCHD were considered false negative in this hypothetical screening. All other subjects were considered true positives. This secondary analysis allowed us to estimate the general effectiveness of the AAP protocol (i.e., false negative vs. true positive) in a cohort of infants with known CCHD at altitude based on retrospective data.

Study data were collected and maintained by using Research Electronic Data Capture (REDCap) tools hosted at the University of Colorado [16]. This study was approved by the Colorado Multiple Institutional Review Board with a full waiver of Health Insurance and Portability and Accountability Act (HIPAA) authorization.

Baseline demographic data are presented as means, standard deviations, and range. Group proportions for categorical variables were statistically assessed using the Fisher exact test. The Shapiro-Wilk test for normality was used to evaluate distributions for all continuous variables. Then, the *t*-test and Wilcoxon-Mann-Whitney test were applied to compare continuous variables between groups for those with normal and non-normal distributions, respectively. Pre- and post-ductal pulse oximetry values collected at 24, 28, 36, and 48 h were summarized as a box-whisker plot showing the mean, median, minimum/maximum values, and interquartile ranges. Mean pulse oximetry readings for various types of clinical support (i.e., PGE, oxygen, both, or none) were compared to each other using the Kruskal-Wallis test due to non-normality of data distribution. Post-hoc analysis was made on groups showing statistical difference. Statistical significance level was set at $p < 0.05$ and 95% CI were calculated for mean pulse oximetry values. All analyses were performed using SAS software (version 9.4; SAS Institute, Cary, NC, USA).

3. Results

3.1. Descriptive Analysis of Study Cohort

Two hundred and fourteen subjects with CCHD were identified. Fifty-six subjects were excluded from data collection due to the following reasons: insufficient pulse oximetry data in the EHR, death prior to 24 h of life, or atrial septostomy or surgery prior to 24 h of life. One hundred and fifty-eight subjects were included in this analysis. The distribution of CCHD anatomic diagnoses between the subjects included and excluded from the study was different (Table 1), but we found no other differences between the groups. The mean pre-ductal pulse oximetry readings at 24, 28, 36, and 48 h were 87.1 ± 7.2% (95% CI 85.6, 88.6), 86.7 ± 7.2% (85.2, 88.2), 86.8 ± 7.6% (85.2, 88.4), and 89.3 ± 6.5% (88.0, 90.6), respectively. The mean post-ductal pulse-oximetry readings were 87.8 ± 6.3% (95% CI 86.6, 89.0), 87.4 ± 7.3% (86.1, 88.8), 88.5 ± 6.7% (87.3, 89.7), and 89.2 ± 6.3% (88.2, 90.3), respectively. Figure 1 summarizes the overall distribution of pre- and post-ductal saturation readings at the four time points. For descriptive purposes, data were also stratified by diagnoses and pulse oximetry readings for each collection time (Figure 2). To evaluate the effects of treatment on pulse oximetry, we compared pulse oximetry data in infants receiving PGE and oxygen supplementation (Table 2). Newborns treated with both PGE and oxygen had lower pre- and post-ductal saturation at 48 h (87.4 ± 7.3% (95% CI 85.0, 89.7) and 86.3 ± 7.0% (84.3, 88.3), respectively, $p < 0.05$) when compared to the other treatment categories (PGE only, oxygen only, or no support).

Table 1. Baseline subject characteristics ($n = 214$).

Characteristics	Study Subjects ($n = 158$)	Excluded Subjects ($n = 56$)	p-Value
Gestational age, weeks (range)	38.2 ± 2.4 (29–45)	38.3 ± 2.4 (30–41.3)	0.379
Birth weight, g (range)	2988.7 ± 579.3 (1230–4165)	3071.0 ± 671.7 (960–4780)	0.277
Male gender, n (%)	101 (63.9)	35 (62.5)	0.849
Race, n (%)			
White/Caucasian	111 (70.3)	37 (66.1)	
Black/African American	10 (6.3)	3 (5.4)	
Hawaiian/Pacific Islander	1 (0.6)	0 (0)	
Asian	1 (0.6)	1 (1.8)	0.470
American Indian/Alaskan Native	3 (3.2)	1 (1.8)	
Other	26 (16.5)	9 (16.1)	
Not specified	4 (2.5)	5 (8.9)	
Ethnicity, n (%)			
Hispanic/Latino	54 (34.2)	15 (26.8)	
Not Hispanic/Latino	100 (63.3)	36 (64.3)	0.088
Not specified	4 (2.5)	5 (8.9)	

Table 1. *Cont.*

Characteristics	Study Subjects (n = 158)	Excluded Subjects (n = 56)	p-Value
Apgar score, score (range)			
1 min	7 ± 2 (0–9)	7 ± 2 (2–8)	0.409
5 min	8 ± 1 (0–9)	8 ± 1 (4–9)	0.212
Prenatal diagnosis of CCHD, n (%)	84 (53.2)	20 (35.7)	0.152
Family history of CCHD, n (%)	18 (11.4)	3 (5.4)	0.361
Genetic diagnosis, n (%)			
Down syndrome	2 (1.3)	0 (0)	0.825
22q11 deletion	6 (3.8)	1 (1.8)	
None specified	150 (94.9)	50 (89.3)	
CCHD diagnosis, n (%)			
HLHS	48 (30.4)	17 (30.4)	
TOF	34 (21.5)	5 (8.9)	
TGA	30 (19.0)	26 (46.4)	
TA	13 (8.2)	2 (3.6)	0.002 *
TAPVR	10 (6.3)	5 (8.9)	
TVA	10 (6.3)	0 (0)	
PA/IVS	7 (4.4)	1 (1.8)	
Combination of above	6 (3.8)	0 (0)	
Maternal age, years (range)	28.1 ± 5.8 (15–42)	26.5 ± 6.0 (15–41)	0.089
Maternal diabetes status, n (%)			
Diabetes (Type I or Type II)	7 (4.5)	0 (0)	0.272
Gestational diabetes	6 (3.8)	3 (5.4)	
Not diabetic	144 (91.7)	53 (94.6)	

Diagnoses are abbreviated: HLHS, hypoplastic left heart syndrome; TOF, tetralogy of Fallot; TGA, transposition of the great arteries; TA, truncus arteriosus; TAPVR, total anomalous pulmonary venous return; TVA, tricuspid valve atresia; PA/IVS, pulmonary valve atresia with intact ventricular septum; CCHD, critical congenital heart disease. * $p < 0.05$.

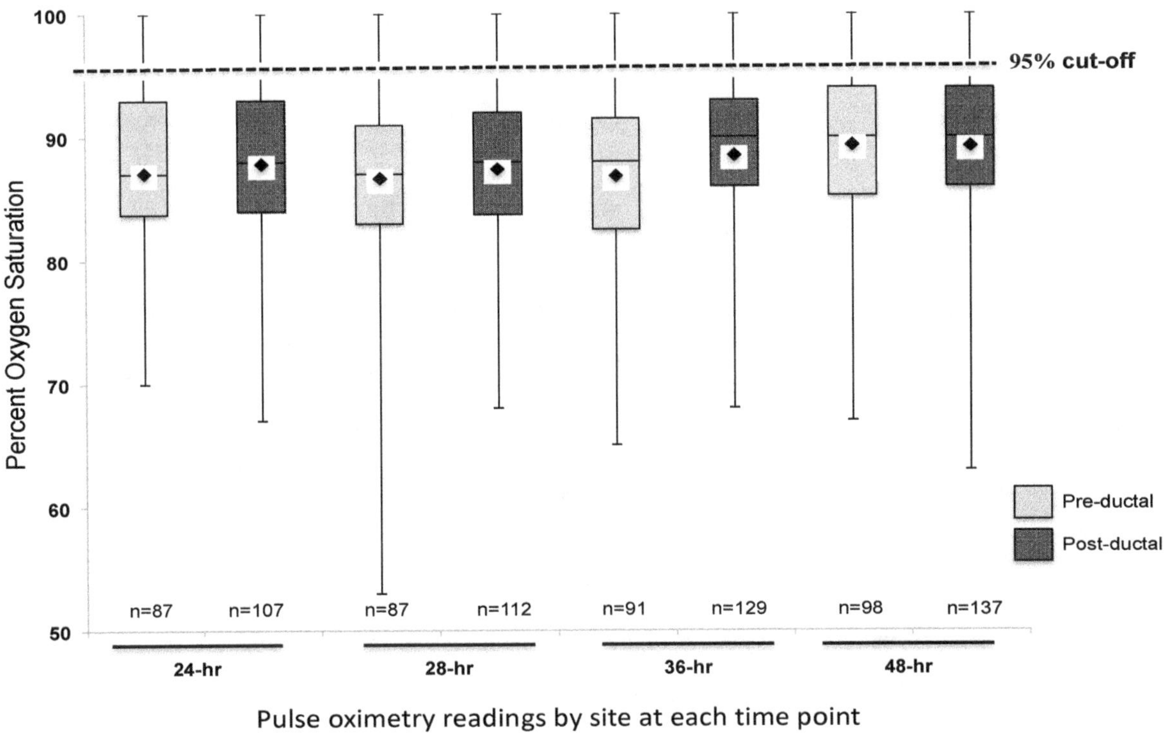

Figure 1. Pre- and post-ductal pulse oximetry data at 24, 28, 36, and 48 h of life (n = 158). Mean saturation at each time point indicated by the diamond on each box plot.

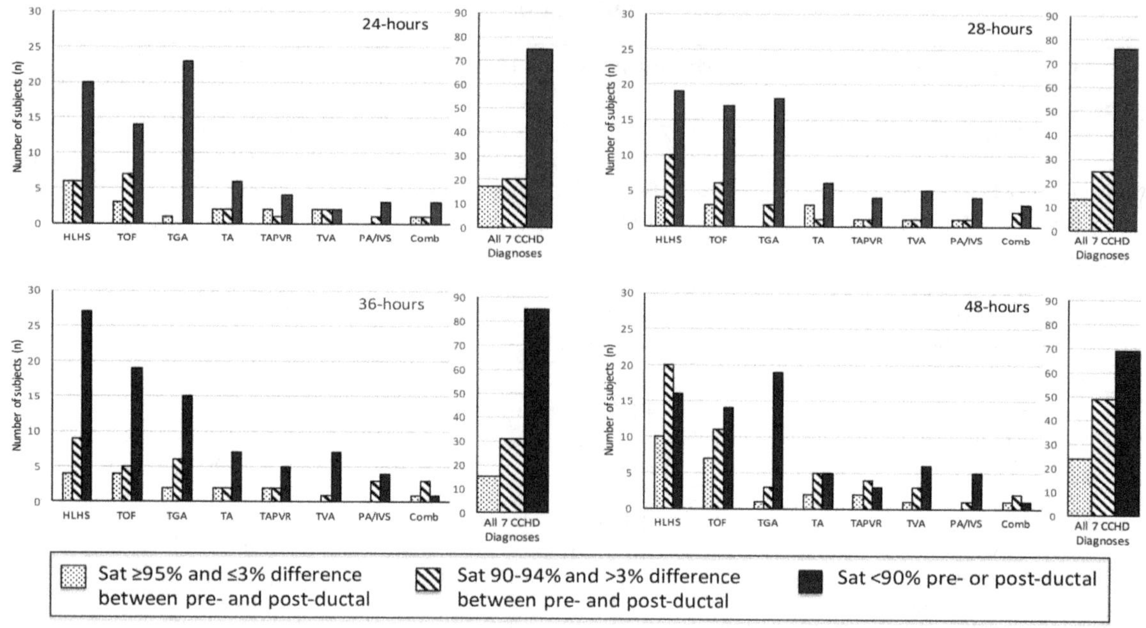

Figure 2. Pulse oximetry by saturation group at 24, 28, 36, and 48 h of life (n = 158).

Table 2. Pre- and post-ductal pulse oximetry readings, PGE administration, and oxygen supplementation data at 24, 28, 36, and 48 h of life (n = 158). * $p < 0.05$.

		No Support	PGE	Oxygen	Both PGE and Oxygen
24-hours	**Pre-ductal**	90.3 ± 7.7 (77–100) (n = 7)	88.6 ± 7.3 (75–100) (n = 30)	86.6 ± 4.3 (80–95) (n = 14)	85.2 ± 7.6 (70–98) (n = 36)
	Post-ductal	89.4 ± 5.4 (80–97) (n = 14)	87.8 ± 6.3 (73–99) (n = 33)	88.9 ± 6.0 (78–97) (n = 18)	86.8 ± 6.6 (67–100) (n = 42)
28-hours	**Pre-ductal**	88.0 ± 5.0 (81–95) (n = 7)	88.3 ± 6.8 (74–100) (n = 28)	84.6 ± 7.1 (72–96) (n = 18)	86.1 ± 7.8 (53–96) (n = 34)
	Post-ductal	90.3 ± 6.2 (78–100) (n = 14)	88.5 ± 7.4 (70–100) (n = 35)	85.7 ± 6.7 (72–95) (n = 20)	86.2 ± 7.6 (68–100) (n = 43)
36-hours	**Pre-ductal**	89.0 ± 9.2 (77–99) (n = 4)	88.4 ± 5.0 (76–100) (n = 33)	86.3 ± 8.0 (65–98) (n = 16)	85.5 ± 8.9 (65–100) (n = 38)
	Post-ductal	90.0 ± 4.9 (82–100) (n = 15)	90.2 ± 4.4 (79–98) (n = 46)	88.9 ± 7.0 (72–100) (n = 22)	86.1 ± 8.2 (68–99) (n = 46)
48-hours	**Pre-ductal**	91.0 ± 5.3 (80–97) (n = 8)	90.4 ± 6.4 (70–100) (n = 42)	89.8 ± 4.5 (81–98) (n = 13)	87.4 ± 7.3 * (67–100) (n = 35)
	Post-ductal	90.3 ± 6.4 (75–100) (n = 21)	90.5 ± 5.2 (75–99) (n = 51)	91.5 ± 4.8 (80–97) (n = 20)	86.3 ± 7.0 * (63–100) (n = 45)

3.2. Secondary Analysis: Hypothetical Screening of Study Cohort

Application of the AAP screening cutoffs to the retrospective data independently at each time point (not allowing for rescreens) would have resulted in 67% failing a screen at 24 h (75 of 112 subjects), 66.7% at 28 h (76 of 114 subjects), 64.9% at 36 h (85 of 131 subjects), and 48.6% at 48 h (69 of 142 subjects). A sequential screening analysis, similar to the AAP protocol, was subsequently applied to 149 subjects as 9 of the 158 subjects were excluded due to an inadequate number of pulse oximetry readings to apply the AAP protocol (Figure 3). Twenty-nine subjects who screened negative with passing pulse oximetry readings resulted in a 19.5% hypothetical false negative screening rate in our cohort. The 29 false negative screened subjects represented all diagnosis categories. The false negative screening rate was 18.8% (n = 80) in subjects with a prenatal concern for CCHD and 20.3% (n = 69) in subjects without a prenatal concern for CCHD.

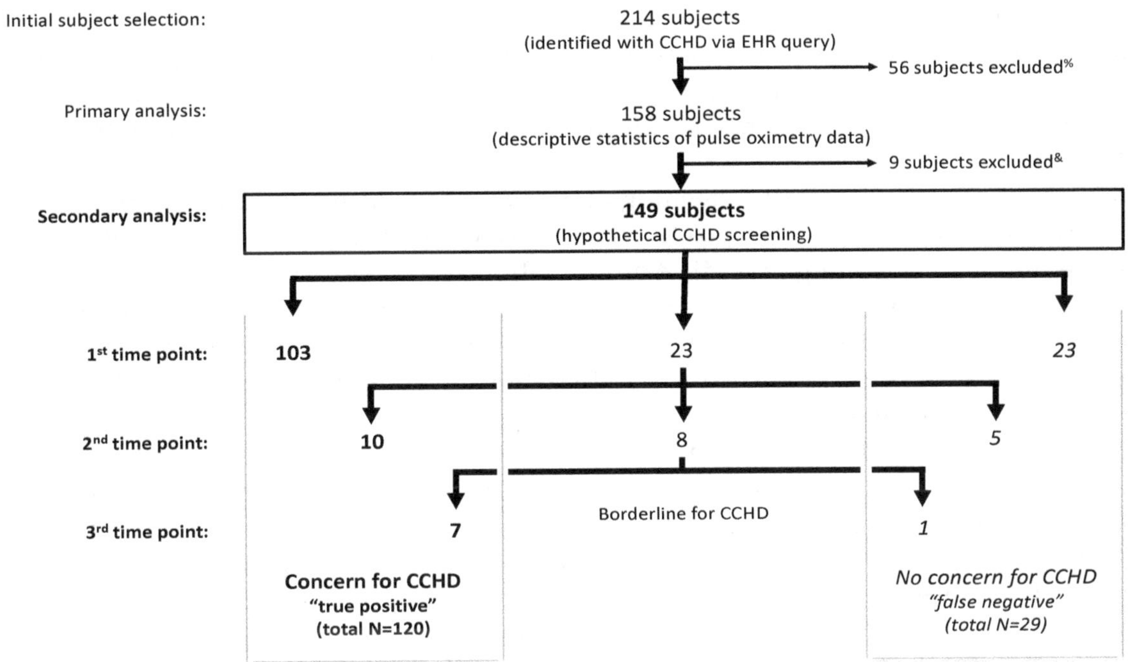

Figure 3. Application of the American Academy of Pediatrics (AAP) protocol to retrospective data in newborns with known CCHD (n = 149) results in 120 true positive screens and 80.5% sensitivity. [%] Exclusion criteria: insufficient pulse oximetry data in the electronic health record (EHR), death prior to 24 h of life, atrial septostomy or surgery prior to 24 h of life. [&] Inadequate number of pulse oximetry readings to complete the AAP protocol.

4. Discussion

In this study, we report mean pulse oximetry readings in a cohort of newborns with CCHD at altitude and thereby demonstrate the expected hypoxemia of the seven targeted CCHD diagnoses. Prior studies of newborn oxygen saturations have suggested a wider range and lower average saturations for infants born at higher altitude compared to those born at sea level [3,13,15]. We demonstrate in our cohort of infants at moderate altitude with the seven CCHD diagnoses targeted by the AAP (HLHS, TGA, TA, TAPVR, TVA, PA/IVS), that the mean pulse oximetry values are lower than recommended cutoffs for newborn screening. Wright and colleagues [3] evaluated the pulse oximetry screening protocol at 5557 feet (1694 m) and reported a mean pre-ductal saturation of 97.2% (±1.9) and a post-ductal saturation of 97.2% (±2.1) in 1003 healthy newborns at approximately 24 h of life (23.8 ± 2.3 h of life, mean ± SD), similar to what would be expected in a healthy newborn cohort at sea level and significantly higher than our cohort of infants with CCHD. Another study performed at a similar altitude demonstrated lower mean saturations of 92% and 93%, at 24 and 48 h, respectively [12]. Additionally, despite similar average saturation measurements, Wright et al. demonstrated a higher rate of screen failure. This variability certainly supports the need for further study of oxygen saturation and the screening protocol at moderate altitude.

In a secondary analysis we evaluated the hypothetical effectiveness of a sequential pulse oximetry screening protocol similar to the AAP-recommended protocol by application in a population of infants with known CCHD. By evaluating a cohort with known CCHD, we were able to demonstrate a 19.5% false negative screening rate, or a true positive screen capture rate of 80.5%, at moderate altitude. Ailes and colleagues sought to address the difficulties in studying this rare disease by simulation of the population [17] and we present an alternative strategy that yields comparable findings. Our findings are comparable to the true positive screening rate found by Thangaratinam and colleagues [18], who performed a meta-analysis in 2012 of 13 studies at sea level evaluating pulse oximetry screening and calculated an overall sensitivity of 76.5% in screening for CCHD. Further, our retrospective evaluation revealed a similar sensitivity to that of two other large prospective studies (65.5% and 75%) [19,20]. Notably, the retrospective study design allowed us to perform this evaluation in a relatively large cohort of patients with CCHD that has not yet been achievable with a prospective study design [18].

Evaluations of pulse oximetry screening of neonates supported in the intensive care unit have raised concerns for increased false positive rates, issues with oxygen supplementation, and the appropriate timing of screening [21–24]. Additionally, a study performed by Lueth and colleagues evaluated a modification to the AAP-recommended screening protocol with transient oxygen supplementation in newborns at moderate altitude. Their intent was to replicate sea-level atmospheric oxygen tension and induce pulmonary vasodilatation to potentiate the neonatal transition [11]. This group found an increase in specificity of screening with a reduction in false positive screens by providing transient supplemental oxygen to newborns with an indeterminate or borderline first screen at moderate altitude [11]. Because low oxygen saturation in CCHD is primarily caused by shunting of de-oxygenated blood to the systemic circulation, oxygen supplementation in clinical practice does not typically normalize the percent saturation to greater than 95% in hypoxemic CCHD. It is difficult to know to what degree oxygen supplementation resulted in an increase in pulse oximetry reading in our study; however, we found no difference in mean oxygen saturation between patients with CCHD treated with supplemental oxygen versus those without supplemental oxygen. Nevertheless, Table 2 shows the range of saturations in both subjects receiving oxygen and those with no support exceeding 95%. Of the 29 false negative subjects in our study, 15 received supplemental oxygen at one or more pulse oximetry readings (14 did not receive oxygen supplementation). It is certainly possible that removal of oxygen support in the subjects in our study with CCHD would induce further hypoxemia and increase the specificity of the screening test, however, we are unable to make this assessment from the data gathered. This question requires further investigation and the effect of oxygen supplementation on the screening protocol remains unclear. Our mean saturation data do provide some support to the findings of Lueth and colleagues suggesting that oxygen supplementation may not have a negative impact on the sensitivity of pulse oximetry screening for CCHD in newborns. We would not advocate for screening of hypoxemic newborns on oxygen supplementation in the intensive care unit at this time as this is not the intent of the screening guideline [6], however, the findings of this study may inform discussion regarding the timing and process for screening of well infants born at moderate-high altitude who frequently require supplemental oxygen therapy in the first days and weeks of life [13,25]. Certainly, any consideration of pulse oximetry screening for CCHD in the context of supplemental oxygen should be taken with scrutiny both of the patient physiology and use of the screening protocol guideline.

Our retrospective application of the AAP screening protocol did not allow us to exactly replicate the timing of the AAP screening protocol (three screens separated by 1 h each). In addition, the AAP screening protocol is meant to evaluate asymptomatic newborns not presenting in the first 24 h of life, whereas we studied newborns diagnosed with known CCHD. We identify both of these as limitations to this study, however, we used this cohort of infants with known CCHD to estimate the sensitivity of the screening protocol. Further, our retrospective approach resulted in 158 subjects while the very large prospective studies yielded 24–29 subjects with congenital heart disease after screening 20,000–40,000 newborns [18]. Certainly, a future direction will be to apply this study design to a larger cohort of infants with CCHD. An additional limitation is that we found a difference in CCHD diagnoses between the subjects included in the study when compared to those excluded. A disproportionate number of the subjects with transposition of the great arteries were excluded because of atrial septostomy performed before 24 h of life (commonly required for infants with TGA). This may suggest that our cohort of subjects is not representative of the general population of newborns with CCHD, however, newborns requiring atrial septostomy early in life are more likely to present in extremis and not require pulse oximetry screening to identify disease. Finally, this retrospective assessment was dependent on the EHR with pulse oximetry readings that were subject to measurement and recording error from the bedside care provider. These values were not taken for formal screening or research purposes, rather, the readings were collected as a part of routine clinical care. However, these subjects all received hourly oximetry readings recorded in the EHR and the standard is for validation and confirmation by a bedside nurse with interpretation of the waveform when the infants were calm. We identify this limitation to the study design and that of measurement and documentation error by the clinical care team in the EHR. Finally, we applied the screening protocol to newborns who received PGE, oxygen, or both PGE and oxygen, to allow comparison with those who did not receive either PGE or oxygen. We recognize the contribution of both PGE and supplemental oxygen in the interpretation of subjects' pulse oximetry data; however, our results suggest that even when oxygen and PGE were administered the infants still had pulse oximetry values that were low and the therapy did not change the outcome of screening with pulse oximetry in these newborns.

We present the first report evaluating the oxygen saturations of a cohort of infants with known CCHD at moderate altitude. Additionally, we present the results of a hypothetical AAP-recommended pulse oximetry screening protocol in this same cohort. We also found that oxygen supplementation did not impact the ability of the screening protocol to identify CCHD in this cohort, which adds to the consideration of screening in neonatal intensive care units and at higher altitudes. We cannot assess the false positive rate of screening at moderate altitude with our cohort and encourage continued efforts for large population-based studies to evaluate pulse oximetry screening for CCHD.

Author Contributions: J.S.K. designed the study, performed data extraction, interpreted data, and was the primary author of the manuscript. M.W.A. performed data extraction, statistical analysis, and revised the manuscript. M.K.S. was the secondary mentor on the project, interpreted data, and revised the manuscript. C.M.R. was the primary mentor on the project, designed the study, interpreted data, and revised the manuscript. All authors approved the final manuscript as submitted and agree to be accountable for all aspects of work.

References

1. Hoffman, J.I.E. It Is Time for Routine Neonatal Screening by Pulse Oximetry. *Neonatology* **2011**, *99*, 1–9. [CrossRef] [PubMed]
2. Wren, C.; Richmond, S.; Donaldson, L. Presentation of Congenital Heart Disease in Infancy: Implications for Routine Examination. *Arch. Dis. Child. Fetal Neonatal Ed.* **1999**, *80*, F49–F53. [CrossRef] [PubMed]
3. Wright, J.; Kohn, M.; Niermeyer, S.; Rausch, C.M. Feasibility of Critical Congenital Heart Disease Newborn Screening at Moderate Altitude. *Pediatrics* **2014**, *133*, e561–e569. [CrossRef] [PubMed]
4. Peterson, C.; Grosse, S.D.; Oster, M.E.; Olney, R.S.; Cassell, C.H. Cost-Effectiveness of Routine Screening for Critical Congenital Heart Disease in US Newborns. *Pediatrics* **2013**, *132*, e595–e603. [CrossRef] [PubMed]
5. Mahle, W.T.; Newburger, J.W.; Matherne, G.P.; Smith, F.C.; Hoke, T.R.; Koppel, R.; Gidding, S.S.; Beekman, R.H.; Grosse, S.D. Role of Pulse Oximetry in Examining Newborns for Congenital Heart Disease: A Scientific Statement from the AHA and AAP. *Pediatrics* **2009**, *124*, 823–836. [CrossRef] [PubMed]
6. Mahle, W.T.; Martin, G.R.; Beekman, R.H.; Morrow, W.R. Section on Cardiology and Cardiac Surgery Executive Committee. Endorsement of Health and Human Services Recommendation for Pulse Oximetry Screening for Critical Congenital Heart Disease. *Pediatrics* **2012** *129*, 190–192. [PubMed]

7. Martin, G.R.; Beekman, R.H.; Mikula, E.B.; Fasules, J.; Garg, L.F.; Kemper, A.R.; Morrow, W.R.; Pearson, G.D.; Mahle, W.T. Implementing Recommended Screening for Critical Congenital Heart Disease. *Pediatrics* **2013**, *132*, e185–e192. [CrossRef] [PubMed]
8. Kemper, A.R.; Mahle, W.T.; Martin, G.R.; Cooley, W.C.; Kumar, P.; Morrow, W.R.; Kelm, K.; Pearson, G.D.; Glidewell, J.; Grosse, S.D.; et al. Strategies for Implementing Screening for Critical Congenital Heart Disease. *Pediatrics* **2011**, *128*, e1259–e1267. [CrossRef] [PubMed]
9. Plana, M.N.; Zamora, J.; Suresh, G.; Fernandez-Pineda, L.; Thangaratinam, S.; Ewer, A.K. Pulse Oximetry Screening for Critical Congenital Heart Defects. *Cochrane Database Syst. Rev.* **2018**, *3*, CD011912. [CrossRef] [PubMed]
10. Oster, M.E.; Aucott, S.W.; Glidewell, J.; Hackell, J.; Kochilas, L.; Martin, G.R.; Phillippi, J.; Pinto, N.M.; Saarinen, A.; Sontag, M.; et al. Lessons Learned from Newborn Screening for Critical Congenital Heart Defects. *Pediatrics* **2016**, *137*, e20154573. [CrossRef] [PubMed]
11. Lueth, E.; Russell, L.; Wright, J.; Duster, M.; Kohn, M.; Miller, J.; Eller, C.; Sontag, M.; Rausch, C. A Novel Approach to Critical Congenital Heart Disease (CCHD) Screening at Moderate Altitude. *IJNS* **2016**, *2*, 4–11. [CrossRef]
12. Thilo, E.H.; Park-Moore, B.; Berman, E.R.; Carson, B.S. Oxygen Saturation by Pulse Oximetry in Healthy Infants at an Altitude of 1610 M (5280 Ft). What Is Normal? *Am. J. Dis. Child.* **1991**, *145*, 1137–1140. [CrossRef] [PubMed]
13. Ravert, P.; Detwiler, T.L.; Dickinson, J.K. Mean Oxygen Saturation in Well Neonates at Altitudes between 4498 and 8150 Feet. *Adv. Neonatal Care* **2011**, *11*, 412–417. [CrossRef] [PubMed]
14. Bakr, A.F.; Habib, H.S. Normal Values of Pulse Oximetry in Newborns at High Altitude. *J. Trop. Pediatr.* **2005**, *51*, 170–173. [CrossRef] [PubMed]
15. Samuel, T.Y.; Bromiker, R.; Mimouni, F.B.; Picard, E.; Lahav, S.; Mandel, D.; Goldberg, S. Newborn Oxygen Saturation at Mild Altitude Versus Sea Level: Implications for Neonatal Screening for Critical Congenital Heart Disease. *Acta Paediatr.* **2013**, *102*, 379–384. [CrossRef] [PubMed]
16. Harris, P.A.; Taylor, R.; Thielke, R.; Payne, J.; Gonzalez, N.; Conde, J.G. Research Electronic Data Capture (REDCap)—A Metadata-Driven Methodology and Workflow Process for Providing Translational Research Informatics Support. *J. Biomed. Inform.* **2009**, *42*, 377–381. [CrossRef] [PubMed]
17. Ailes, E.C.; Gilboa, S.M.; Honein, M.A.; Oster, M.E. Estimated Number of Infants Detected and Missed by Critical Congenital Heart Defect Screening. *Pediatrics* **2015**, *135*, 1000–1008. [CrossRef] [PubMed]
18. Thangaratinam, S.; Brown, K.; Zamora, J.; Khan, K.S.; Ewer, A.K. Pulse Oximetry Screening for Critical Congenital Heart Defects in Asymptomatic Newborn Babies: A Systematic Review and Meta-Analysis. *Lancet* **2012**, *379*, 2459–2464. [CrossRef]
19. De-Wahl Granelli, A.; Wennergren, M.; Sandberg, K.; Mellander, M.; Bejlum, C.; Inganäs, L.; Eriksson, M.; Segerdahl, N.; Agren, A.; Ekman-Joelsson, B.-M.; et al. Impact of Pulse Oximetry Screening on the Detection of Duct Dependent Congenital Heart Disease: A Swedish Prospective Screening Study in 39,821 Newborns. *BMJ* **2009**, *338*, a3037. [CrossRef] [PubMed]
20. Ewer, A.K.; Middleton, L.J.; Furmston, A.T.; Bhoyar, A.; Daniels, J.P.; Thangaratinam, S.; Deeks, J.J.; Khan, K.S. PulseOx Study Group. Pulse Oximetry Screening for Congenital Heart Defects in Newborn Infants (PulseOx): A Test Accuracy Study. *Lancet* **2011**, *378*, 785–794. [CrossRef]
21. Manja, V.; Mathew, B.; Carrion, V.; Lakshminrusimha, S. Critical Congenital Heart Disease Screening by Pulse Oximetry in a Neonatal Intensive Care Unit. *J. Perinatol.* **2015**, *35*, 67–71. [CrossRef] [PubMed]
22. Hu, X.-J.; Zhao, Q.-M.; Ma, X.-J.; Yan, W.-L.; Ge, X.-L.; Jia, B.; Liu, F.; Wu, L.; Ye, M.; Huang, G.-Y. Pulse Oximetry Could Significantly Enhance the Early Detection of Critical Congenital Heart Disease in Neonatal Intensive Care Units. *Acta Paediatr.* **2016**, *105*, e499–e505. [CrossRef] [PubMed]
23. Goetz, E.M.; Magnuson, K.M.; Eickhoff, J.C.; Porte, M.A.; Hokanson, J.S. Pulse Oximetry Screening for Critical Congenital Heart Disease in the Neonatal Intensive Care Unit. *J. Perinatol.* **2016**, *36*, 52–56. [CrossRef] [PubMed]
24. Van Naarden Braun, K.; Grazel, R.; Koppel, R.; Lakshminrusimha, S.; Lohr, J.; Kumar, P.; Govindaswami, B.; Giuliano, M.; Cohen, M.; Spillane, N.; et al. Evaluation of Critical Congenital Heart Defects Screening Using Pulse Oximetry in the Neonatal Intensive Care Unit. *J. Perinatol.* **2017**, *37*, 1117–1123. [CrossRef] [PubMed]
25. Niermeyer, S.; Shaffer, E.M.; Thilo, E.; Corbin, C.; Moore, L.G. Arterial Oxygenation and Pulmonary Arterial Pressure in Healthy Neonates and Infants at High Altitude. *J. Pediatr.* **1993**, *123*, 767–772. [CrossRef]

4

The Neonatal Screening Program in Brazil, Focus on Sickle Cell Disease (SCD)

Ana C. Silva-Pinto [1,2,*], Maria Cândida Alencar de Queiroz [2], Paula Juliana Antoniazzo Zamaro [3], Miranete Arruda [1,4] and Helena Pimentel dos Santos [1,5]

1 Policy of Integral Attention to People with Sickle Cell Disease (PIAPSCD), Technical Advisory Council for Sickle Cell Disease (TAC-SCD), CGSH/DAET/SAS, Ministry of Health, Asa Norte Brasília 70719-040, Brazil; miranetearruda1@gmail.com (M.A.); helena.pimentel@apaesalvador.org.br (H.P.d.S.)
2 Regional Blood Center of Ribeirão Preto, HC-FMRP, University of Sao Paulo (USP), Campus Universitário, Ribeirão Preto 14049-900, Brazil; maria.candida@saude.gov.br
3 National Newborn Screening Program Policy (NNSPP)/CGSH/SAS, Ministry of Health, Asa Norte Brasília 70719-040, Brazil; triagemneonatal@saude.gov.br
4 State Health Secretariat, State of Pernambuco, Recife 50751-530, Brazil
5 Newborn Screening Program, APAE-Salvador, Salvador 41830-141, Brazil
* Correspondence: acristina@hemocentro.fmrp.usp.br;

Abstract: Since 2001, the Brazilian Ministry of Health has been coordinating a National Neonatal Screening Program (NNSP) that now covers all the 26 states and the Federal District of the Brazilian Republic and targets six diseases including sickle cell disease (SCD) and other hemoglobinopathies. In 2005, the program coverage reached 80% of the total live births. Since then, it has oscillated between 80% and 84% globally with disparities from one state to another (>95% in São Paulo State). The Ministry of Health has also published several Guidelines for clinical follow-up and treatment for the diseases comprised by the neonatal screening program. The main challenge was, and still is, to organize the public health network (SUS), from diagnosis and basic care to reference centers in order to provide comprehensive care for patients diagnosed by neonatal screening, especially for SCD patients. Considerable gains have already been achieved, including the implementation of a network within SUS and the addition of scientific and technological progress to treatment protocols. The goals for the care of SCD patients are the intensification of information provided to health care professionals and patients, measures to prevent complications, and care and health promotion, considering these patients in a global and integrated way, to reduce mortality and enhance their quality of life.

Keywords: neonatal screening; sickle cell disease; hemoglobinopathies

---

1. Background

The Brazilian population is currently estimated at over 208 million people. For the most part, three distinct peoples form the ethnic backgrounds of this population: the Native Americans (Indians), the Portuguese, and the Africans. Population data from the 2010 Demographic Census showed that 50.7% of the Brazilian population is made up of Afro-Americans, 47.7% Caucasians, and 0.7% Indians (0.9% unspecified). Since the population is broadly miscegenated, all national programs must be universalized and not directed at a specific portion of the population. Therefore, the neonatal screening program is national and universal, aiming to reach 100% of live births in the country [1].

2. The Neonatal Screening Program

The history of neonatal screening (NS) in Brazil goes back to 1976, when APAE-São Paulo began neonatal screening for phenylketonuria (PKU). Several pilot NS initiatives were then initiated independently without coordination nor standardization among Brazilian states. In 1992, the screening for PKU and congenital hypothyroidism (CH) was included in the public health system, known as SUS [2]. In 1998, the State of Minas Gerais was the first to introduce a universal State NS Program for sickle cell disease (SCD) in the already existing programs for PK and CH [3].

However, the recognition of NS as a specific public health program only happened in 2001 after the founding of the National Neonatal Screening Program (NNSP) coordinated by the Ministry of Health [4]. The program led to the definition of standards and protocols for the whole country, and placed screening as a global health action aimed at preventing child health problems not only through testing to detect the disease but also the active search of suspected cases, diagnostic confirmation, treatment, and follow-up of patients [5]. The NNSP initially focused on PKU, CH, cystic fibrosis, SCD, and other hemoglobinopathies. In 2014, the program was extended to screening for biotinidase deficiency and congenital adrenal hyperplasia.

The Ministry of Health defined priorities and divided the program into four phases, accrediting the states according to each one's capacity. From 2001 onward, reference services were certified sequentially in one of the four phases of the NNSP. Table 1 shows the years at which each of the phases reached universal implementation in all the states and the Federal District.

Figure 1 illustrates the sequential expansion of the neonatal screening program in the various states of Brazil between 2010 and 2014.

Table 1. The implementation of neonatal screening divided into phases, and its year of universalization.

Phases	Diseases	Year of National Implementation
Phase I	Phenylketonuria and congenital hypothyroidism	2006
Phase II	Sickle cell disease and other hemoglobinopathies	2013
Phase III	Cystic fibrosis	2013
Phase IV	Congenital adrenal hyperplasia and biotinidase deficiency	2014

The coverage rate of the program (percentage of the screened live births) varied over the years (Figure 2). Since 2006, it has remained above 85% at the national level, with few variations. This figure relates to variations in the health care network capacity from state to state and to variations in the population's access to it. In São Paulo State, for example, the percentage of coverage reaches over 95%.

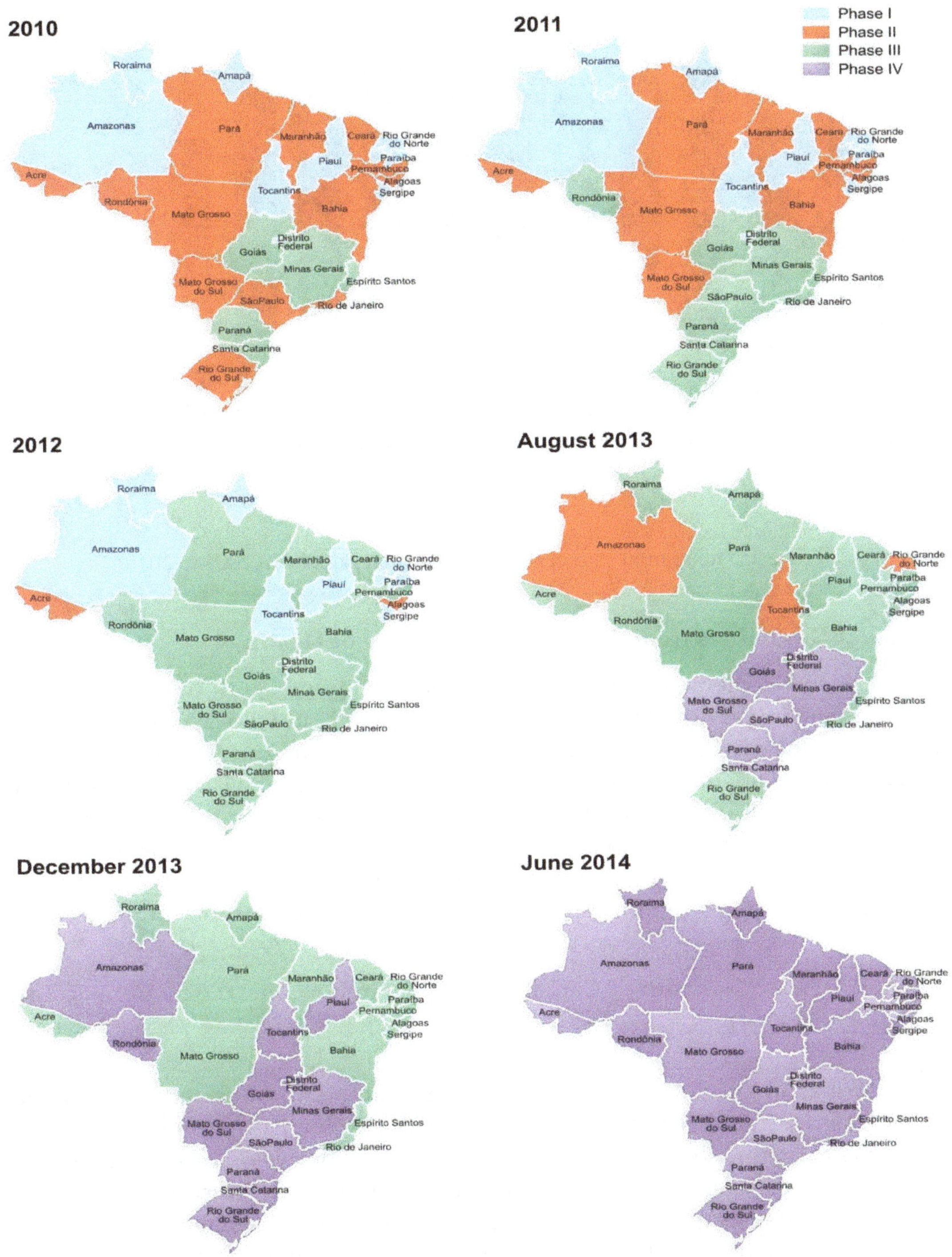

Figure 1. Expansion of the neonatal screening program in Brazil from 2010 to 2014 regarding the four phases of the National Neonatal Screening Program (NNSP).

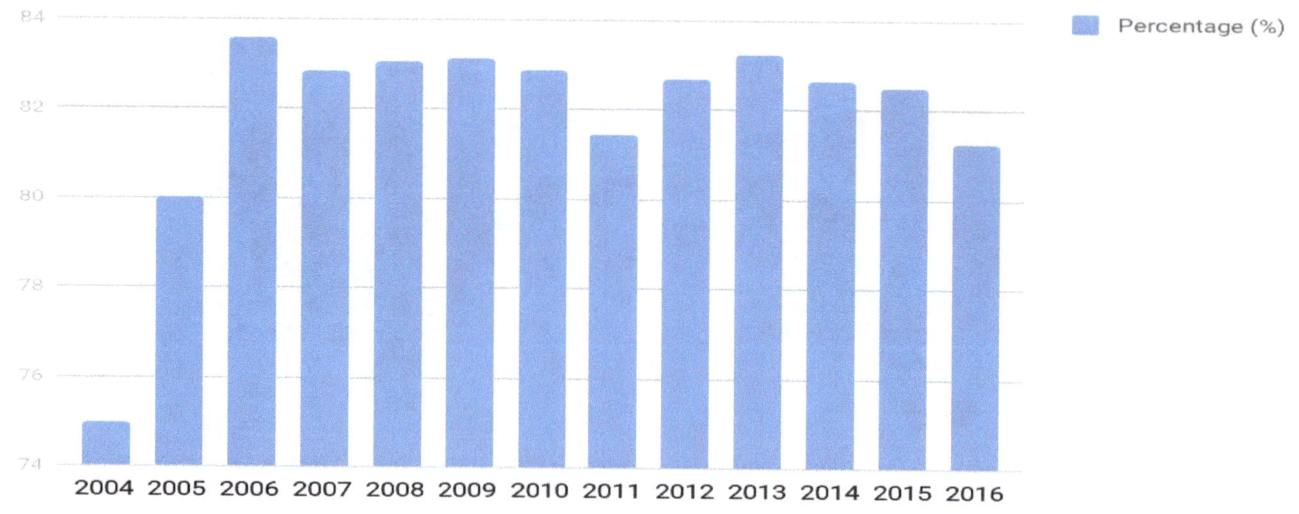

Figure 2. The annual rate of the program coverage from 2004 to 2016.

3. Resolutions and Guidelines from the Brazilian Ministry of Health

In addition to the implementation of neonatal screening and with the goal of standardizing standards of care, the Ministry of Health has published several guidelines for clinical follow-up and treatment for each of the diseases included in the neonatal screening program (see, for example, the Clinical Protocol and Therapeutic Guidelines for Sickle Cell Disease [6]). These include the description of the general concepts for each disease, diagnostic criteria, inclusion and exclusion criteria, treatment and mechanisms of regulation, and control and treatment evaluation. Altogether, they establish a national policy and should be used by the state and municipal Health Secretariats for the regulation of care access, authorization, registration, and reimbursement of the corresponding procedures.

4. The Sickle Cell Disease Network of Care Inside SUS: From Neonatal Screening to Follow-Up in Reference Centers

Health is inscribed in the national Constitution as a right for everyone and a duty of the Brazilian Republic. This was the framework for the creation of the Unified Health System, known as SUS, which contemplates the guidelines for health promotion and provision of services and establishes the community participation and transfer of federal resources to other jurisdictions [7,8]. Despite the great barriers that SUS has faced since its conception, it has managed to establish itself as a system that proposes to be an institutional redistributive model, guaranteeing universal coverage. In this context, the inclusion of sickle cell disease (SCD) and other hemoglobinopathies in the National Neonatal Screening Program (NNSP) instituted by the SUS in 2001 shows recognition of this group of pathologies as a national public health issue [9].

The proportion of live births with SCD varies widely among the states, being more frequent in states with a higher concentration of African descendants. For example, in Bahia for every 650 births, 1 child has SCD, followed by Rio de Janeiro (1:1200) and then Pernambuco, Maranhão, and Minas Gerais, with 1:1400. Table 2 shows the incidence of newborns affected by SCD in 12 states representative of the four most populated regions of Brazil (the fifth region being the North that covers the Amazonian forest).

Table 2. Incidence of sickle cell disease and sickle cell trait in some Brazilian states.

Regions of Brazil	State	Incidence/Live Births	Incidence of the S Mutation
Northeast	Maranhão	1:1400	1:23
	Pernambuco	1:1400	1:23
	Bahia	1:650	1:17
Center-west	Goiás	1:1400	1:28
	Mato Grosso do Sul	1:8300	1:70
Southeast	Minas Gerais	1:1400	1:30
	Espírito Santo	1:1800	1:28
	Rio de Janeiro	1:1200	1:21
	São Paulo	1:4000	1:35
South	Paraná	1:13,000	1:65
	Santa Catarina	1:13,000	1:65
	Rio Grande do Sul	1:13,500	1:65

Building up the current network and system of care for the people with SCD in Brazil has been a long process, in some ways reminiscent of the 1970s struggle for civil rights and equality for access to care in the USA that led to the US *National Sickle Cell Anemia Control Act* in 1972 [10,11]. In the 1980s, Brazilian representative entities for the the defense of the rights of family and people with SCD took the first steps to formulate claims, initially at the local level, and then expanded their coordination with the formation in 2001 of the National Federation of Associations of People with Sickle Diseases (FENAFAL). The march Zumbi dos Palmares against Racism, for Citizenship and for Life, held in Brasilia in 1995, was an important milestone in the struggle of black people against the Brazilian State for affirmative action and against racism in terms of health care. From this action, important policies emerged, including the Policy of Integral Attention to People with Sickle Cell Disease (PIAPSCD) [12]. The major goals were to change the natural history of SCD in Brazil, by reducing morbidity and mortality, promoting greater survival, and improving the quality of life for people with SCD. Commitments were made to provide genetic guidance, safeguarding reproductive rights of people with the sickle cell trait, and to disseminate information about SCD to the general population.

In 2006, the Ministry of Health established a Technical Advisory Council for Sickle Cell Disease (TAC-SCD) to help states and municipalities organize their programs of care for people with SCD. TAC is composed of specialists, managers of state and municipal jurisdictions of SUS, and representatives of educational, research, and assistance institutions involved in the care of people with SCD who are invited to act voluntarily. There is also a representation of the users chosen by FENAFAL. TAC is responsible for producing the guidelines for the management of SCD and its complications, genetic guidelines, family guidelines, guidelines for oral health and on the role of nursing, which are printed and distributed in the reference centers and in the basic SUS network. These materials are available electronically in the SUS Virtual Library (VL). The members of TAC also conduct training courses, workshops, and symposia on SCD in all regions of the country, contributing to the continuing education of health professionals.

Within SUS, the standardized attention to people with SCD encompasses all levels from early diagnosis to bone marrow transplantation. Assistance begins in basic care with the early diagnosis free of charge through the NNSP that links the affected child to the basic health unit, responsible for the first procedures of prevention such as prophylaxis with penicillin initiated in the first month of life, immunobiological approaches, and then referral to the regional Specialized Care Service. In most states, the reference center is the Blood Center, which is normally integrated with the local health network to meet other health needs, such as the use of hydroxyurea, transcranial Doppler, and all procedures of greater complexity. The implementation of the SCD network in all the states is intended to guarantee decentralized care beginning with diagnosis, with the assistance of a multi-professional and multidisciplinary team, providing health education with a focus on self-management and access to specialized and high complexity care in all the 26 states and the Federal District [13].

5. Challenges for the Full Implementation of the SCD Care Network

Despite major advances, the organization of a robust health care network for people with SCD is still a major challenge to SUS. Only a network with the potential for the collective construction of solutions is able to cope with the complexity of demands and to guarantee the promotion of autonomy and citizenship to people with SCD. The disease has not yet reached the level of visibility pursued that is necessary to provide its target population with the right to health they deserve to extend their life horizon with personal and social well-being.

Notably, considerable gains have already been achieved, including the implementation of neonatal screening at the national level together with scientific and technological progress with respect to treatment. Preliminary data on the effect of hydroxyurea treatment and mortality rates have been published [14–16]. However, more precise epidemiological data covering the entire country are still needed. A national registry for SCD patients is being set up to collect more reliable information to evaluate the system: percentage of new cases that actually enter follow-up at reference centers, immunization rate, percentage of patients that started pneumococcal prophylaxis, rate of children screened with transcranial Doppler, use of hydroxyurea, and death rates at the country level. What is sought to bring attention to people with SCD is the intensification of information provided, measures to prevent injuries, and care and health promotion, considering these patients in a global and integrated way, to reduce mortality and enhance their quality of life.

Author Contributions: All authors contributed equally to the manuscript: A.C.S.-P. was responsible for the design, writing, and review of the manuscript; M.C.A.d.Q. was responsible for the SCD network writing and review; P.J.A.Z. was responsible for the newborn screening data and figures; M.A. was responsible for SCD epidemiological data and the review of the final version; and H.P.d.S. was responsible for the newborn screening background and review of the manuscript.

References

1. Brasil, IBGE. Demographic Census 2010. Available online: https://www.ibge.gov.br/ (accessed on 17 September 2018).
2. Brasil, Ministério da Saúde. Portaria GM/MS n°22 de 15/01/1992—triagem para fenilcetonúria e hipotireoidismo Congênito. *Diário Oficial da União*, 15 January 1992.
3. Paixão, M.C.; Cunha Ferraz, M.H.; Januário, J.N.; Viana, M.B.; Lima, J.M. Reliability of isoelectrofocusing for the detection of Hb S, Hb C, and HB D in a pioneering population-based program of newborn screening in Brazil. *Hemoglobin* **2001**, *25*, 297–303. [CrossRef] [PubMed]
4. Brasil, Ministério da saúde. Portaria GM/MS n° 822 de 06 de junho de 2001—Programa de triagem neonatal no Brasil. *Diário Oficial da União*, 6 June 2001.
5. Carvalho, T.M.; Santos, H.P.; Santos, I.C.G.P.; Vargas, P.R.; Pedrosa, J. Newborn screening: A national public health programme in Brazil. *J. Inherit. Metab. Dis.* **2007**, *30*, 615. [CrossRef] [PubMed]
6. Brasil, Ministério da saúde. Portaria SAS/MS N° 55 de 29 de janeiro de 2010—Protocolo Clínico e Diretrizes Terapêuticas para Doença Falciforme". *Diário Oficial da União*, 29 January 2010.
7. Brasil, Ministério da saúde. Lei n° 8.080, de 19 de setembro de 1990, criação do SUS—Sistema Único de Saúde. *Diário Oficial da União*, 19 September 1990.
8. Seta, M.H.; Oliveira, C.V.D.S.; Pepe, V.L.E. Health protection in Brazil: the National Sanitary Surveillance System. *Cien Saude Colet* **2017**, *22*, 3225–3234. [CrossRef] [PubMed]
9. Ramalho, A.S.; Magna, L.A.; Paiva-Silva, R.B. A portaria n° 822/01 do Ministério da Saúde e as peculiaridades das hemoglobinopatias em saúde pública no Brasil. *Cad. Saúde Pública* **2003**, *19*, 1195–1199. [CrossRef] [PubMed]

10. Vichinsky, E. Sickle cell disease and thalassemia: disorders of globin production. (2008) pages 3-5, in Special anniversary brochure, American Society of Hematology: 50 Years in Hematology: Research That Revolutionized Patient Care. Available online: http://www.hematology.org/About/History/50-Years/1533.aspx (accessed on 13 January 2019).
11. Bassett, M.T. Beyond Berets: The Black Panthers as Health Activists. *Am. J. Public Health* **2016**, *106*, 1741–1743. [CrossRef] [PubMed]
12. Brasil, Ministério da saúde. Portaria de nº 1391 de 16 de agosto de 2005—Diretrizes para a Política Nacional de Atenção Integral às Pessoas com Doença Falciforme e outras Hemoglobinopatias. *Diário Oficial da União*, 16 August 2005.
13. Cançado, R.D.; Jesus, J.A. A doença falciforme no Brasil. *Rev. Bras. Hematol. Hemoter.* **2007**, *29*, 204–206. [CrossRef]
14. Lobo, C.L.; Pinto, J.F.; Nascimento, E.M.; Moura, P.G.; Cardoso, G.P.; Hankins, J.S. The effect of hydroxcarbamide therapy on survival of children with sickle cell disease. *Br. J. Haematol.* **2013**, *161*, 852–860. [CrossRef] [PubMed]
15. Fernandes, A.P.; Januário, J.N.; Cangussu, C.B.; Macedo, D.L.; Viana, M.B. Mortality of children with sickle cell disease: A population study. *J. Pediatr. (Rio J).* **2010**, *86*, 279–284. [CrossRef]
16. Lobo, C.L.C.; Nascimento, E.M.D.; Jesus, L.J.C.; Freitas, T.G.; Lugon, J.R.; Ballas, S.K. Mortality in children, adolescents and adults with sickle cell anemia in Rio de Janeiro, Brazil. *Rev. Bras. Hematol. Hemoter.* **2018**, *40*, 37–42. [CrossRef] [PubMed]

5

Establishing Pompe Disease Newborn Screening: The Role of Industry

Joan M. Keutzer †

Sanofi Genzyme, Cambridge, MA 02142, USA; keutzer@verizon.net
† Retired.

Abstract: When clinical trials for enzyme replacement therapy for Pompe disease commenced, a need for newborn screening (NBS) for Pompe disease was recognized. Two methods for NBS for Pompe disease by measuring acid α-glucosidase in dried blood spots on filter paper were developed in an international collaborative research effort led by Genzyme. Both methods were used successfully in NBS pilot programs to demonstrate the feasibility of NBS for Pompe disease. Since 2009, all babies born in Taiwan have been screened for Pompe disease. Pompe disease was added to the Recommended Uniform (Newborn) Screening Panel in the United States in 2015. NBS for Pompe disease is possible because of the unprecedented and selfless collaborations of countless international experts who shared their thoughts and data freely with the common goal of establishing NBS for Pompe disease expeditiously.

Keywords: newborn screening; Pompe disease; acid α-glucosidase

---

1. Introduction

We frequently hear that "it takes a village" to get things done. In the case of Pompe disease newborn screening (NBS), "it took the world". NBS for Pompe disease resulted from an unprecedented international collaboration among patients with Pompe disease, the Pompe disease medical and scientific communities, government agencies, and industry. Starting in 1999, the baton was passed between research groups who acted urgently to generate the data required, develop methods for newborn screening for Pompe disease, and begin to establish newborn screening for Pompe disease.

In 1998, Genzyme (now Sanofi Genzyme) initiated a clinical development program for enzyme replacement therapy (ERT) for Pompe disease. During meetings to plan the clinical trials, physicians voiced concerns about the ability of patients with Pompe disease to get an early and accurate diagnosis. They cautioned that if the deficiencies in diagnostic testing were not addressed, that Genzyme would not be able to conduct successful clinical trials with ERT in Pompe disease because some symptoms would be irreversible. Thus, diagnostic delays could result in the inability to determine if ERT for Pompe disease was a viable treatment option. Patients with later-onset Pompe disease (LOPD) referred to the test as unreliable and invasive. Some patients told Genzyme that they had three muscle biopsies before they received a diagnosis. Parents of patients with infantile-onset Pompe disease (IOPD) mentioned waiting two grueling months after the collection of a skin biopsy to get a diagnosis. There was no assay that could use blood samples to diagnose Pompe disease.

In response, I assembled a team of Genzyme colleagues to determine if there was a role that we could play in improving diagnostics for Pompe disease. The team consisted of members from Research and Development, Genzyme Diagnostics, Genzyme Genetics, Regulatory Affairs, and the Pompe disease Clinical Development Team. The team interviewed multiple Pompe disease stakeholders, including patients, physicians, and diagnostic laboratories. Ultimately, Henri Termeer, the CEO of Genzyme, decided to sponsor international research to develop assays useful for NBS, diagnosis using blood samples, patient monitoring, and genotyping for Pompe disease. This decision was not supported unanimously internally. Some felt very strongly that it created a conflict of interest if a company was developing therapeutic and diagnostic testing for the same disease. Several healthy conversations about our role in patient diagnosis ensued and led to a commitment to keep our involvement in assay development scientific and make the resultant intellectual property and methodologies available to all. Much of the work was co-sponsored or sponsored by Genzyme. In 2003, Genzyme established an R&D lab to optimize, validate, and transfer methodology. The team was active through 2016.

2. Early Attempts to Develop Newborn Screening Assays

We hoped that NBS for Pompe disease could replicate what was done for other enzyme deficiencies, like PKU, and measure the accumulation of the enzyme's substrate in dried bloodspots on filter paper (DBS) in a multiplex assay that could screen for multiple treatable lysosomal storage disorders (LSDs) simultaneously. In 2000, we started to collaborate with Sarah Young and David Millington on work they had initiated earlier. They developed the urine Hex4 assay, which is an indirect measure of elevated glycogen. The assay did not translate into an assay for DBS, but it is useful for monitoring patients with Pompe disease [1].

We knew that the measurement of acid α-glucosidase enzyme activity in mixed leukocytes and whole blood was complicated by the presence of another alpha-glucosidase, maltase glucoamylase (MGA), which is active at an acid pH and masks the deficiency of acid α-glucosidase; therefore, we sponsored the search for an inhibitor of MGA so that acid α-glucosidase could be quantitated in blood. For the first two years, no one found a useful inhibitor, but labs in Europe, Asia, and the United States kept trying. At International Conference on Inborn Errors of Metabolism (ICIEM) in Cambridge, UK in September 2000, Nestor Chamoles from the Laboratorio Chamoles in Buenos Aires, Argentina presented a poster that demonstrated that it was possible to measure the lysosomal enzyme alpha-L-iduronidase in DBS and differentiate DBS from patients with MPS I from DBS from obligate heterozygotes and healthy individuals [2]. We encouraged Chamoles to try to create an assay for acid α-glucosidase in DBS using 4-methylumbelliferyl-α-D-glucopyranoside (4-MUG) as the substrate.

3. Measuring Acid α-Glucosidase in Dried Bloodspots on Filter Paper

We knew that NBS was relying more heavily on multiplex assays, so we continued to search for technologies that could be used in a multiplex assay for LSDs. Our assumption was that like the other multiplex assays in NBS, the assay would measure analytes (substrates of the missing enzymes) in DBS, but that changed to wanting to measure several enzyme activities in a multiplex assay. At the same ICIEM meeting in Cambridge, UK in September 2000, Frantisek Turecek, C. Ronald Scott, and Michael H. Gelb from the University of Washington presented an assay that measured acid sphingomyelinase and β-galactocerebrosidase in skin fibroblast homogenates for clinical laboratory diagnosis [3]. The assay used novel biotinylated substrate conjugates, purification of the products on streptavidin agarose beads, and quantification of products using electrospray ionization mass spectrometry with stable-isotope-labeled internal standards that were chemically identical to the products of the enzymatic reactions. We invited them to join the efforts and their initial goal was to develop a multiplex assay for six lysosomal storage disorders Pompe disease, MPS I, Fabry disease, Gaucher disease, Krabbe disease, and Niemann–Pick disease types A and B.

In 2003, Gabriella Niizawa from the Chamoles lab developed a fluorometric assay using 4-methylumbelliferyl-α-D-glucopyranoside (4-MUG) as the substrate that could differentiate DBS from patients with IOPD from obligate heterozygotes and healthy individuals. The method used maltose to inhibit MGA since MGA has a higher affinity for maltose than acid α-glucosidase [4]. Chamoles invited X. Kate Zhang and me to his lab to run the assay and in June 2003, and allowed us to take his protocol into the Genzyme LSD assay development lab so we could try to optimize the protocol and adapt it from one using 1.5 mL microcentrifuge tubes to one that uses in 96-well plates and could be automated. Our activities were limited by the paucity of samples from patients previously diagnosed with Pompe disease.

In September 2003, Genzyme received a phone call from a father from Peru. He wanted to know how to access treatment for Pompe disease because his 4-month-old baby was suspected of having the disease because her brother died from Pompe disease. The baby did not have a confirmed diagnosis. We talked to Chamoles who said he was not ready to use the DBS assay for suspected cases but would test and report a result if Genzyme tested duplicate samples blinded and the results concurred. We requested duplicate DBS from the baby, the mother, the father, and someone unrelated. Peru did not have an NBS program, so we had to use a courier to deliver DBS cards to the clinic. Chamoles and Genzyme had similar results. Samples from both parents and the unrelated donor were in the normal range and the sample from the baby was consistent with a diagnosis of Pompe disease. The child and her family relocated to Durham, NC to participate in the ongoing clinical trial at Duke University Medical Center. The diagnosis of Pompe disease was confirmed at Duke using an assay in fibroblasts. This patient was the first identified with Pompe disease using the new blood-based assay and we gained confidence in the methodology.

Chamoles, Gelb, and the Genzyme R&D Team met at ICIEM in Brisbane in September 2003 where Chamoles presented data on maltose inhibition of MGA. We agreed to meet as soon as possible to discuss sharing lab methods. At the time, Gelb did not have a DBS assay for Pompe disease. In January 2004, Genzyme hosted a mini symposium to generate a collaborative research agenda. At that meeting, Gelb and Turecek revealed that they identified 80 μM acarbose (a drug used to control blood glucose levels in type 2 diabetes) to inhibit MGA [5]. However, all three labs had issues with sample availability. Chamoles had a limited number of samples because he collected DBS from patients undergoing diagnostic evaluation for Pompe disease and from their parents who were considered obligate carriers, but he shared them. Genzyme agreed that they would adapt both methods that used microcentrifuge tubes to 96-well dishes so that the relative effectiveness of maltose and acarbose could be studied more easily.

4. Optimizing the Methods

During the adaptation, optimization and validation activities led by Helmut Kallwass, the Genzyme R&D team, determined that acarbose was superior to maltose in the assay and that 8 μM acarbose was superior to 80 μM acarbose. Although 8 μM and 80 μM acarbose selectively blocked MGA over acid α-glucosidase, use of 8 uM acarbose inhibited less acid α-glucosidase (i.e., acarbose does have finite affinity for acid α-glucosidase but has higher affinity for MGA). However, we thought it was important to compare the DBS assay to the fibroblast assay in matched samples. Fortunately, in anticipation of evaluating the DBS assay, the R&D group at Duke University under the leadership of Deeksha Bali collected DBS from some IOPD patients for which they had fibroblast cultures. Bali's team saw discrimination between patients with IOPD, obligate heterozygotes, and controls using 8 μM acarbose and the results using acarbose compared well with those using the skin fibroblast assay in the patients [6].

The Genzyme Clinical Development Team assisted in sample collection. In 2003, the informed consent and protocol for the pivotal Phase 3 clinical trial for patients with IOPD (A Study of the Safety and Efficacy of rhGAA in Patients with Infantile-onset Pompe Disease (NCT00059280)) were amended to include collecting DBS for developing DBS enzyme activity assays for acid α-glucosidase. In 2004, a Prospective, Observational Study in Patients with Late-Onset Pompe Disease (NCT00077662) included an optional request for DBS samples. In 2005, A Placebo-Controlled Study of Safety and Effectiveness of Myozyme (alglucosidase alfa) in Patients with Late-Onset Pompe Disease called the Late-Onset Treatment Study [LOTS] (NCT00158600) included an optional request for DBS samples during screening. There was virtually 100% patient participation in donating DBS in the three clinical trials. Without these samples, we could not have progressed in developing NBS or blood-based diagnostic testing for Pompe disease.

The DBS assay consistently differentiated the 24 previously diagnosed IOPD and 100 patients screened for LOTS from controls. Testing DBS samples from 61 patients from LOPOS previously diagnosed with LOPD revealed that 58 had results consistent with a diagnosis of Pompe disease and three had results in the normal range. Measuring acid α-glucosidase enzyme activity in fibroblasts and acid α-glucosidase gene (*GAA*) sequence analysis confirmed that the three patients with a neuromuscular disease were misdiagnosed with Pompe disease [7]. Four fibroblast samples had ≤1% residual enzyme activity so results from fibroblasts cannot be used to predict disease phenotype in cases identified by newborn screening. The results in the DBS assay were similar for IOPD and LOPD, so the DBS assay cannot be used to predict disease phenotype.

It is worth noting that all participating DBS collection sites were trained on how to make DBS via conference call and none of the DBS received from the clinical sites were unsatisfactory for use in assay development; this suggested that it might be feasible to use DBS samples for clinical diagnosis. DBS sampling permits access to testing for metabolic diseases in remote areas; DBS samples can be conveniently collected and shipped through the mail to a distant laboratory for analysis.

5. Early Experience with the Acid α-Glucosidase Enzyme Assay

Paul (Wuh-Liang) Hwu and Nancy (Yin-Hsiu) Chien invited Chamoles and I to a meeting at the Asian Regional International NBS Meeting in September 2004. They proposed that they were uniquely situated to conduct the first large-scale Pompe disease NBS pilot. They described a plan to treat those diagnosed with IOPD immediately and follow the patients' outcomes using the protocols identical to the pivotal alglucosidase alfa clinical trial in IOPD, since they were a clinical trial site. We transferred that methodology from our Genzyme R&D lab to the National Taiwan University Hospital (NTUH) NBS Center in October 2004. NTUH introduced the word's first Pompe disease NBS pilot program at the end of 2005 [8]. Yuan-Tsong Chen from Academia Sinica in Taipei, Taiwan collaborated in the design and execution of the program.

Initially, the NTUH lab ran three separate fluorometric assays to measure acid α-glucosidase, neutral α-glucosidase (NAG), and maltase-glucoamylase (MGA) activities. NAG and MGA were used to differentiate cases of Pompe disease from false positive cases. As the pilot progressed and the lab had more experience, cautious and methodical adjustments of assay cut-offs were used to minimize the risk of false positive and false negative test results. During the pilot, NTUH identified the high prevalence of the *GAA* pseudodeficiency allele (p.G576S) and the increase in phenotype severity when the polymorphism is in cis [9]. Since 2009, all newborns in Taiwan have been screened for Pompe disease. In 2015, NTUH adopted the tandem mass spectrometry-based multiplex LSD enzyme assay.

Today, it seems obvious that the DBS assay with acarbose is useful in diagnosing Pompe disease since all assays for Pompe disease using samples from blood include acarbose, but previous experiences with Pompe disease diagnoses and misdiagnoses left many skeptical of the new method in its early days. In December 2006, Genzyme sponsored a meeting of The Pompe Disease Diagnostic Working Group in London to establish a consensus regarding the application of these new assays for the laboratory diagnosis of Pompe disease. The Working Group consisted of scientists, geneticists, and clinicians working in the field of Pompe disease. The group agreed that cultured skin fibroblasts had been the gold standard, but was rapidly being replaced by assays in blood samples because they are less invasive, more rapid, and are easier to standardize [10]. The meeting was an important step in bringing laboratories and clinicians together to agree that the DBS assay using acarbose to inhibit MGA was useful to get a presumptive positive diagnoses for Pompe disease and that at least one secondary positive test (for example, *GAA* sequence analysis) would support a biochemical diagnosis of Pompe disease. Genzyme's R&D team made the DBS assay protocol available to anyone who requested it and trained labs at Genzyme and remotely as requested. This hastened the adoption of the fluorescent assay to measure acid α-glucosidase enzyme activity and increased the number of patients being diagnosed with Pompe disease worldwide.

While the team at NTUH was using the Genzyme R&D adaptation of the Chamoles lab assay in their NBS program, the Genzyme R&D team that was led by Zhang was adapting the tandem mass spectrometry-based assay for multiple LSD enzymes from the University of Washington [5] to a high-throughput method. However, Genzyme did not have any experience in NBS, so we asked each NBS lab in the United States to answer a survey about the published assay and its suitability for use in NBS. For each survey returned, Genzyme made a donation to the Association of Public Health Laboratories. Based on the responses from NBS labs, Genzyme transformed the assay into a robust high throughput 96-well plate format assay using a robotic liquid handling system for sample transfer and minimizing the detergent burden on the mass spectrometer by replacing Triton X-100 with CHAPS. We addressed the environmental concerns of the NBS labs by replacing chloroform with ethyl acetate [11]. We created a reliable supply of the substrates and internal standards manufactured in our GMP facility using validated manufacturing processes.

We facilitated the use of the assay in NBS through a ten year (2006–2016) donation and grant agreement with the Centers for Disease Control and Prevention (CDC) Foundation so that (1) the reagents could be distributed without charge to NBS labs before they were commercially available, (2) NBS labs could be trained on lysosomal storage disorder NBS methods, and (3) quality control and external quality assurance samples were available for use in NBS [12]. The reagents were manufactured at Genzyme Pharmaceuticals in Liestal, Switzerland and tested for quality and distributed to the CDC by Genzyme Diagnostics in Framingham, Massachusetts.

6. Pompe Disease and the Recommended Uniform (Newborn) Screening Panel

In May 2006, Priya Kishnani nominated Pompe disease for inclusion in the Recommended Uniform (Newborn) Screening Panel (RUSP) in the United States. In October 2008, the nomination was denied. The Advisory Committee recommended additional studies before the condition could be re-nominated. The response to the nomination stated that "the initial test specificity for Pompe disease alone should be improved in comparison to the data shown by the Taiwan study, further evaluation of alternative screenings methods that could be multiplexed to target additional conditions (for example, other Lysosomal Storage Disease conditions) in order to decrease the burden on public health laboratories, and a standardized method of diagnosis after a positive newborn screen is required [13].

The Pompe disease community and Genzyme were disappointed by the response, but Genzyme remained staunch and committed to two additional efforts: funding an NBS study in Washington state and sponsoring an expert group to generate guidance for NBS for Pompe disease for practitioners around the world.

Fortuitously, the team in Washington had just developed a true triplex enzyme assay for Pompe disease, Fabry disease, and MPS I in which the enzymatic activities of acid α-glucosidase, α-galactosidase A, and α-L-iduronidase were quantified in DBS using a single assay buffer [14]. The validated triplex assay was transferred expeditiously to the Washington State NBS Lab and used to measure enzyme activities in approximately 110,000 DBS that had been stored at 18 °C for 8–10 months after collection. The word approximately is used because the study started before the reagents for Fabry disease and MPS I were ready for distribution by the CDC and results were not reported for tests done using research grade reagents, so the number of results reported vary by disease [15]. The study was anonymous but confirmed the diagnosis by DNA sequencing using a duplicate punch from the same sample. The positive predictive values for Pompe disease, Fabry disease, and MPS I were 0.24, 0.43, and 0.33, respectively. The false positive rates were 1/8600, 1/12,100, and 1/17,500, respectively.

The Washington State NBS data generated a lot of hope in the MPS I and Pompe disease communities. In late 2011, cross-functional teams of patient advocacy groups, diagnostic experts, disease experts, and NBS experts were established for MPS I and Pompe disease. MPS I and Pompe disease were nominated for inclusion in the RUSP in 2012; and the nominations were approved for formal data review. Evidence review for Pompe disease preceded evidence review for MPS I because the Advisory Committee budget could not support parallel evidence reviews. In 2013, the Advisory Committee recommend adding Pompe Disease to the RUSP. In 2015, Pompe disease was added to the RUSP [16]. In 2015, the Advisory Committee recommended adding MPS I to the RUSP. In 2016, MPS I was added to the RUSP [16].

Recognizing the importance of consistency in NBS, Sanofi Genzyme facilitated and provided financial support for the meeting of the Pompe Disease NBS Working Group, which was led by Hwu and Kishnani to discuss and develop a general guidance document for NBS for Pompe disease for practitioners around the world. The guidance was published in a supplement in Pediatrics [17]. Sub-teams from the Working Group authored guidelines for NBS for Pompe Disease; the initial evaluation of patients after positive NBS and recommended algorithms leading to a confirmed diagnosis of Pompe disease; management of confirmed newborn-screened patients with Pompe disease across the disease spectrum; and the role of genetic counseling in Pompe disease after patients are identified through NBS.

NBS for Pompe disease is possible because of the unprecedented and selfless collaborations of countless international experts who shared their thoughts and data without delay so that the next step in the process could be initiated during the lag required for preparation of publications. NBS for Pompe disease was facilitated by the financial, organizational, and technical contributions from Genzyme and Sanofi Genzyme.

Acknowledgments: The author is grateful to each patient with Pompe disease who donated samples for these studies and to the numerous physicians, scientists, and Genzyme colleagues who participated in all aspects of this work. Their trust was empowering. Henri Termeer is recognized for his unwavering support and pioneering vision, and Nestor Chamoles for his passion and deep commitment. Please note that I referenced the first paper for each major milestone, but recognize that these efforts have culminated in many, many more publications.

References

1. An, Y.; Young, S.P.; Kishnani, P.S.; Millington, D.S.; Amalfitano, A.; Corz, D.; Chen, Y.T. Glucose tetrasaccharide as a biomarker for monitoring the therapeutic response to enzyme replacement therapy for Pompe disease. *Mol. Genet. Metab.* **2005**, *85*, 247–254. [CrossRef] [PubMed]
2. Chamoles, N.A.; Blanco, M.; Gaggioli, D. Diagnosis of alpha-L-iduronidase deficiency in dried blood spots on filter paper: The possibility of newborn diagnosis. *Clin. Chem.* **2001**, *47*, 780–781. [CrossRef] [PubMed]
3. Zhou, X.; Turecek, F.; Scott, C.R.; Gelb, M.H. Quantification of cellular acid sphingomyelinase and galactocerebroside beta-galactosidase activities by electrospray ionization mass spectrometry. *Clin. Chem.* **2001**, *47*, 874–881. [CrossRef] [PubMed]
4. Chamoles, N.A.; Niizawa, G.; Blanco, M.; Gaggioli, D.; Casentini, C. Glycogen storage disease type II: Enzymatic screening in dried blood spots on filter paper. *Clin. Chim. Acta.* **2004**, *347*, 97–102. [CrossRef] [PubMed]
5. Li, Y.; Scott, C.R.; Chamoles, N.A.; Ghavami, A.; Pinto, B.M.; Turecek, F.; Gelb, M.H. Direct multiplex assay of lysosomal enzymes in dried blood spots for newborn screening. *Clin. Chem.* **2004**, *50*, 1785–1796. [CrossRef] [PubMed]
6. Zhang, H.; Kallwass, H.; Young, S.P.; Carr, C.; Dai, J.; Kishnani, P.S.; Millington, D.S.; Keutzer, J.; Chen, Y.T.; Bali, D. Comparison of maltose and acarbose as inhibitors of maltase-glucoamylase activity in assaying acid alpha-glucosidase activity in dried blood spots for the diagnosis of infantile Pompe disease. *Genet. Med.* **2006**, *8*, 302–306. [CrossRef] [PubMed]
7. Kallwass, H.; Carr, C.; Gerrein, J.; Titlow, M.; Pomponio, R.; Bali, D.; Dai, J.; Kishnani, P.; Skrinar, A.; Corzo, D.; et al. Rapid diagnosis of late-onset Pompe disease by fluorometric assay of alpha-glucosidase activities in dried blood spots. *Mol. Genet. Metab.* **2007**, *90*, 449–452. [CrossRef] [PubMed]
8. Chien, Y.H.; Chiang, S.C.; Zhang, X.K.; Keutzer, J.; Lee, N.C.; Huang, A.C.; Chen, C.A.; Wu, M.H.; Huang, P.H.; Tsai, F.J.; et al. Early detection of Pompe disease by newborn screening is feasible: Results from the Taiwan screening program. *Pediatrics* **2008**, *122*, e39–e45. [CrossRef] [PubMed]
9. Chiang, S.C.; Hwu, W.L.; Lee, N.C.; Hsu, L.W.; Chien, Y.H. Algorithm for Pompe disease newborn screening: Results from the Taiwan screening program. *Mol. Genet. Metab.* **2012**, *106*, 281–286. [CrossRef] [PubMed]

10. Pompe Disease Diagnostic Working Group; Winchester, B.; Bali, D.; Bodamer, O.A.; Caillaud, C.; Christensen, E.; Cooper, A.; Cupler, E.; Deschauer, M.; Fumić, K.; et al. Methods for a prompt and reliable laboratory diagnosis of Pompe disease: Report from an international consensus meeting. *Mol. Genet. Metab.* **2008**, *93*, 275–281. [CrossRef]
11. Zhang, X.K.; Elbin, C.S.; Chuang, W.L.; Cooper, S.K.; Marashio, C.A.; Beauregard, C.; Keutzer, J.M. Multiplex enzyme assay screening of dried blood spots for lysosomal storage disorders by using tandem mass spectrometry. *Clin. Chem.* **2008**, *54*, 1725–1728. [CrossRef] [PubMed]
12. De Jesus, V.R.; Zhang, X.K.; Keutzer, J.; Bodamer, O.A.; Mühl, A.; Orsini, J.J.; Caggana, M.; Vogt, R.F.; Hannon, W.H. Development and evaluation of quality control dried blood spot materials in newborn screening for lysosomal storage disorders. *Clin. Chem.* **2009**, *55*, 158–164. [CrossRef] [PubMed]
13. Advisory Committee on Heritable Disorders in Newborns and Children's response to Dr Kishnani. Available online: https://www.hrsa.gov/sites/default/files/hrsa/advisory-committees/heritable-disorders/rusp/previous-nominations/pompe-letter-from-committee-2008.pdf (accessed on 19 May 2020).
14. Duffey, T.A.; Bellamy, G.; Elliott, S.; Fox, A.C.; Glass, M.; Turecek, F.; Gelb, M.H.; Scott, C.R. A tandem mass spectrometry triplex assay for the detection of Fabry, Pompe, and mucopolysaccharidosis-I (Hurler). *Clin. Chem.* **2010**, *56*, 1854–1861. [CrossRef] [PubMed]
15. Scott, C.R.; Elliott, S.; Buroker, N.; Thomas, L.I.; Keutzer, J.; Glass, M.; Gelb, M.H.; Turecek, F. Identification of infants at risk for developing Fabry, Pompe, or mucopolysaccharidosis-I from newborn blood spots by tandem mass spectrometry. *J. Pediatr.* **2013**, *163*, 498–503. [CrossRef] [PubMed]
16. Advisory Committee on Heritable Disorders in Newborns and Children: Previously Nominated Conditions. Available online: https://www.hrsa.gov/advisory-committees/heritable-disorders/rusp/previous-nominations.html (accessed on 19 May 2020).
17. Newborn Screening, Diagnosis, and Treatment for Pompe Disease. Available online: https://pediatrics.aappublications.org/content/140/Supplement_1 (accessed on 19 May 2020).

6

Newborn Screening for Pompe Disease in Illinois: Experience with 684,290 Infants

Barbara K. Burton [1,2,*], Joel Charrow [1,2], George E. Hoganson [3], Julie Fleischer [4], Dorothy K. Grange [5], Stephen R. Braddock [6], Lauren Hitchins [2], Rachel Hickey [2], Katherine M. Christensen [6], Daniel Groepper [4], Heather Shryock [7], Pamela Smith [7], Rong Shao [8] and Khaja Basheeruddin [8]

1 Department of Pediatrics, Feinberg School of Medicine of Northwestern University, Chicago, IL 60611, USA; JCharrow@luriechildrens.org
2 Department of Pediatrics, Ann and Robert H. Lurie Children's Hospital of Chicago, Chicago, IL 60611, USA; lhitchins@luriechildrens.org (L.H.); rahickey@luriechildrens.org (R.H.)
3 Department of Pediatrics, University of Illinois College of Medicine, Chicago, IL 60612, USA; geh@uic.edu
4 Department of Pediatrics, Southern Illinois University School of Medicine, Springfield, IL 62701, USA; jfleischer95@siumed.edu (J.F.); dgroepper@siumed.edu (D.G.)
5 Department of Pediatrics, Washington University School of Medicine and St. Louis Children's Hospital, St. Louis, MO 63110, USA; grange_d@kids.wustl.edu
6 Department of Pediatrics, Saint Louis University, St. Louis, MO 63104, USA; braddock@slu.edu (S.R.B.); katherine.christensen@health.slu.edu (K.M.C.)
7 Office of Health Promotion, Illinois Department of Public Health, Springfield, IL 62761, USA; Heather.Shryock@Illinois.gov (H.S.); Pamela.E.Smith@illinois.gov (P.S.)
8 Newborn Screening Laboratory, Illinois Department of Public Health, Chicago, IL 60603, USA; Rong.Shao@Illinois.gov (R.S.); Khaja.Basheeruddin@Illinois.gov (K.B.)
* Correspondence: bburton@luriechildrens.org

Abstract: Statewide newborn screening for Pompe disease began in Illinois in 2015. As of 30 September 2019, a total of 684,290 infants had been screened and 395 infants (0.06%) were screen positive. A total of 29 cases of Pompe disease were identified (3 infantile, 26 late-onset). While many of the remainder were found to have normal alpha-glucosidase activity on the follow-up testing (234 of 395), other findings included 62 carriers, 39 infants with pseudodeficiency, and eight infants who could not be given a definitive diagnosis due to inconclusive follow-up testing.

Keywords: Pompe disease; newborn screening

1. Introduction

Pompe disease is an autosomal recessive lysosomal storage disorder resulting from the deficiency of acid alpha-glucosidase (GAA). The deficiency of enzyme activity results in the lysosomal accumulation of glycogen and multisystemic clinical manifestations, including prominent skeletal muscle weakness. Patients with the most severe form of the disorder, referred to as infantile onset Pompe disease (IOPD), also have cardiac involvement manifested as hypertrophic cardiomyopathy. In the absence of treatment, patients with IOPD rarely survive beyond two years of age. Patients with late onset Pompe disease (LOPD) may develop clinical manifestations at any age from early childhood through adult life. Progressive limb girdle muscle weakness is the hallmark of the disorder, with disproportionate involvement of the respiratory muscles often leading to respiratory insufficiency. Cardiac involvement is rare in patients with LOPD. There are patients who exhibit an intermediate phenotype with onset of muscle weakness and motor delay in the first year of life without cardiomyopathy. These patients are variably referred to as having either LOPD or atypical IOPD. Enzyme replacement therapy with alglucosidase alfa has been available for both IOPD and LOPD since 2006 and has significantly changed the natural history of the disorder. In patients with IOPD, it prolongs ventilator-free survival and often results in resolution of cardiomyopathy [1]. A subset of patients with IOPD, particularly those who are cross-reacting material (CRIM) negative, are at high risk of developing high titer antibodies to the enzyme, however, with subsequent loss of efficacy [2]. Immune modulation protocols have been developed and have shown to be effective in preventing the development of high titer antibodies in these patients [3]. In patients with LOPD, treatment with alglucosidase alfa may result in improved endurance as measured on the 6-min walk test and stabilization of motor and pulmonary function [4].

Patients with IOPD invariably exhibit elevated levels of serum creatine kinase (CK), whether diagnosed clinically or through newborn screening [5]. Patients with LOPD often, but not always, have elevated CK levels as well. In all patients with elevated levels, a decline is typically observed after initiation of enzyme replacement therapy. A second biomarker that is useful in the diagnosis and monitoring of Pompe disease is a specific urinary glucose tetrasaccharide (Glc4 or Hex4) [6]. In the newborn screening setting, levels of this tetrasaccharide have been reported to be consistently elevated in patients with IOPD but normal in those with LOPD who do not require therapy prior to three years of age [7].

Pseudodeficiency for the GAA enzyme has been well-described and is particularly common in Asian populations [8]. Patients with pseudodeficiency have low levels of GAA measured in vitro, at times as low as those observed in affected individuals but have no evidence of clinical disease or glycogen storage in tissues. Common alleles associated with pseudodeficiency have been identified.

The rapidly progressive nature of IOPD and the availability of disease-modifying therapy was the impetus for the initiation of a pilot screening program for Pompe disease in Taiwan in 2005. Newborn screening for this disorder was shown to not only be feasible [9], but to also improve the prognosis for infantile onset Pompe disease through the earlier implementation of enzyme replacement therapy [10]. Missouri became the first state in the United States to implement newborn screening for Pompe disease in 2013 using the digital microfluidic method [11]. The data from both Taiwan and Missouri were instrumental in securing the addition of Pompe disease to the Recommended Uniform Screening Panel (RUSP) in the US in 2015.

Illinois was the second state in the United Sates to implement statewide newborn screening for Pompe disease and the first to do so using tandem mass spectrometry. Pilot screening in selected hospitals began in November 2014 and was expanded statewide in June 2015. Results from the initial 15 months of screening were previously reported [12]. The purpose of this communication was to extend the initial report and describe the outcome of Pompe newborn screening through September 2019.

2. Materials and Methods

Newborn screening for Pompe disease is performed by determination of alpha-glucosidase enzyme activity in dried blood spots by liquid chromatography–mass spectrometry (LC–MS) using a multiplex assay with reagents from PerkinElmer®. The method and testing cutoffs have been previously described [12]. All infants born in the state of Illinois have been tested since June 2015. Parents can opt out of any newborn screening but cannot selectively opt out of testing for specific disorders. In practice, the opt-out option is virtually never utilized. Infants with a positive screen are urgently referred to one of several referral centers for diagnostic evaluation. A protocol for follow-up (Figure 1) was developed by a working group prior to the initiation of screening and is generally followed by all of the referral centers but is not mandatory and the specific testing ordered is at the discretion of each consulting provider. All centers obtain blood for creatinine kinase (CK) and alpha-glucosidase activity at the time of initial assessment, as well as cardiac studies including chest radiograph and electrocardiogram with echocardiogram in many cases. When deficient enzyme activity is confirmed, molecular analysis is performed at one of several reference laboratories. When two or more mutations or variants are detected, it is recommended that parental testing be performed for phasing. However, the results of parental testing are not routinely collected by the screening program. Many clinicians obtain urine glucose or hexose tetrasaccharide (Glc4, Hex4) at the initial assessment and some include a full metabolic panel and brain natriuretic peptide (BNP). Over time, most centers have obtained fewer follow-up cardiac assessments than recommended on the algorithm on those infants with no initial evidence of cardiac disease. In particular, most infants who have the common c.-32-13T>G mutation do not undergo additional cardiac evaluation since the incidence of cardiac disease in association with this mutation has been shown to be very low [13]. Follow-up echocardiography for infants with other mutations is variable and at the discretion of the clinician.

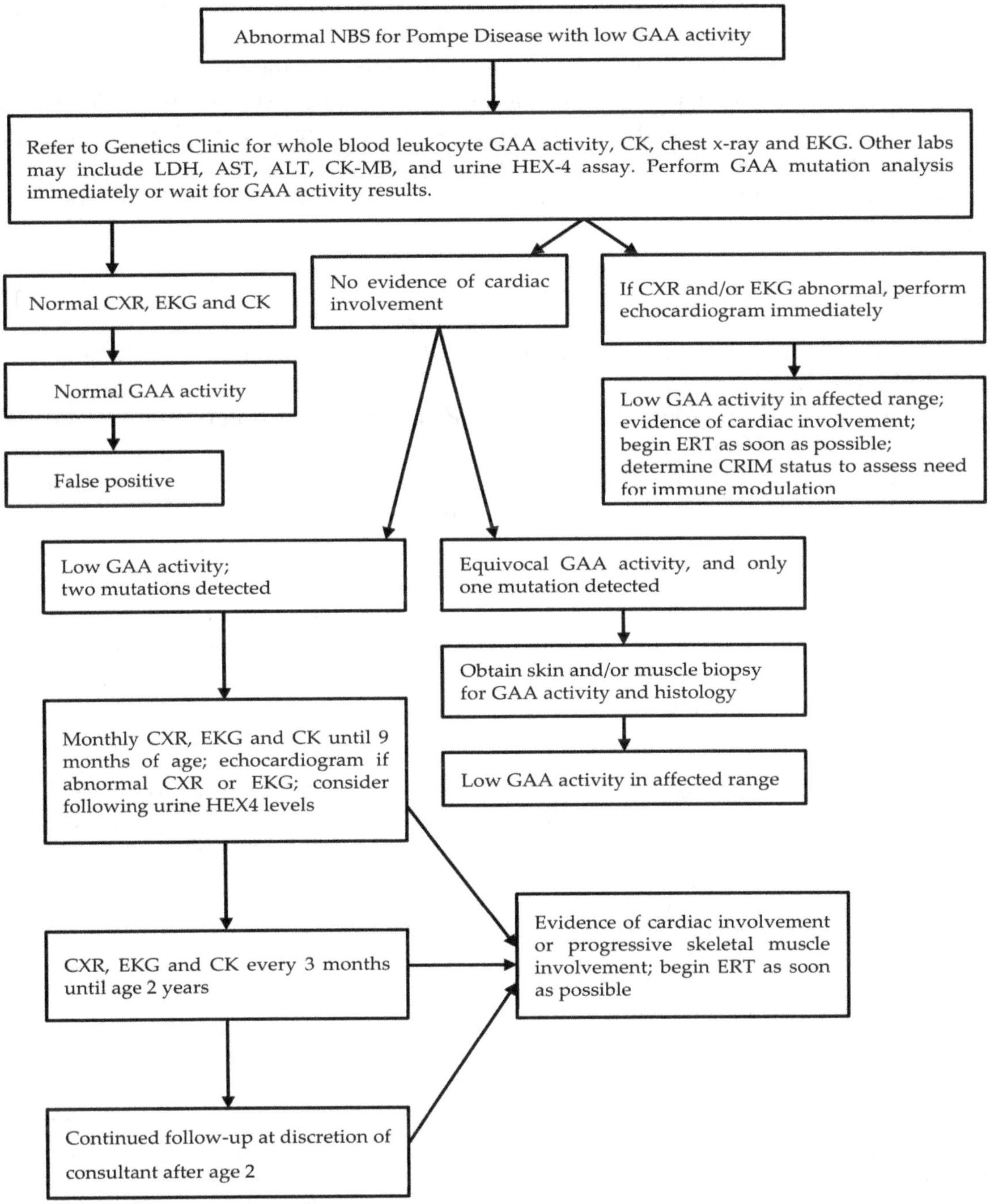

Figure 1. Pompe Disease Algorithm.

Affected infants are classified as having infantile onset Pompe disease (IOPD) if they have evidence of cardiomyopathy in the first year of life. All other definitely affected infants are classified as having late onset Pompe disease (LOPD). The latter category includes infants found to have hypotonia, motor delay or muscle weakness in the first year of life. Infants who have no evidence of cardiac disease but have alpha-glucosidase activity in the affected range and have one pathogenic mutation and one variant of unknown significance (VUS) or two VUS are referred to as having possible LOPD or undetermined status. It is recognized that these infants may not be affected since the variants of unknown significance could be benign, but follow-up is recommended nonetheless, similar to what is provided to infants with definite LOPD.

In the case of infants diagnosed with late onset Pompe disease (LOPD), or possible LOPD defined as low enzyme activity with one pathogenic mutation and one variant of undetermined significance (VUS) or two VUSs in trans, follow-up assessments are typically performed in the first year of life at 3 month intervals and include history and physical examination, developmental assessment, serum CK, and, in some cases, a complete metabolic panel and/or BNP, and urine Glc4. The undetermined cases are followed in the same manner as those with definite LOPD. For patients doing well, the interval between assessments is typically increased to 6 months to a year after one year of age. When LOPD or possible LOPD is diagnosed in an infant, older siblings born prior to the onset of newborn screening are routinely tested.

3. Results

A total of 684,290 infants were screened between 3 November 2014 and 30 September 2019. Three hundred and ninety-seven of these (0.06%), or 1 in 1724, screened positive for Pompe disease and were referred for diagnostic assessment. The outcome of the evaluation of these infants is seen in Table 1. A total of 29 infants had a definitive diagnosis of Pompe disease for a minimum incidence in the population of 1 in 23,596. Of these 29, 26 infants (90%) were found to have late onset Pompe disease. An additional 8 infants were defined as having an undetermined phenotype or "possible" Pompe disease. These were infants with low enzyme activity and two variants in the GAA gene, one or both of which were of unknown significance. Since it is likely that some of these infants will go on to develop Pompe disease, the incidence in the population is likely higher than the 1 in 23,596 calculated from the definite cases. Since screening was initiated, there have been no reports of infants diagnosed with Pompe disease who were missed by newborn screening. There have also been no infants with GAA activity in the affected range with only a single variant detected in the gene.

Table 1. Outcome of follow-up in infants screen positive for Pompe disease (n = 395).

Category	Number of Infants Identified
Infantile Pompe disease	3
Late onset Pompe disease	26
Normal enzyme activity	234
Carrier [1]	62
Pseudodeficiency [2]	39
Phenotype undetermined [3]	8
Loss to follow-up or refused	7
Died prior to follow-up [4]	1
Pending	15

[1] Infants with one pathogenic variant, or one VUS, with or without pseudodeficiency alleles were classified as carriers. [2] Infants in this category had only pseudodeficiency allelesc.1726G>A, c.2065G>A, and/or c.271G>A. 38 of 39 infants in this group were of Asian descent. [3] Infants in this category had one pathogenic variant and one or two VUS. [4] This was a premature infant who had multiple complications of prematurity but no findings to suggest Pompe disease.

Three infants had evidence of cardiomyopathy at the time of their initial assessment and were diagnosed with infantile onset Pompe disease (IOPD). All three were determined to be CRIM positive based on molecular analysis. Two were started on enzyme replacement therapy (ERT) with no immune modulation at 4 and 6 weeks of age. The third infant was also CRIM positive but had a mutation previously found to confer high risk for the development of high titer antibodies and had very severe cardiomyopathy requiring treatment in an intensive care unit from day 1 of life. He was treated with ERT beginning at 10 days of age and was simultaneously treated with rituximab, methotrexate, and intravenous immunoglobulin [14]. All three infants are currently doing well, all are ambulatory, and none of the three required any ventilatory support at the last follow-up. There were no infants who had a normal cardiac assessment initially who were later found to have evidence of cardiomyopathy.

Thus far, only one infant with LOPD has been started on ERT (Table 2, Case 25). This was an infant who, at the time of initial assessment, was found to have a CK of 555 international units per liter (IU/L) but no evidence of cardiomyopathy. At two months of age, head lag and mild hypotonia were noted but physical therapy assessment revealed a normal Alberta infant motor scale (AIMS) score at the 85th percentile for age. Multiple additional measurements of CK continued to be in the range of 550–650 U/L. Development appeared to progress normally for several months but by 9 months of age, significant hip laxity and gross motor delay were evident. The AIMS score had decreased to below the 5th percentile for age. A decision was made to initiate treatment and ERT was started at ten months of age, along with short term methotrexate [15]. After three months of therapy, the patient was making motor progress but continued to exhibit significant weakness so the dose of alglucosidase alfa was increased from the label dose of 20 mg/kg every two weeks to 40 mg/kg every two weeks. No other infants or children identified through newborn screening as having LOPD have been reported to have persistent clinical symptoms, although elevations of CK are common at diagnosis, as seen in Table 2.

Table 2. Follow-up data on infants with definite or "possible" Pompe disease.

Case	Genotype	Phenotype	GAA Activity [a] Result (nl)	CK (IU/L) Result (nl)	Urine Glc4 or Hex4 [b] Result (nl)	Cardiac Findings	Other Clinical Findings
1	c.2560C>T, c.1211A>T, c.2161G>C	IOPD	0.02 (>3.0)	1064 (35–232)	NR	HCM	Hypotonia
2	c.1437+1G>A, c.2227C>T	IOPD	0.8 (>3.88)	566 (32–250)	NR	HCM	Hypotonia; Motor delay
3	c.2560C>T, c.2459_2461del	IOPD	1.6 (>3.88)	3488 (30–279)	Glc4 14.9 (0.14–1.29)	HCM	Initial hypotonia [c]
4–16	c.-32-13T>G homozygous	LOPD	0.0–2.8	153–669 (8/17 elevated)	See footnote [d]	Normal [e]	None
17	c.-32-13T>G, c.1655T>C	LOPD	0.8 (>3.0)	550	Normal	ASD	Mild hypotonia
18	c.-32-13T>G, c.2238G>C	LOPD	2.55 (>3.88)	86 (29–168)	Normal	None	None
19	c.-32-13T>G, c.1839G>A	LOPD	1.5 (>3.88)	641 (30–279)	Glc4 7.59 (0.14–1.29)	None	None
20	c.-32-13T>G, c.258DPC	LOPD	0.3 (>3.0)	NR	NR	None	None
21	c.-32-13T>G, c.2238G>C, c.2065G>A	LOPD	1.0 (>3.0)	NR	Hex4 41.6 (<20)	RVH on ECG; PFO on echo	None
22	c.-32-13T>G, c.2297A>G	LOPD [f]	2.3 (>3.88)	168 (55–170)	Glc4 1.21 (0.08–1.37)	Normal	None
23	c.307T>G, c.1375G>C, c.271G>A	LOPD [f]	1.6 (>3.88)	Normal	Glc4 2.0 (1.14–1.29)	Normal	None
24	c.1637-3_1637-4delinsG, c.1831G>A	LOPD	2.4 (>3.88)	93 (30–279)	Glc4 12.98 (0.14–1.29)	Normal	None

Table 2. *Cont.*

Case	Genotype	Phenotype	GAA Activity [a] Result (nl)	CK (IU/L) Result (nl)	Urine Glc4 or Hex4 [b] Result (nl)	Cardiac Findings	Other Clinical Findings
25	c.-32-12T>G, c.2219-2220delTG	LOPD [g]	2.0 (>3.88)	555 (30–279)	Glc4 11.79 (0.14–1.29)	PFO	Hypotonia; gross motor delay
26	c.2238G>C, c.2242dupG	LOPD [f]	2.9 (>3.88)	142 (30–279)	Glc4 6.54 (0.14–1.29)	Normal	None
27	c.2173delC, c.858+17-858+23delCGGGGCGG	LOPD	2.9 (>3.88)	272 (30–279)	NR	Normal	None
28	c.1121G>T, c.885C>T	LOPD	0.3 (>3.0)	NR	NR	Normal	None
29	c.307T>G, c.525delT	LOPD	0.5 (>3.0)	193 (55–170)	NR	Normal	None
30	c.655G>A, c.1418G>C	UND	3.0 (>7.4)	73 (39–308)	Hex4 11.2 (<20)	PFO	None
31	c.525delT, c.265C>T	UND [f]	2.9 (>3.88)	74 (30–279)	Glc4 6.76 (0.14–1.29)	PFO [h]	None
32	c.1942G>A, c.1346C>T, c.2065G>A, c.1726G>A	UND	0.2 (>3.0)	167 (39–308)	NR	Normal	None
33	c.664G>A, c.1346C>T	UND	0.0 (>3.88)	101 (30–279)	NR	Normal	None
34	c.726G>A, c.1357G>A	UND	0.7 (>3.0)	NR	NR	Normal	None
35	c.1631T>A, c.2509C>T, c.2065G>A	UND	UND	0.7 (>3.0)	NR	NR	Normal
36	c.307T>G, c.265C>T	UND	2.1 (>3.88)	152 (30–279)	NR	NR	Normal
37	c.1781G>A, c.1194+3G>C	UND	3.5 (>3.88)	571 (30–279)	Glc4 3.46 (0.14–1.29)	Normal	None

[a] GAA activity units: pmol/punch/h. [b] Urine Glc4 or Hex4 activity units: mmol/mol creatinine. [c] Initial hypotonia and hypoventilation during sleep; resolved by 10 months of age. [d] 13 Cases: NR for 7; Glc4 5.42–9.83 (0.142–1.29) for 4; Hex4 6.8 and 13.2 (<20) for 2. [e] One case with left ventricular hypertrophy on ECG, with normal echo; all others normal. [f] Older sibling, born prior to newborn screening, has same genotype. [g] Symptomatic at 9 months of age, started on ERT. [h] Also had mildly dilated ascending aorta. ASD = Atrial septal defect. CK = creatine kinase. GAA activity = dried blood spot alpha-glucosidase activity determined at time of diagnostic evaluation. Glc4 = glucose tetrasaccharide. HCM = Hypertrophic cardiomyopathy. Hex4 = hexose tetrasaccharide. IOPD = Infantile onset Pompe disease. LOPD = Late onset Pompe disease. nl = Normal. NR = Not reported. PFO = Patent foramen ovale. RVH = Right ventricular hypertrophy. UND = Undetermined.

For patients with more than two variants, clinical significance of all variants was not always evident. There were patients who had two pathogenic variants and either pseudodeficiency alleles or variants of unknown significance. All of the variants in the patients with definite or possible Pompe disease are listed in Table 2.

The results of the clinical and laboratory assessments performed on affected infants at the time of initial evaluation are seen in Table 2. It should be noted that these data are obtained from the consulting physicians by the Illinois department of public health and reporting may be incomplete in some cases. Due to privacy restrictions restricting release of identifying information, original records on all of these infants were not available to the authors. If a result is listed as NR (not reported), it may not have been done or may simply not have been reported, even if it was done. After the initial data were gathered following diagnosis, a follow-up questionnaire was sent annually to consulting physicians for each patient. The length of follow-up for the patients reported ranges from several months to 4 years.

4. Discussion

Pompe disease newborn screening has been successfully implemented in the state of Illinois over the past 5 years. As reported from other states [16], the overall incidence of Pompe disease was found to be higher than previously estimated, with the large majority of cases being of the late onset type. In addition, there were patients in whom a definitive diagnosis could not be established, who will require ongoing follow-up.

The patients identified through newborn screening who are now on treatment have thus far had an excellent outcome and experience elsewhere has documented the benefits of treatment initiation prior to the onset of overt clinical symptoms [17]. Questions remain regarding the optimal follow-up of infants diagnosed with LOPD and the optimal time for initiation of treatment. It is anticipated that the collective experience of the many states now performing screening will shed light on these issues in the coming years. In the meantime, a method of systemic data collection to enable long-term assessment of outcomes and best practices is critically needed. Although there is an industry-sponsored registry for patients with confirmed Pompe disease [18], it is not ideal for the inclusion of asymptomatic patients, particularly those with genotypes that do not permit a definitive diagnosis ("possible" Pompe patients) and is not accessible by all treating physicians. A similar need exists for other disorders, including other lysosomal disorders, recently added to newborn screening since many are associated with phenotypes that may not become evident until much later in childhood or even in adult life.

5. Conclusions

Pompe newborn screening in the state of Illinois has been ongoing for 5 years and has led to the diagnosis of 3 infants with IOPD, 26 with LOPD, and eight with an undetermined diagnosis.

Author Contributions: B.K.B., J.C., G.E.H., J.F., S.R.B., D.K.G., R.H., L.H., D.G., and K.M.C. were involved in evaluation of patients with positive newborn screening tests and in treatment of those patients with a definitive diagnosis. P.S. and H.S. obtained and collated follow-up data on infants with a positive newborn screening test. R.S. and K.B. performed and analyzed the newborn screening tests. B.K.B. curated data obtained from the Department of Public Health and wrote the first draft of the manuscript. All authors have read and agreed to the published version of the manuscript.

Acknowledgments: The authors would like to acknowledge Vera Shively for her expert editorial assistance.

References

1. Kishnani, P.S.; Corzo, D.; Leslie, N.D.; Gruskin, D.; van der Ploeg, A.; Clancy, J.P.; Parini, R.; Morin, G.; Beck, M.; Bauer, M.S.; et al. Early treatment with alglucosidase alfa prolongs long-term survival in infants with Pompe disease. *Pediatr. Res.* **2009**, *66*, 329–335. [CrossRef] [PubMed]
2. Kishnani, P.S.; Goldenberg, P.C.; DeArmey, S.L.; Heller, J.; Benjamin, D.; Young, S.; Bali, D.; Smith, S.A.; Li, J.S.; Mandel, H.; et al. Cross-reactive immunologic material status affects treatment outcomes in Pompe disease infants. *Mol. Genet. Metab.* **2010**, *99*, 26–33. [CrossRef] [PubMed]
3. Messinger, Y.H.; Mendelsohn, N.J.; Rhead, W.; Dimmock, D.; Hershkovitz, E.; Champion, M.; Jones, S.A.; Olson, R.; White, A.; Wells, C.; et al. Successful immune tolerance induction to enzyme replacement therapy in CRIM-negative infants with Pompe disease. *Mol. Genet. Metab.* **2012**, *14*, 135–142.
4. Van der Ploeg, A.T.; Clemens, P.R.; Corzo, D.; Escolar, D.M.; Florence, J.; Groeneveld, G.J.; Herson, S.; Kishnani, P.S.; Laforet, P.; Lake, S.L.; et al. A randomized study of alglucosidase alfa in late-onset Pompe disease. *N. Engl. J. Med.* **2010**, *362*, 1396–1406. [CrossRef] [PubMed]
5. Kishnani, P.S.; Steiner, R.D.; Bali, D.; Berger, K.; Byrne, B.J.; Case, L.E.; Crowley, J.F.; Downs, S.; Howell, R.R.; Kravitz, R.M.; et al. Pompe disease diagnosis and management guidelines. *Genet. Med.* **2006**, *8*, 267–288. [CrossRef] [PubMed]
6. Young, S.P.; Piraud, M.; Goldstein, J.L.; Zhang, H.; Rehder, C.; Laforet, P.; Kishnani, P.S.; Millington, D.S.; Bashir, M.R.; Bali, D.S. Assessing disease severity in Pompe disease: The roles of a urine glucose tetrasaccharide

biomarker and imaging techniques. *Am. J. Med. Genet. C Semin. Med. Genet.* **2012**, *160C*, 50–58. [CrossRef] [PubMed]

7. Chien, Y.H.; Goldstein, J.L.; Hwu, W.L.; Smith, P.B.; Lee, N.C.; Chiang, S.C.; Tolun, A.A.; Zhang, H.; Vaisnins, A.E.; Millington, D.S.; et al. Baseline urine glucose tetrasaccharide concentrations in patients with infantile- and late-onset Pompe disease identified by newborn screening. *JIMD Rep.* **2015**, *19*, 67–73. [PubMed]
8. Kumamoto, S.; Katafuchi, T.; Nakamura, K.; Endo, F.; Oda, E.; Okuyama, T.; Kroos, M.A.; Reuser, A.J.; Okumiya, T. High frequency of acid alpha-glucosidase pseudodeficiency complicating newborn screening for glycogen storage disease type II in the Japanese population. *Mol. Genet. Metab.* **2009**, *99*, 190–195. [CrossRef] [PubMed]
9. Chien, Y.H.; Chiang, S.C.; Zhang, X.K.; Keutzer, J.; Lee, N.C.; Huang, A.C.; Chen, C.A.; Wu, M.H.; Huang, P.H.; Tsai, F.J.; et al. Early detection of Pompe disease by newborn screening is feasible: Results from the Taiwan screening program. *Pediatrics* **2008**, *122*, e39–e45. [CrossRef] [PubMed]
10. Chien, Y.H.; Lee, N.C.; Thurberg, B.L.; Chiang, S.C.; Zhang, X.K.; Keutzer, J.; Huang, A.C.; Wu, M.H.; Huang, P.H.; Tsai, F.J.; et al. Pompe disease in infants: Improving the prognosis by newborn screening and early treatment. *Pediatrics* **2009**, *124*, e1116–e1125. [CrossRef] [PubMed]
11. Hopkins, P.V.; Campbell, C.; Klug, T.; Rogers, S.; Raburn-Miller, J.; Kiesling, J. Lysosomal storage disorder newborn screening implementation: Findings from the first six months of full population pilot testing in Missouri. *J. Pediatr.* **2015**, *166*, 172–177. [CrossRef] [PubMed]
12. Burton, B.K.; Charrow, J.; Hoganson, G.E.; Waggoner, D.; Tinkle, B.; Braddock, S.R.; Schneider, M.; Grange, D.K.; Nash, C.; Shryock, H.; et al. Newborn screening for lysosomal storage disorders in Illinois: The initial 15-month experience. *J. Pediatr.* **2017**, *190*, 130–135. [CrossRef] [PubMed]
13. Herbert, M.; Cope, H.; Li, J.S.; Kishnani, P.S. Severe cardiac involvement is rare in patients with late-onset Pompe disease and the common c.-32-13T>G variant: Implications for newborn screening. *J. Pediatr.* **2018**, *198*, 308–312. [CrossRef] [PubMed]
14. Kazi, Z.B.; Desai, A.K.; Berrier, K.L.; Troxler, R.B.; Wang, R.Y.; Abdul-Rahman, O.A.; Tanpaiboon, P.; Mendelsohn, N.J.; Herskovitz, E.; Kronn, D.; et al. Sustained immune tolerance induction in enzyme replacement therapy-treated CRIM-negative patients with infantile Pompe disease. *JCI Insight* **2017**, *2*, e94328. [CrossRef] [PubMed]
15. Kazi, Z.B.; Desai, A.K.; Troxler, R.B.; Kronn, D.; Packman, S.; Sabbadini, M.; Rizzo, W.B.; Scherer, K.; Abdul-Rahman, O.; Tanpaiboon, P.; et al. An immune tolerance approach using transient low-dose methotrexate in ERT-naïve setting of patients treated with a therapeutic protein: Experience in infantile-onset Pompe disease. *Genet. Med.* **2019**, *21*, 887–895. [CrossRef] [PubMed]
16. Hopkins, P.V.; Klug, T.; Vermette, L.; Raburn-Miller, J.; Kiesling, J.; Rogers, S. Incidence of 4 lysosomal storage disorders from 4 years of newborn screening. *JAMA Pediatr.* **2018**, *172*, 696–697. [CrossRef] [PubMed]
17. Yang, C.F.; Yang, C.C.; Liao, H.C.; Huang, L.Y.; Chiang, C.C.; Ho, H.C.; Lai, C.J.; Chu, T.H.; Yang, T.F.; Hsu, T.R.; et al. Very early treatment for infantile-onset Pompe disease contributes to better outcomes. *J. Pediatr.* **2016**, *169*, 174–180. [CrossRef] [PubMed]
18. Reuser, A.J.J.; van der Ploeg, A.T.; Chien, Y.H.; Llerena, J., Jr.; Abbott, M.A.; Clemens, P.R.; Kimonis, V.E.; Leslie, N.; Maruti, S.S.; Sanson, B.J.; et al. GAA variants and phenotypes amount 1,079 patients with Pompe disease; data from the Pompe Registry. *Hum. Mutat.* **2019**, *40*, 2146–2164. [CrossRef] [PubMed]

7

Newborn Screening for Sickle Cell Disease in Europe

Yvonne Daniel [1,†,*], Jacques Elion [2,†], Bichr Allaf [3], Catherine Badens [4], Marelle J. Bouva [5], Ian Brincat [6], Elena Cela [7], Cathy Coppinger [1], Mariane de Montalembert [8], Béatrice Gulbis [9], Joan Henthorn [1], Olivier Ketelslegers [10], Corrina McMahon [11], Allison Streetly [12,13], Raffaella Colombatti [14,†] and Stephan Lobitz [15,†]

1 Public Health England, NHS Sickle Cell and Thalassemia Screening Programme, London SE16LH, UK; Cathy.Coppinger@phe.gov.uk (C.C.); joan.henthorn@gmail.com (J.H.)
2 Laboratoire d'Excellence GR-Ex, UMR_S1134, Inserm, Université Paris Diderot, Sorbonne Paris Cité, Institut National de la Transfusion Sanguine, 75015 Paris, France; jacques.elion@inserm.fr
3 NBS Laboratory for Haemoglobinopathies, Hôpital Universitaire Robert-Debré, 75019 Paris, France; bichr.allaf@aphp.fr
4 Département de génétique médicale, Aix-Marseille Université, Hôpital de la Timone, 13385 Marseille, France; catherine.badens@ap-hm.fr
5 National Institute for Public Health and the Environment, Centre for Health Protection, 3720 Bilthoven, The Netherlands; marelle.bouva@rivm.nl
6 Pediatric Medicine Laboratory, Department of Pathology, Mater Dei Hospital, Triq Tal-Qroqq, MSD2090 Msida, Malta; ian.brincat@gov.mt
7 Department of Pediatric Oncology/Hematology, Hospital Universitario General Gregorio Marañón, Facultad de Medicina, Universidad Complutense Madrid, 28007 Madrid, Spain; elena.cela@salud.madrid.org
8 Department of Pediatrics, Reference Center for Sickle Cell Disease, AP-HP Hôpital Universitaire Necker-Enfants Malades, 75743 Paris, France; mariane.demontal@aphp.fr
9 Department of Clinical Chemistry, Cliniques Universitaires de Bruxelles, Hôpital Erasme—ULB, 1070 Bruxelles, Belgium; beatrice.gulbis@erasme.ulb.ac.be
10 Laboratoire—Biologie Clinique, Centre Hospitalier Régional de la Citadelle, 4000 Liège, Belgium; Olivier.ketelslegers@chrcitadelle.be
11 Our Lady's Children's Hospital, Crumlin, D12V004 Dublin, Ireland; corrina.mcmahon@olchc.ie
12 School of Population Health and Environmental Sciences, Faculty of Life Sciences & Medicine, King's College London, London WC2R2LS, UK; allison.streetly@phe.gov.uk
13 Division of Healthcare Public Health, Health Protection and Medical Directorate, Public Health England, London SE18UG, UK
14 Department of Child and Maternal Health, Clinic of Pediatric Hematology/Oncology, Azienda Ospedaliera-Università di Padova, 35129 Padova, Italy; rcolombatti@gmail.com
15 Department of Pediatric Oncology/Hematology, Kinderkrankenhaus Amsterdamer Straße, 50735 Cologne, Germany; lobitzs@kliniken-koeln.de
* Correspondence: yvonne.a.daniel@kcl.ac.uk
† These authors contributed equally to the manuscript.

Abstract: The history of newborn screening (NBS) for sickle cell disease (SCD) in Europe goes back almost 40 years. However, most European countries have not established it to date. The European screening map is surprisingly heterogenous. The first countries to introduce sickle cell screening on a national scale were France and England. The French West Indies started to screen their newborns for SCD as early as 1983/84. To this day, all countries of the United Kingdom of Great Britain and Northern Ireland have added SCD as a target disease to their NBS programs. The Netherlands, Spain and Malta also have national programs. Belgium screens regionally in the Brussels and Liège regions, Ireland has been running a pilot for many years that has become quasi-official. However, the Belgian and Irish programs are not publicly funded. Italy and Germany have completed several pilot studies but are still in the preparatory phase of national NBS programs for SCD, although both countries have well-established concepts for metabolic and endocrine disorders. This article will give a brief overview of the situation in Europe and put a focus on the programs of the two pioneers of the continent, England and France.

Keywords: screening; sickle cell disease; newborn

---

1. England

1.1. Historical Background

Newborn screening (NBS) for sickle cell disease (SCD) was implemented in England between 2002 and 2005. Migration to the United Kingdom (UK) after 1945 had led to an increase in the population at risk from SCD, whilst the 1972 USA National Sickle Cell Anemia Control Act [1] had resulted in increased recognition and politicization of the disorder. The 1986 randomized trial of penicillin in SCD children aged less than 5 by Gaston et al. [2] demonstrated improved outcomes and provided a clear justification for NBS for SCD. Pockets of NBS had been implemented locally in some high prevalence areas in the 1970s but these were not systematic and resulted in inequitable policies throughout the country. These factors led to a major review by a Health Technology Assessment [3] working party which formed the basis for subsequent policy decisions. Political commitment was achieved via the National Health Service (NHS) plan in 2000 [4] and this led to the formation of a small team to plan and drive implementation of a linked newborn and antenatal screening program.

At this time, despite political commitment there were no policies and no financial resources had been allocated. Funding was only able to be sourced once an implementation plan had been developed. The working group had to resolve the controversy and sensitivities associated with implementing a genetic test in a minority group along with resistance from some who questioned the value of the program. There was also conflict between the desires of stakeholders and what could realistically be achieved. Initially overseas practices were reviewed, and a survey of local practices was carried out to inform decisions. A steering group was established in 2001, comprised of key health professionals, users and representatives from patient groups to endorse the policy decisions put forward by the expert working sub groups. Sub groups were developed to work on specific issues such as training, laboratory practices, education and information for users and professionals. The UK National Screening Committee makes recommendations to ministers about all decisions regarding screening policy in the UK and in 2002 approval was given for universal screening of SCD in children. The techniques in use also detected other hemoglobinopathies including beta thalassemia disease (defined clinically as transfusion dependent beta thalassemia or non-transfusion dependent beta thalassemia or HbE/beta thalassemia) thus it was also agreed that these cases along with all other hemoglobin variants detected would be reported. Policy was subsequently updated following review in 2011 such that the only other haemoglobins now reported are beta thalassemia disease, hemoglobins S, C, D, E and O^{Arab}, along with any variant co-inherited with Hb S. The four countries which form the UK operate semi-autonomously and screening in Scotland, Northern Ireland and Wales was adopted later. Scotland and Northern Ireland broadly follow the English policy whilst Wales implemented screening much later and has its own strategy [5].

1.2. Implementation

Along with stakeholder engagement, initial work was related to the development of policies for implementation. These covered areas such as sample type, technology to be used, testing protocols, reporting, delivery of results and referral into care. It was agreed that the blood spot sample already collected for metabolic screening would be used and that the program would be incorporated into the newborn blood spot screening pathway. Following reorganization there were 13 laboratories performing NBS in England, and thus implementation required policies which ensured consistency as well as a significant training investment. A two-stage testing protocol was implemented to increase the robustness of data with only high-performance liquid chromatography (HPLC) and iso-electric focusing (IEF) recognized as acceptable techniques (https://www.gov.uk/government/publications/sickle-cell-and-thalassemia-screening-handbook-for-laboratories). Counselling was aligned with genetics and different models were developed to fit with local prevalence of the conditions, resources and practices. Areas with high incidence had dedicated counsellors. Clinical policies and standards were developed, and these were subsequently published (https://www.gov.uk/government/publications/sickle-cell-disease-in-children-standards-for-clinical-care). Some funds were provided towards the development of initiatives such as transcranial Doppler scanning. Standards and the key performance indicators to measure performance against these standards were introduced (https://www.gov.uk/government/publications/standards-for-sickle-cell-and-thalassaemia-screening). The standards have evolved over time and are now reviewed annually to ensure they remain fit for purpose. A communication strategy is an important aspect to ensure engagement in the process. Educational materials such as booklets and leaflets for professionals, parents and the public (available in different languages) were developed. More recently blogs and other online resources have been used. Information and educational resources were developed for professionals and a variety of education and training for NHS screening staff is available (https://www.gov.uk/guidance/sickle-cell-and-thalassaemia-screening-education-and-training#haemoglobinopathies-sct-screening-programme-update).

Annual data collection and reporting has been developed and the information is used to inform decisions and to monitor trends, performance and the effect of changes in practice. Quality assurance of the whole pathway via peer review and inspection has been an important factor in ensuring consistency and maintaining standards. The ongoing evaluation present since the program's inception has led to the development of initiatives such as a failsafe to ensure samples are received on all babies and provision for the testing of babies who have been transfused. An initiative to measure outcomes from early detection of SCD in England was commenced in 2010 and has subsequently reported [6].

1.3. Results

More than 8 million babies have now been screened in the England; 3686 screen positive babies were identified between 2005 and 31 March 2017 [6], a summary of results is shown in Table 1.

Table 1. Screen positive babies between 2005 and 31 March 2017.

Screening Result	Number	Percentage
FS	2580	70.0%
FSC	927	25.1%
FS + other hemoglobin variant *	179	4.9%

* Refers to Hb D, E, O^{Arab} and any other rare variants detected.

The recently published newborn outcomes project which assessed timeliness of entry into care and treatment, antenatal screening history, and mortality reported on 1313 screen positive infants [6]. The paper concludes that the screening program accurately identifies babies with SCD, enrolment into care is timely but does not meet program standards, and despite mortality being low deaths still occur from invasive pneumococcal disease with adherence to antibiotics remaining important.

1.4. Summary

The long road from the first pockets of screening to full implementation of universal NBS for SCD in the whole of the UK took almost 30 years. Initially implementation was in England followed by Scotland, Northern Ireland and eventually Wales in 2014. Implementation was driven by increasing immigration and public pressure for inclusion in health care strategy. Testing for SCD is now firmly embedded in newborn blood spot screening which is assessed as a complete pathway rather than individual components. Additionally as part of linked antenatal and newborn screening, the program acts as a quality measure for antenatal screening with any apparent discrepancies being investigated. A key element in the success of the program has been the input of the small team who have driven the process, and ensured and maintained stakeholder engagement and development and implementation of policies. Ongoing evaluation and assessment is an essential aspect to ensure the program is fit for purpose. The program has proven itself to be adaptable, for example by adopting new technologies such as mass spectrometry testing [7,8]. The use of the new technology to withhold detection of carrier conditions has led to differing strategies in the UK. Within England, consistency has been maintained despite some adoption of this technique. Balancing all stakeholder expectations and requirements continues to be a challenge in the program.

The newborn outcomes project has shown that the program accurately identifies babies with SCD but there are some issues including acceptance of penicillin and delays between babies' positive screening results and enrolment into care and mortality associated with invasive pneumococcal disease. A detailed review into all aspects of the process and stakeholder requirements (a discovery process), identified a lack of a centralized view of the baby's progress along the pathway, lack of feedback to data providers, and duplication of data entry. A new improved system has been developed which will:

1. Automate the process of referring screen-positive babies into treatment centres and record their health outcomes;
2. Help ensure affected babies are treated as early as possible;
3. Provide oversight of the progress along the pathway to prevent babies getting 'lost' in the system;
4. Improve the process of collecting and sharing data;
5. Remove the need for clinicians to enter the same data twice;
6. Integrate with the National Hemoglobinopathy Register and National Congenital Anomalies and Rare Disorders Registration Service.

Beta thalassemia continues to be reported when found in NBS for SCD, and this has been due to lack of available evidence on the efficacy of detection and the clinical justification for early detection. There is now improved evidence on the sensitivity and specificity of the test [9,10]. However published clinical evidence remains scarce.

In conclusion, over 10 years' experience in England has shown this to be a robust program, which benefits from technical expertise along with strong stakeholder engagement. A key aspect of the program's success has been the development of clinical care pathways to ensure screen positive babies receive appropriate care in a timely manner.

2. France

2.1. Historical Background and Implementation

The first pilot study on NBS for SCD in France was conducted on the Caribbean island of Guadeloupe in 1983 and led to a universal screening program in Guadeloupe within one year [11]. The program was rapidly extended to Martinique, and in 1986 the first pilot studies in Metropolitan France (Paris and Marseille) were started.

In 1995, SCD became an additional target disease of the national NBS program in France (together with phenylketonuria, congenital hypothyroidism, congenital adrenal hyperplasia and cystic fibrosis). However, although the French NBS is universal in nature, screening for SCD in Metropolitan France is targeted at couples at risk to date, while in French overseas territories SCD screening is universal [12].

NBS for SCD is centralized in France and performed in five reference laboratories. Three of these are located in Metropolitan France (Paris, Marseille, Lille) and two are run on the Caribbean islands of Guadeloupe and Martinique. Since the year 2000, all French maternity clinics (public and private) are covered by the program which receives funding from the French social security system.

2.2. Methods

NBS for SCD in France is done in a two-tier strategy from heel prick dried blood spots. Initially, IEF was the method of choice. Today, the first-tier methods are HPLC, capillary electrophoresis (CE) and very recently MALDI-TOF mass spectrometry found its way into NBS in one laboratory. Second-tier testing is done with an established method different from the first one (e.g., first-tier: HPLC; second-tier: CE). The United Kingdom National External Quality Assessment Service (UK NEQAS) provides the external quality control assessment for the French NBS program. Absolute numbers of new cases, incidence, coverage and genotypes are collected and published annually globally and for each of the French regions (http://www.afdphe.org/sites/default/files/bilan_afdphe_2016.pdf). Screening results consistent with SCD are communicated to the families by a trained pediatrician of the national care program. Parents of carriers are informed by mail and offered information by a physician or a genetic counsellor. Testing of the father is recommended to identify couples at risk of having a significant disorder of hemoglobin. In this latter context, genetic counselling including extended information on SCD is provided and the opportunities of having prenatal or preimplantation genetic diagnosis are mentioned. A psychologist will participate in the process whenever necessary.

2.3. Results

Between the beginning of the national program in 1995 and 2016, 5.4 million newborns have been screened and 7,644 of tested newborns were diagnosed with SCD. A summary of results is shown in Table 2.

Table 2. Screen positive babies between 1995 and 2016.

Screening Result	Number	Percentage
FS	6015	78.7%
FSC	1600	20.9%
FS + other hemoglobin variant *	29	0.4%

* Refers to Hb D, E, O^{Arab} and any other rare variants detected.

In 2016, 431 cases of SCD were identified by NBS which corresponded with a birth prevalence of 1 in 1836, i.e., the highest among all target diseases tested in the French national NBS program. 356 of these 431 cases were diagnosed in Metropolitan France, and 218 of the 356 cases in Metropolitan France were diagnosed in the Ile de France, i.e., in the Parisian area. This translated into a birth prevalence of 1 in 824 in the Ile de France. In the French Overseas, 75 babies were affected by SCD. This was a mean birth prevalence of 1 in 525, varying from 1 in 1968 on the Island of Réunion and 1 in 206 in French Guiana (http://www.afdphe.org/sites/default/files/bilan_afdphe_2016.pdf).

The birth coverage by universal NBS in the French Overseas is over 98%. In the targeted program of Metropolitan France, a mean of 38.9% of all newborns was screened in 2016 (minimum: 9.1% in the Brittany region; maximum: 73.6% in the Ile de France). Only 277 parents (0.035%) refused to participate to the French NBS program in 2016. Between 2006 and 2016, there was a significant increase of couples at risk that led to a subsequent increase of the newborns screened in the targeted program in Metropolitan France from 27 to 38.9% (see above). In the same period, the prevalence of affected newborns rose by 24%.

The targeted SCD NBS in Metropolitan France is probably more cost-effective than a universal approach. The present cost per test is EUR 3.06. This equals to total costs of EUR 1.02 million per year for the whole program or EUR 2,359 per newborn identified. However, there are several drawbacks: most importantly, about 2% of affected newborns are missed, because they are not screened for various reasons [13]. Hence, patients' associations and most of the concerned medical health care professionals advocate a universal screening approach. Beyond missed cases, arguments in favor of universal screening include putative discrimination and inequality to the access to care. Still, in its December

2013 orientation report the *Haute Autorité de Santé* concluded that there is currently no evidence to justify universal NBS for SCD in Metropolitan France.

2.4. Follow-Up and Organization of Care

The first French Sickle Cell Disease Comprehensive Care Center was established in Guadeloupe in 1990 [11]. In 2005, a pioneering national program on rare diseases was started in France. Its objectives include the definition of pathways to access to care, the prevention of diagnostic wavering, the establishment of reference centers, the organization of specialized training for health care professionals, the development of information platforms for patients, relatives, health care professionals and the community, and the promotion of research.

During the first phase of this program (2005–2008), two accredited reference centers for SCD (Ile de France and French Antilles), one reference center for thalassemia (Marseille) and a network of reference laboratories were founded. The mission of these institutions was to establish clear healthcare channels for the patients through the formation of a national network of qualified centers. In 2005, national treatment guidelines for SCD were published online.

In the second phase of the national program for rare diseases (2011–2014), 13 constitutive reference centers and 46 competence centers in addition to the coordination reference centers were established to ensure a dense and comprehensive coverage of the whole French national territory.

A national registry for thalassemias has been established that included 692 patients (beta thalassemia: 612; alpha thalassemia: 80) in 2016, but a national registry for SCD is only now being established. (Definitions: beta thalassemia = transfusion dependent beta thalassemia or non-transfusion dependent beta thalassemia or HbE/beta thalassemia; alpha thalassemia = alpha thalassemia hydrops fetalis syndrome, HbH disease and HbH-Constant Spring disease.)

The whole network was certified in 2017 for five years. The program is evaluated regularly for its efficiency by health authorities and through published studies [14,15] and the next turn of certification is to occur in 2022.

In addition, local networks have been established at the initiative of some dedicated physicians, like RoFSED (*Réseau Francilien de Soin des Enfants Drépanocytaires*) in the Parisian area, and supported by public funds to connect the national health care system with proximity stakeholders, e.g., general practitioners, local health care and social professionals and school personnel. They are essential actors in terms of therapeutic education of the patients and parents and information of the general public (e.g., brochures, educational sessions and tools, games, films etc.; for examples, please see: http://www.rofsed.fr).

3. The Netherlands

The Netherlands has had a national NBS since 1974. Participation is voluntary, but virtually all of the newborns (approximately 175,000 annually) are tested. Since 2015 also newborns from the Dutch Caribbean, Bonaire, St Eustatius and Saba (200–250 children), are screened. For this, the specimens are sent to one of the five designated NBS laboratories in The Netherlands. Specimens are heel prick dried blood spots that are currently examined for 19 conditions. 16 of which are endocrine and metabolic disorders. The other three are blood disorders. NBS for SCD was introduced in 2007 [16,17] and in 2017 the program was extended to include beta thalassemia major and hemoglobin H disease [18,19].

An inquiry performed in 2002 resulted in the estimation of 50 sickle cell patients born annually and at least 800 SCD patients in total [20]. The total number of SCD patients, adults and children, in The Netherlands is now estimated to be in an order of 1500–2000. This number is based on expert opinion only, but clinicians and researchers are working together to set up a national registry.

NBS for hemoglobinopathies is universal, i.e., without any preselection on the basis of the putative ethnic origin of the baby. The method of choice to analyze dried blood spots is HPLC. A distinctive feature of the Dutch program is that there is no second-tier method in place. Children with positive screening tests are referred to pediatric hematologists for confirmation. In spite of this practice, only five false positives were reported in the first 10 years of screening. Almost all of these false positives were carriers of HbS or had another hemoglobinopathy. The first year of screening resulted in 40 diagnoses of SCD [21]. The 2016 annual bulletin reported 30 referrals for SCD and 30 referrals for alpha and beta thalassemia combined (https://www.rivm.nl/sites/default/files/2018-11/HielprikMon2016-Engels-def.pdf). In addition 800–850 carriers are detected every year [22]. The carrier state is reported routinely to the general practitioner to facilitate family testing if parents do not object to knowing the carrier status of their child.

4. Spain

A national universal newborn screening program has been available in Spain since 1978. It is on a voluntary basis, but has a nearly 100% coverage. Universal screening for hemoglobinopathies started in the Madrid region in 2003, in the Basque country in 2011, in Valencia in 2012, and was extended nationwide in 2015. More than 400,000 neonates were screened in 2016 with 48 cases of SCD identified [23]. HPLC is the first test used in most of the regions. Confirmatory testing is done with HPLC on the same dried blood spot and on a new capillary sample before the age of three months.

5. Belgium

Belgium does not screen for hemoglobinopathies on a national level. However, there are currently three regional programs in place [24]. The *Cliniques Universitaires de Bruxelles, hôpital Erasme* (currently the LHUB-ULB) are responsible for the Brussels region. They were the first institutions to introduce NBS for SCD in Belgium in 1994 [25–28] and the only institutions to receive public funding until 2015.

Both of the other two screening projects are located in Liège at the *Centre Hospitalier Régional de la Citadelle* (CHR Citadelle), which started NBS for SCD solely in its own institution in 2002 [27] and the *Centre Hospitalier Universitaire de Liège* (CHU de Liège) that covers 14 maternity wards in Wallonia since 2007 [29,30]. SCD screening in the Liège region has a quasi-official status, but is not reimbursed by the insurance companies. It is financed through hospital funding.

Since 2008, Belgium has been running a registry for SCD patients. From the academic point-of-view it is interesting that all patients diagnosed with SCD in Belgium are reported to this registry. While some of them have been identified through NBS, others have been identified later in life on the basis of clinical symptoms. By comparing the two populations, the Belgian group was able to demonstrate that NBS for SCD improves clinical outcome by a significant reduction of bacteremia and hospitalization [31,32].

To complement the screening data from the well-established programs in Brussels and Liège, two thirds (n = 39,599) of all Belgian newborns were screened in a six-month pilot study [24]. The highest incidences were found in urban areas. However, in total, SCD was more common than any other target disease in the Belgian NBS program. 17 babies (1:2329) were diagnosed with sickling disorders. 1 in 77 was demonstrated to be heterozygous for hemoglobin S.

In terms of the methodology, the Belgian programs are heterogenous. While LHUB-ULB and CHR Citadelle used to screen by CE from liquid cord blood, CHU de Liège applied tandem mass spectrometry to dried blood spots on heel prick filter paper. HPLC and molecular genetics are used as confirmatory methods. In the pilot study, dried blood spots were examined by capillary electrophoresis. Positive results were confirmed by either HPLC or IEF. All Belgian projects have in common that all newborns were screened without any preselection on the basis of their putative ethnic origin (i.e., universal screening).

6. Italy

A National Newborn Screening Program (NBS) has been present in Italy since the nineties and around 500,000 babies are born every year. The National Health System is organized on a regional basis and, therefore, every region can organize its own NBS. Therefore, there are significant differences in the regional legislations regulating NBS and in the development of the regional NBS programs in terms of the diseases to be included, funding allocated and program organization (http://www.aismme.org/images/Linee_guida_05.08.pdf). The screening is mandatory but does not include hemoglobinopathies. Nevertheless, since the end of 2000, due to the increase of patients with SCD as a result of immigration, several scientific societies have started to raise the issue of NBS for SCD: the Italian Association of Pediatric Hematology Oncology (AIEOP) highly recommended NBS for SCD in its guidelines published in 2012 in Italian and 2013 in English [33] and in 2017 the AIEOP together with the Italian Society of Thalassemia and Hemoglobinopathies (SITE) issued a joint document for the recommendation of NBS for SCD in Italy (http://www.site-italia.org/file/collana_scientifica/libretto_5_2017/index.php). These efforts have led to the development of six NBS pilot programs [34–39], three of which are currently active [35,38,39] and one is being scaled up [37]. Two programs are universal [37,39] and the remaining are targeted [35]; one is antenatal. Methodologies and techniques vary: some use cord blood, others dried blood spot, HPLC is usually the first test whilst the confirmatory test can be molecular biology or IEF. Overall, the results of the universal programs are in line with those of other European countries with high immigration, with 1.16% incidence of positive tests (0.07% with SCD, 0.68% with sickle cell trait) [37].

7. Germany

NBS in Germany started in 1969 with nationwide testing of all newborns for phenylketonuria. Over the years, the number of targeted diseases rose to 16 with cystic fibrosis and tyrosinemia being the last implemented in 2016 and 2017, respectively. All target diseases are endocrine or metabolic disorders. NBS in Germany is offered to every family, but participation is voluntary. However, coverage is very close to 100%. In 2015, 737,575 babies were born in Germany and 539 confirmed diagnoses of NBS target diseases were made (1:1368).

SCD is not a target disease of the German NBS program. Principally, this is owing to the fact that the disease has not been endemic in Germany in the past. It has thus been neglected over decades, although a significant and steady increase of diagnoses was observed by Kohne and Kleihauer as early as in the late 1960s [40,41]. The first systematic attempt to identify newborns suffering from SCD was made by Genzel who started a targeted pilot project in her Department of Obstetrics in Munich [42]. One affected baby was diagnosed in a targeted screening approach of 306 children born to Sub-Saharan African mothers.

With the formation of the *GPOH-Konsortium Sichelzellkrankheit* and its official assignment by the German Society for Pediatric Oncology and Hematology (GPOH) to develop a management program for children and adolescents with SCD, awareness and care improved dramatically. To date, members of this consortium have completed four regional pilot studies on NBS for SCD [43–47]. Two have been done in the Berlin NBS laboratory and one in the Hamburg and the Heidelberg NBS laboratory, respectively. Another study in Berlin is currently recruiting patients and a joint German–Polish pilot project has recently been started.

Altogether, dried blood spot samples of 118,019 newborns have been investigated in the four published studies and 32 affected babies (1:3688) were identified as having SCD. These results led the authors to the conclusion that NBS for SCD is clearly indicated in Germany.

The formal application to introduce NBS for SCD was assessed by the *Gemeinsamer Bundesausschuss* (GBA) in May 2018 for the first time. The GBA is the political body that decides what the public health insurance companies have to pay for. It consists of representatives of the different interest groups in the German healthcare system (e.g., patients, doctors, insurance companies etc.). The GBA has admitted the application for the highly formal decision-making process. A result is not expected before May 2021.

8. Ireland

Ireland has had a national NBS program since 1966, for metabolic and endocrine diseases using heel prick and dried blood spot analysis. Participation is mandatory but opting out is possible.

Currently the program captures 99.9% of all newborn infants. Targeted and voluntary national hemoglobinopathy screening has been available since 2003. Currently, it is performed on cord blood using CE as first line testing and HPLC/IEF as a confirmatory test [48]. The number of newborns diagnosed by NBS with SCD or beta thalassemia major is 10–15/year and all are referred to a single pediatric hemoglobinopathy center.

9. Malta

In Malta, all newborn are screened for SCD (universal NBS program). In 2017, 4370 babies were tested, none of which suffered from the disorder. However, eight carriers were detected. As in many other countries, a two-tier strategy is applied. IEF serves as the first tier method. Any sample containing Hb S (i.e., heterozygous, homozygous or compound heterozygous, respectively) is re-examined by HPLC to confirm the first-tier result. In case of a positive result, the screening laboratory notifies the thalassemia and sickle cell clinic who in turn will notify the parents and an appointment is given for a follow up. If requested, parents and siblings are screened (personal communication).

10. Closing Remarks

Despite all these varieties, there is broad consensus among European NBS and SCD experts on the fundamental standards that a state-of-the-art NBS program for SCD should fulfil. These standards have recently been defined in a two-day consensus conference of more than 50 experts from 13 European countries and published elsewhere [49,50]. Future intensification of this collaboration will hopefully lead to a harmonization of NBS programs for SCD in Europe.

References

1. National Sickle Cell Anemia Control Act. Available online: https://www.govinfo.gov/content/pkg/STATUTE-86/pdf/STATUTE-86-Pg136-2.pdf (accessed on 9 February 2019).
2. Gaston, M.H.; Verter, J.I.; Woods, G.; Pegelow, C.; Kelleher, J.; Presbury, G.; Zarkowsky, H.; Vichinsky, E.; Iyer, R.; Lobel, J.S.; et al. Prophylaxis with oral penicillin in children with sickle cell anemia. A randomized trial. *N. Engl. J. Med.* **1986**, *314*, 1593–1599. [CrossRef] [PubMed]
3. Zeuner, D.; Ades, A.E.; Karnon, J.; Brown, J.; Dezateux, C.; Anionwu, E.N. Antenatal and neonatal haemoglobinopathy screening in the UK: Review and economic analysis. *Health Technol. Assess.* **1999**, *3*, 1–186.
4. *The NHS Plan: A Plan for Investment, A Plan for Reform*; Department of Health: London, UK, 2000.
5. Moat, S.J.; Rees, D.; King, L.; Ifederu, A.; Harvey, K.; Hall, K.; Lloyd, G.; Morrell, C.; Hillier, S. Newborn blood spot screening for sickle cell disease by using tandem mass spectrometry: Implementation of a protocol to identify only the disease states of sickle cell disease. *Clin. Chem.* **2014**, *60*, 373–380. [CrossRef] [PubMed]
6. Streetly, A.; Sisodia, R.; Dick, M.; Latinovic, R.; Hounsell, K.; Dormandy, E. Evaluation of newborn sickle cell screening programme in England: 2010-2016. *Arch. Dis Child.* **2018**, *103*, 648–653. [CrossRef] [PubMed]
7. Daniel, Y.; Henthorn, J. *Tandem Mass Spectrometry for Sickle Cell and Thalassaemia Newborn Screening Pilot Study*; Public Health England: London, UK, 2015.
8. Daniel, Y.A.; Henthorn, J. Newborn screening for sickling and other haemoglobin disorders using tandem mass spectrometry: A pilot study of methodology in laboratories in England. *J. Med. Screen.* **2016**, *23*, 175–178. [CrossRef] [PubMed]
9. Daniel, Y.; Henthorn, J. Reliability of the current newborn screening action value for beta thalassaemia disease detection in England: A prospective study. *J. Med. Screen.* **2018**. [CrossRef] [PubMed]
10. Streetly, A.; Latinovic, R.; Henthorn, J.; Daniel, Y.; Dormandy, E.; Darbyshire, P.; Mantio, D.; Fraser, L.; Farrar, L.; Will, A.; et al. Newborn bloodspot results: Predictive value of screen positive test for thalassaemia major. *J. Med. Screen* **2013**, *20*, 183–187. [CrossRef] [PubMed]
11. Saint-Martin, C.; Romana, M.; Bibrac, A.; Brudey, K.; Tarer, V.; Divialle-Doumdo, L.; Petras, M.; Keclard-Christophe, L.; Lamothe, S.; Broquere, C.; et al. Universal newborn screening for haemoglobinopathies in Guadeloupe (French West Indies): A 27-year experience. *J. Med. Screen.* **2013**, *20*, 177–182. [CrossRef] [PubMed]

12. Bardakdjian-Michau, J.; Bahuau, M.; Hurtrel, D.; Godart, C.; Riou, J.; Mathis, M.; Goossens, M.; Badens, C.; Ducrocq, R.; Elion, J.; et al. Neonatal screening for sickle cell disease in France. *J. Clin. Pathol.* **2009**, *62*, 31–33. [CrossRef] [PubMed]
13. Thuret, I.; Sarles, J.; Merono, F.; Suzineau, E.; Collomb, J.; Lena-Russo, D.; Levy, N.; Bardakdjian, J.; Badens, C. Neonatal screening for sickle cell disease in France: Evaluation of the selective process. *J. Clin. Pathol.* **2010**, *63*, 548–551. [CrossRef] [PubMed]
14. Bardakdjian-Michau, J.; Guilloud-Batailie, M.; Maier-Redelsperger, M.; Elion, J.; Girot, R.; Feingold, J.; Galacteros, F.; de Montalembert, M. Decreased morbidity in homozygous sickle cell disease detected at birth. *Hemoglobin* **2002**, *26*, 211–217. [CrossRef] [PubMed]
15. Couque, N.; Girard, D.; Ducrocq, R.; Boizeau, P.; Haouari, Z.; Missud, F.; Holvoet, L.; Ithier, G.; Belloy, M.; Odievre, M.H.; et al. Improvement of medical care in a cohort of newborns with sickle-cell disease in North Paris: Impact of national guidelines. *Br. J. Haematol.* **2016**, *173*, 927–937. [CrossRef] [PubMed]
16. Bouva, M.J.; Mohrmann, K.; Brinkman, H.B.; Kemper-Proper, E.A.; Elvers, B.; Loeber, J.G.; Verheul, F.E.; Giordano, P.C. Implementing neonatal screening for haemoglobinopathies in the Netherlands. *J. Med. Screen.* **2010**, *17*, 58–65. [CrossRef] [PubMed]
17. *Neonatal Screening*; Health Council of the Netherlands: The Hague, The Netherlands, 2005.
18. Bouva, M.J.; Sollaino, C.; Perseu, L.; Galanello, R.; Giordano, P.C.; Harteveld, C.L.; Cnossen, M.H.; Schielen, P.C.; Elvers, L.H.; Peters, M. Relationship between neonatal screening results by HPLC and the number of alpha-thalassaemia gene mutations; consequences for the cut-off value. *J. Med. Screen.* **2011**, *18*, 182–186. [CrossRef] [PubMed]
19. *Neonatal Screening: New Recommendations*; Health Council of the Netherlands: The Hague, The Netherlands, 2015.
20. Giordano, P.C.; Bouva, M.J.; Harteveld, C.L. A confidential inquiry estimating the number of patients affected with sickle cell disease and thalassemia major confirms the need for a prevention strategy in the Netherlands. *Hemoglobin* **2004**, *28*, 287–296. [CrossRef] [PubMed]
21. Peter, M.; Appel, I.M.; Cnossen, M.H.; Breuning-Boers, J.M.; Heijboer, H. Sickle cell disease in heel prick screening. I. *Ned. Tijdschr. Geneeskd.* **2009**, *153*, 854–857.
22. Vansenne, F.; de Borgie, C.; Bouva, M.J.; Legdeur, M.A.; van Zwieten, R.; Petrij, F.; Peters, M. Sickle cell disease in heel prick screening. II. *Ned. Tijdschr. Geneeskd.* **2009**, *153*, 858–861. [PubMed]
23. Cela, E.; Bellon, J.M.; de la Cruz, M.; Belendez, C.; Berrueco, R.; Ruiz, A.; Elorza, I.; Diaz de Heredia, C.; Cervera, A.; Valles, G.; et al. National registry of hemoglobinopathies in Spain (REPHem). *Pediatr. Blood Cancer* **2017**, *64*. [CrossRef] [PubMed]
24. Ketelslegers, O.; Eyskens, F.; Boemer, F.; Bours, V.; Minon, J.-M.; Gulbis, B. Epidemiological data on sickle cell disease in Belgium. *Belg. J. Hematol.* **2015**, *6*, 135–141.
25. Gulbis, B.; Tshilolo, L.; Cotton, F.; Lin, C.; Vertongen, F. Newborn screening for haemoglobinopathies: The Brussels experience. *J. Med. Screen.* **1999**, *6*, 11–15. [CrossRef] [PubMed]
26. Gulbis, B.; Ferster, A.; Cotton, F.; Lebouchard, M.P.; Cochaux, P.; Vertongen, F. Neonatal haemoglobinopathy screening: Review of a 10-year programme in Brussels. *J. Med. Screen.* **2006**, *13*, 76–78. [CrossRef] [PubMed]
27. Gulbis, B.; Cotton, F.; Ferster, A.; Ketelslegers, O.; Dresse, M.F.; Ronge-Collard, E.; Minon, J.M.; Le, P.Q.; Vertongen, F. Neonatal haemoglobinopathy screening in Belgium. *J. Clin. Pathol.* **2009**, *62*, 49–52. [CrossRef] [PubMed]
28. Wolff, F.; Cotton, F.; Gulbis, B. Screening for haemoglobinopathies on cord blood: Laboratory and clinical experience. *J. Med. Screen.* **2012**, *19*, 116–122. [CrossRef] [PubMed]
29. Boemer, F.; Cornet, Y.; Libioulle, C.; Segers, K.; Bours, V.; Schoos, R. 3-years experience review of neonatal screening for hemoglobin disorders using tandem mass spectrometry. *Clin. Chim. Acta* **2011**, *412*, 1476–1479. [CrossRef] [PubMed]
30. Boemer, F.; Ketelslegers, O.; Minon, J.M.; Bours, V.; Schoos, R. Newborn screening for sickle cell disease using tandem mass spectrometry. *Clin. Chem.* **2008**, *54*, 2036–2041. [CrossRef] [PubMed]
31. Le, P.Q.; Ferster, A.; Cotton, F.; Vertongen, F.; Vermylen, C.; Vanderfaeillie, A.; Dedeken, L.; Heijmans, C.; Ketelslegers, O.; Dresse, M.F.; et al. Sickle cell disease from Africa to Belgium, from neonatal screening to clinical management. *Med. Trop.* **2010**, *70*, 467–470.
32. Le, P.Q.; Ferster, A.; Dedeken, L.; Vermylen, C.; Vanderfaeillie, A.; Rozen, L.; Heijmans, C.; Huybrechts, S.;

Devalck, C.; Cotton, F.; et al. Neonatal screening improves sickle cell disease clinical outcome in Belgium. *J. Med. Screen.* **2017**, *25*, 57–63. [CrossRef] [PubMed]

33. Colombatti, R.; Perrotta, S.; Samperi, P.; Casale, M.; Masera, N.; Palazzi, G.; Sainati, L.; Russo, G.; Italian Association of Pediatric Hematology-Oncology Sickle Cell Disease Working Group. Organizing national responses for rare blood disorders: The Italian experience with sickle cell disease in childhood. *Orphanet J. Rare Dis.* **2013**, *8*, 169. [CrossRef] [PubMed]
34. Rolla, R.; Castagno, M.; Zaffaroni, M.; Grigollo, B.; Colombo, S.; Piccotti, S.; Dellora, C.; Bona, G.; Bellomo, G. Neonatal screening for sickle cell disease and other hemoglobinopathies in "the changing Europe". *Clin. Lab.* **2014**, *60*, 2089–2093. [CrossRef] [PubMed]
35. Venturelli, D.; Lodi, M.; Palazzi, G.; Bergonzini, G.; Doretto, G.; Zini, A.; Monica, C.; Cano, M.C.; Ilaria, M.; Montagnani, G.; et al. Sickle cell disease in areas of immigration of high-risk populations: A low cost and reproducible method of screening in northern Italy. *Blood Transfus.* **2014**, *12*, 346–351. [CrossRef] [PubMed]
36. Ballardini, E.; Tarocco, A.; Marsella, M.; Bernardoni, R.; Carandina, G.; Melandri, C.; Guerra, G.; Patella, A.; Zucchelli, M.; Ferlini, A.; et al. Universal neonatal screening for sickle cell disease and other haemoglobinopathies in Ferrara, Italy. *Blood Transfus.* **2013**, *11*, 245–249. [CrossRef] [PubMed]
37. Martella, M.; Cattaneo, L.; Viola, G.; Azzena, S.; Cappellari, A.; Baraldi, E.; Zorloni, C.; Masera, N.; Biondi, A.; Basso, G.; et al. Universal Newborn Screening for Sickle Cell Disease: Preliminary Results of the First Year of a Multicentric Italian Project. In Proceedings of the 22nd Annual Congress of the European Hematology Association, Madrid, spain, June 2017; pp. 22–25.
38. De Zen, L.; Dall'Amico, R.; Sainati, L.; Colombatti, R.; Testa, E.R.; Catapano, R.; Zanolli, F. Screening neonatale per le emoglobinopatie su Dried Blood Spot. In Proceedings of the XXXVI. Congresso Nazionale Associazione Italiana Ematologia Oncologia Pediatrica (AIEOP), Pisa, Italy, June 2010; pp. 6–8.
39. Mandrile, G.; Cavazzuti, C.; Gaglioti, C.M.; Cociglio, S.; Lux, C.M.; Chiavilli, F.; Piga, A. 40 anni di screening delle emoglobinopatie: l'esperienza di Rovigo. In Proceedings of the X. Congresso Nazionale SITE, Rome, Italy, September 2018; pp. 27–29.
40. Kohne, E.; Kleihauer, E. Häufigkeit und Formen von anomalen Hämoglobinen und Thalassämie-Syndromen in der deutschen Bevölkerung. *Klinische Wochenschrift* **1974**, *52*, 1003–1010. [CrossRef]
41. Kohne, E.; Kleihauer, E. Hemoglobinopathies: A longitudinal study over four decades. *Dtsch. Arztebl. Int.* **2010**, *107*, 65–71. [CrossRef] [PubMed]
42. Dickerhoff, R.; Genzel-Boroviczeny, O.; Kohne, E. Haemoglobinopathies and newborn haemoglobinopathy screening in Germany. *J. Clin. Pathol.* **2009**, *62*, 34. [CrossRef] [PubMed]
43. Lobitz, S.; Klein, J.; Brose, A.; Blankenstein, O.; Frommel, C. Newborn screening by tandem mass spectrometry confirms the high prevalence of sickle cell disease among German newborns. *Ann. Hematol.* **2018**. [CrossRef] [PubMed]
44. Lobitz, S.; Frommel, C.; Brose, A.; Klein, J.; Blankenstein, O. Incidence of sickle cell disease in an unselected cohort of neonates born in Berlin, Germany. *Eur. J. Hum. Genet.* **2014**, *22*, 1051–1053. [CrossRef] [PubMed]
45. Frommel, C.; Brose, A.; Klein, J.; Blankenstein, O.; Lobitz, S. Newborn screening for sickle cell disease: Technical and legal aspects of a German pilot study with 38,220 participants. *BioMed Res. Int.* **2014**, *2014*, 695828. [CrossRef] [PubMed]
46. Kunz, J.B.; Awad, S.; Happich, M.; Muckenthaler, L.; Lindner, M.; Gramer, G.; Okun, J.G.; Hoffmann, G.F.; Bruckner, T.; Muckenthaler, M.U.; et al. Significant prevalence of sickle cell disease in Southwest Germany: Results from a birth cohort study indicate the necessity for newborn screening. *Ann. Hematol.* **2016**, *95*, 397–402. [CrossRef] [PubMed]
47. Grosse, R.; Lukacs, Z.; Cobos, P.N.; Oyen, F.; Ehmen, C.; Muntau, B.; Timmann, C.; Noack, B. The Prevalence of Sickle Cell Disease and Its Implication for Newborn Screening in Germany (Hamburg Metropolitan Area). *Pediatr. Blood Cancer* **2015**. [CrossRef] [PubMed]
48. Gibbons, C.; Geoghegan, R.; Conroy, H.; Lippacott, S.; O'Brien, D.; Lynam, P.; Langabeer, L.; Cotter, M.; Smith, O.; McMahon, C. Sickle cell disease: Time for a targeted neonatal screening programme. *Ir. Med. J.* **2015**, *108*, 43–45. [PubMed]
49. Shook, L.M.; Ware, R.E. Sickle cell screening in Europe: The time has come. *Br. J. Haematol.* **2018**, *183*, 534–535. [CrossRef] [PubMed]
50. Lobitz, S.; Telfer, P.; Cela, E.; Allaf, B.; Angastiniotis, M.; Backman Johansson, C.; Badens, C.; Bento, C.; Bouva, M.J.; Canatan, D.; et al. Newborn screening for sickle cell disease in Europe: Recommendations from a Pan-European Consensus Conference. *Br. J. Haematol.* **2018**, *183*, 648–660. [CrossRef] [PubMed]

8

Congenital Critical Heart Defect Screening in a Health Area of the Community of Valencia (Spain)

Elena Cubells [1], Begoña Torres [2], Antonio Nuñez-Ramiro [1], Manuel Sánchez-Luna [3], Isabel Izquierdo [1] and Máximo Vento [1,2,*]

[1] Division of Neonatology, Hospital Universitario y Politécnico La Fe, 46026 Valencia, Spain; cubecha@hotmail.com (E.C.); aguillermo9nr@hotmail.com (A.N.-R.); izquierdo_isamac@gva.es (I.I.)
[2] Instituto de Investigación Sanitaria La Fe, 46026 Valencia, Spain; bego.torresg@gmail.com
[3] Division of Neonatology, Hospital Universitario Gregorio Marañón, 28007 Madrid, Spain; msluna@salud.madrid.org
* Correspondence: maximo.vento@uv.es or vento_max@gva.es;

Abstract: Despite the progress in the fetal echocardiographic detection of congenital critical heart defects and neonatal physical examination, a significant number of newborn infants are discharged and readmitted to the hospital in severe condition due to cardiac failure or collapse. The aim of this study was to assess the incidence of undetected critical congenital heart disease (CCHD) by a pulse oximetry-screening program in the maternity wards of hospitals with Perinatal Services in a specific geographic area. This is a prospective observational study performed in in the health area corresponding to the city of Valencia. Eligible infants were consecutively admitted newborn infants in the maternities of the participating hospitals with negative fetal echocardiography after normal physical examination in the delivery room. All patients were screened following a specific pulse oximetry protocol before discharge. A total of 8856 newborn infants were screened. A total of three babies presented with severe congenital cardiac malformation and two babies presented with early onset sepsis. Sensitivity was 100% and specificity was 99.97%, with a positive predictive value of 60% and negative predictive value of 100%. Pulse oximetry screening programs in the early neonatal period constitute a valuable tool to avoid inadvertent hospital discharge of severe cardiac malformations and the subsequent life-threatening complications derived.

Keywords: oxygen saturation; pulse oximetry; critical congenital heart disease; screening; newborn

---

1. Introduction

Congenital critical heart defects (CCHD), defined as those needing invasive medical intervention or those that can produce death within the first 30 days after delivery [1], may in many cases exhibit signs and symptoms that develop after hospital discharge, potentially resulting in collapse and death. Today, prenatal fetal heart ultrasound can detect many such cases, but still some of them can be missed [2]. In addition, both physical examination of the neonate after birth can further detect congenital cardiac malformations, but not all are found [3,4]. Moreover, low oxygen saturation can also be missed clinically [5,6]. Under these circumstances, pulse oximetry appears to be a reliable screening technique in neonates before hospital discharge. It is simple, noninvasive, low-cost, and very reliable in the detection of hypoxemia, and therefore has been recommended as a screening tool [7,8]. Upon adding neonatal pulse oximetry screening to prenatal ultrasound detection and postnatal clinical exam, the diagnosis rate of CCHD increases [9] and thus the undiagnosed cases of CCHD are reduced to less than 10% of total CCHD [10].

In September 2011, the US Health and Human Services (HHS) Secretary's Advisory Committee on Heritable Disorders in Newborns and Children recommended that critical congenital heart diseases (CCHD) to be added to the neonatal screening panel based on the evidence of a large number of newborns screened in Sweden and England [11–13].

In a large meta-analysis in 2012, 13 eligible studies with data for 229,421 newborn babies were analyzed. Pulse oximetry was demonstrated to be highly specific for the detection of critical congenital heart defects with moderate sensitivity [14]. More recently, in a Chinese multicenter study, 122,738 consecutive newborn babies (120,707 asymptomatic and 2031 symptomatic) were screened, detecting congenital heart disease in 1071 (157 critical and 330 major) [15].

We aimed to assess the relevance of universal screening for critical congenital heart disease (CCHD) in a specific health area (Valencia, Spain) where fetal detection of cardiac malformations by echocardiography had been substantially implemented in recent years.

2. Population and Methods

This is a prospective observational pilot study performed in the health area of Valencia (Spain). The study protocol was approved by the Internal Review Board (IRB) of the Hospital Universitario y Politécnico La Fe (Valencia, Spain). Parents/guardians of all recruited patients gave informed consent. A total of 12 hospitals, including level I (rural hospital, n = 5), level II (medium sized city hospital, n = 5), and level III hospitals [2], were included for a 6-month period. Eligible infants were newborn babies admitted to the maternity wards with normal fetal ultrasound evaluation for CCDH and normal newborn examination by a neonatologist in the delivery room. Babies with suspicious fetal echocardiography or abnormalities in the physical examination (color, murmurs, pulse abnormalities) were evaluated by a pediatric cardiologist and disregarded for the study.

Included patients were screened between 24–48 h after birth, following the protocol shown in Figure 1. Newborn infants with a positive or doubtful screening were admitted to the Neonatal Intensive Care Unit (NICU) where the clinical, analytical, and echocardiographic study was completed by neonatologists and pediatric cardiologists. After reaching a diagnosis, babies remained in the NICU for treatment or were discharged home.

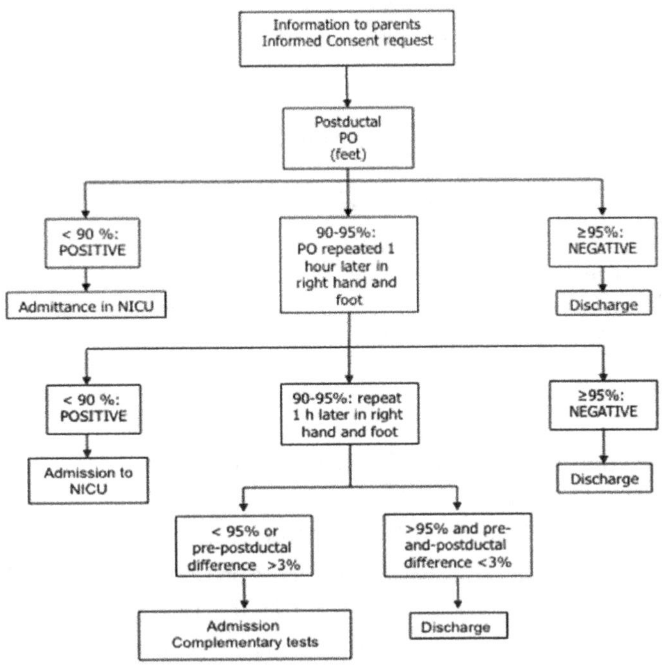

Figure 1. Flow diagram describing the protocol of the Pulsimat study for the screening of critical congenital heart disease. PO: pulse oximetry.

3. Results

Figure 2 shows the flow diagram of the study. From a total of 11,531 newborn infants born in the participating hospitals, 66 babies were diagnosed with CCHD, representing 5.8 per thousand newborn infants. Out of these, 36 patients had CCHD detected in utero and confirmed at birth (3.1 per 1000 births), 27 were diagnosed after birth based on clinical symptoms and echocardiography (2.3 per 1000 births), and three were detected by pulse oximetry screening at discharge (0.26 per thousand live births). A total of 8856 representing 78.6% of all births were screened for critical CCHD. Out of these, five had a positive pulse oximetry screen. However, two cases were caused by respiratory distress secondary to early onset sepsis; thus, only the remaining three cases were due to CCDH, specifically, total anomalous venous return.

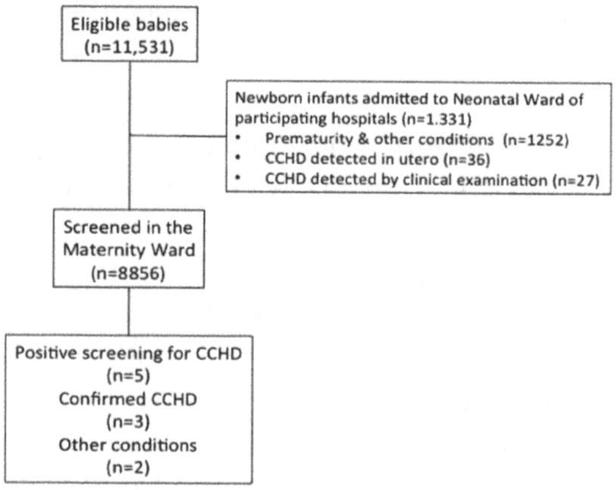

Figure 2. Consort diagram describing eligible patients, disregarded, and finally screened for critical congenital heart disease (CCHD) in the Pulsimat study.

Hence, in the 6-month study period, a total of 66 babies were diagnosed with CCHD; 36 in utero (54.5%), 27 (41.6%) ex utero by clinical examination, and three by pulse oximetry screening at discharge, representing 4.5% of the total instances of CCHD.

Table 1 shows the values for sensitivity, specificity, positive predictive value, and negative predictive value.

Table 1. Screening for congenital cardiac heart defects: analysis of results.

	Echocardiography		
Pulse oximetry	Positive	Negative	Total
Positive	3	2	5
Negative	0	8851	8851
Total	3	8853	8856

4. Discussion

It has been estimated that 30% of all CCHD patients have a late diagnosis and could benefit from neonatal screening [16]. As most previous studies demonstrated that non-cardiac conditions could also be detected by pulse oximetry, false positive detection can represent another advantage of the screening [13,17]. In our study, the detection of CCHD in utero (fetal echocardiography) plus ex utero after clinical examination represented 95.5% of the total, while 4.5% of the babies with CCHD were detected by pre-discharge screening. Interestingly, two patients that would have been discharged home with early onset sepsis had a positive screening and were admitted to the NICU. In June 2013, an international group of neonatologists and cardiologists met in Torino (Italy) with the chief investigators from two European screening studies of pulse oximetry to discuss strategies to develop Europe-wide recommendations for CCHD screening. They concluded that there is a need for a European Consensus on CCDH screening in Europe [18]. Recently, a panel from The European Pulse Oximetry Screening Workgroup investigating pulse oximetry screening for critical congenital heart defects published a European consensus statement that recommended the use of pulse oximetry for the early detection of CCDH in all European countries, using new-generation equipment that is motion tolerant; screening after 6 h of delivery and before discharge from the birth center, preferably within the 24 h after birth; and using two extremities, the right hand and either foot [19]. In addition, guidelines for the management of CCDH have been implemented, including practical aspects and nomograms to facilitate the management of these babies [20]. Finally, the Committee on Standards of the Spanish Neonatal Society (SENeo) has very recently published the National Guidelines for the Screening of Critical Congenital Heart Defects [21]. SENeo recommends performing the screening at >24 h after birth; however, each center should analyze its owns circumstances; in some centers performing screening at <12 h after birth could be preferable, despite the increase in false positives. If express discharge is performed, then any time after birth is recommended. It is also recommended to perform pre- and post-ductal pulse oximetry with motion tolerant devices that are also reliable at low saturations. The ranges of normality are similar to those defined by the European Consensus, with an absolute positivity with SpO2 values <90% and negativity with values ≥95% in any extremity, and a difference ≥3% between pre- and post-ductal pulses. In this scenario, we encourage every European country to implement the guideline that best suits their health organization and characteristics of the population.

Our study has obvious limitations. The number of patients and the geographical area are both small, and thus do not represent the entire Valencian community with 55,000 deliveries per year. However, it reveals that despite the excellent prenatal and postnatal detection of CCHD, approximately 5% of these babies would have been discharged home from the hospital. We could speculate that if we translate these numbers to the entire population of our community, at least 15 newborn infants could have been discharged yearly with a life-threatening condition, although the data obtained in our study do not support this conclusion. We did not see any false negative cases, although they have been described in other studies. Unluckily, the number of patients included in our study was relatively small and hindered the possibility of detecting such cases. In addition, our study revealed that it is feasible to systematically perform pulse oximetry screening in the maternity ward without implying a relevant additional workload for the nursing staff. Finally, it is worth mentioning that pulse oximetry screening can also promptly detect other severe conditions, such as early onset sepsis, that went undiagnosed in the routine clinical examination. The Spanish Neonatal Society (SENeo) is very soon going to put forward a protocol for the screening of CCHD that will be adopted by all the maternity wards in our country [21].

Author Contributions: Elena Cubells, Begoña Torres, Antonio-Nuñez Ramiro recruited the patients, introduced the data in the electronic registry, and performed the statistics. Manuel Sánchez-Luna, Isabel Izquierdo and Maximo Vento conceived the study, designed the study protocol and drafted and approved the final version of the manuscript.

References

1. Schultz, A.H.; Localio, A.R.; Clark, B.J.; Ravishankar, C.; Videon, N.; Kimmel, S.E. Epidemiologic features of the presentation of critical congenital heart disease: Implications for screening. *Pediatrics* **2008**, *121*, 751–757. [CrossRef] [PubMed]
2. Liu, H.; Zhou, J.; Feng, Q.L.; Gu, H.T.; Wan, G.; Zhang, H.M.; Xie, Y.J.; Li, X.S. Fetal echocardiography for congenital heart disease diagnosis: A meta-analysis, power analysis and missing data analysis. *Eur. J. Prev. Cardiol.* **2015**, *22*, 1531–1547. [CrossRef] [PubMed]
3. Górska-Kot, A.; Błaz, W.; Pszeniczna, E.; Rusin, J.; Materna-Kiryluk, A.; Homa, E.; Hejda, G.; Franus, J. Trends in diagnosis and prevalence of critical congenital heart defects in the Podkarpacie province in 2002–2004,

based on data from the Polish Registry of Congenital Malformations. *J. Appl. Genet.* **2006**, *47*, 191–194. [CrossRef] [PubMed]

4. Meberg, A.; Andreassen, A.; Brunvand, L.; Markestad, T.; Moster, D.; Nietsch, L.; Silberg, I.E.; Skålevik, J.E. Pulse oximetry screening as a complementary strategy to detect critical congenital heart defects. *Acta Paediatr.* **2009**, *98*, 682–686. [CrossRef] [PubMed]
5. Hoffman, J.I. It is time for routine neonatal screening by pulse oximetry. *Neonatology* **2011**, *99*, 1–9. [CrossRef] [PubMed]
6. O'Donnell, C.P.; Kamlin, C.O.; Davis, P.G.; Carlin, J.B.; Morley, C.J. Clinical assessment of infant colour at delivery. *Arch. Dis. Child. Fetal Neonatal Ed.* **2007**, *92*, F465–F467. [CrossRef] [PubMed]
7. Mikrou, P.; Singh, A.; Ewer, A.K. Pulse oximetery screening for critical congenital heart defects: A repeat UK national survey. *Arch Dis. Child. Fetal Neonatal. Ed.* **2017**, *10*, F558–F559.
8. Mahle, W.T.; Martin, G.R.; Beekman, R.H., III; Morrow, W.R. Section on Cardiology and Cardiac Surgery Executive Committee. Endorsement of Health and Human Services recommendation for pulse oximetry screening for critical congenital heart disease. *Pediatrics* **2012**, *129*, 190–192. [PubMed]
9. Riede, F.T.; Wörner, C.; Dähnert, I.; Möckel, A.; Kostelka, M.; Schneider, P. Effectiveness of neonatal pulse oximetry screening for detection of critical congenital heart disease in daily clinical routine—Results from a prospective multicenter study. *Eur. J. Pediatr.* **2010**, *169*, 975–981. [CrossRef] [PubMed]
10. Ewer, A.K. Pulse oximetry screening: Do we have enough evidence now? *Lancet* **2014**, *384*, 725–726. [CrossRef]
11. Sebelius, K. *Secretary of Health and Human Services Recommendation for Pulse Oximetry Screening*; Department of Health and Human Services: Washington, DC, USA, 2011. Available online: http://www.hrsa.gov/advisorycommittees/mchbadvisory/heritabledisorders/recommendations/correspondence/cyanoticheartsecre09212011.pdf (accessed on 27 November 2017).
12. De-Wahl Granelli, A.; Wennergren, M.; Sandberg, K.; Mellander, M.; Bejlum, C.; Inganäs, L.; Eriksson, M.; Segerdahl, N.; Agren, A.; Ekman-Joelsson, B.M.; et al. Impact of pulse oximetry screening on the detection of duct dependent congenital heart disease: A Swedish prospective screening study in 39,821 newborns. *BMJ* **2009**, *338*, a3037. [CrossRef] [PubMed]
13. Ewer, A.K.; Middleton, L.J.; Furmston, A.T.; Bhoyar, A.; Daniels, J.P.; Thangaratinam, S.; Deeks, J.J.; Khan, K.S.; PulseOx Study Group. Pulse oximetry screening for congenital heart defects in newborn infants (PulseOx): A test accuracy study. *Lancet* **2011**, *378*, 785–794. [CrossRef]
14. Thangaratinam, S.; Brown, K.; Zamora, J.; Khan, K.S.; Ewer, A.K. Pulse oximetry screening for critical congenital heart defects in asymptomatic newborn babies: A systematic review and meta-analysis. *Lancet* **2012**, *379*, 2459–2464. [CrossRef]
15. Zhao, Q.M.; Ma, X.J.; Ge, X.L.; Liu, F.; Yan, W.L.; Wu, L.; Ye, M.; Zhang, J.; Gao, Y.; Jia, B.; et al. Pulse oximetry with clinical assessment to screen for congenital heart disease in neonates in China: A prospective study. *Lancet* **2014**, *384*, 747–754. [CrossRef]
16. Peterson, C.; Ailes, E.; Riehle-Colarusso, T.; Oster, M.E.; Olney, R.S.; Cassell, C.H.; Fixler, D.E.; Carmichael, S.L.; Shaw, G.M.; Gilboa, S.M.; et al. Late detection of critical congenital heart disease among US infants: Estimation of the potential impact of proposed universal screening using pulse oximetry. *JAMA Pediatr.* **2014**, *168*, 361–370. [CrossRef] [PubMed]
17. De-Wahl Granelli, A.; Meberg, A.; Ojala, T.; Steensberg, J.; Oskarsson, G.; Mellander, M. Nordic pulse oximetry screening—Implementation status and proposal for uniform guidelines. *Acta Paediatr.* **2014**, *103*, 1136–1142. [CrossRef] [PubMed]
18. Ewer, A.K.; Granelli, A.D.; Manzoni, P.; Sánchez Luna, M.; Martin, G.R. Pulse oximetry screening for congenital heart defects. *Lancet* **2013**, *382*, 856–857. [CrossRef]
19. Manzoni, P.; Martin, G.R.; Luna, M.S.; Mestrovic, J.; Simeoni, U.; Zimmermann, L.; Ewer, A.K. Pulse oximetry screening for critical congenital heart defects: a European consensus statement. *Lancet Child Adolesc. Health* **2017**, *1*, 88–90. [CrossRef]
20. Haas, N.A.; Franke, J. Mangement of a child with cyanosis. Guidelines for the management of congenital heart disease. *Cardiol. Young* **2017**, *27* (Suppl. 3), S3–S4.
21. Sánchez Luna, M.; Pérez Muñuzuri, A.; Sanz López, E.; Leante Castellanos, J.L.; Benavente Fernández, I.; Ruiz Campillo, C.W.; Sánchez Redondo, M.D.; Vento Torres, M.; Rite Gracia, S. Pulse oximetry screening of critical congenital heart defects in the neonatal period. The Spanish National Neonatal Society recommendation. *An. Pediatr.* **2017**. [CrossRef]

9

A Newborn Screening, Presymptomatically Identified Infant with Late-Onset Pompe Disease: Case Report, Parental Experience and Recommendations

Raymond Y. Wang [1,2,†]

1 Division of Metabolic Disorders, CHOC Children's Specialists, Orange, CA 92868, USA; rawang@choc.org
2 Department of Pediatrics, University of California-Irvine School of Medicine, Orange, CA 92868, USA
† The parents of the proposita presented firmly state their desire to maintain anonymity. However, they have provided written consent for publication of the proposita's details and their commentary.

Abstract: Pompe disease is an inherited lysosomal storage disorder caused by acid alpha-glucosidase (GAA) enzyme deficiency, resulting in muscle and neuron intralysosomal glycogen storage. Clinical symptoms vary from the severe, infantile-onset form with hypertrophic cardiomyopathy, gross motor delay, and early death from respiratory insufficiency; to a late-onset form with variable onset of proximal muscle weakness and progressive respiratory insufficiency. Newborn screening programs have been instituted to presymptomatically identify neonates with infantile-onset Pompe disease for early initiation of treatment. However, infants with late-onset Pompe disease are also identified, leaving families and physicians in a state of uncertainty regarding prognosis, necessity, and timing of treatment initiation. This report presents a 31 5/7 weeks' gestational age premature infant flagged positive for Pompe disease with low dried blood spot GAA activity; sequencing identified biparental c.-32-13T>G/c.29delA *GAA* variants predicting late-onset Pompe disease. The infant's parents' initial reactions to the positive newborn screen, subsequent experience during confirmatory testing, and post-confirmation reflections are also reported. While uncertainties regarding natural history and prognosis of presymptomatically-identified late-onset Pompe disease infants will be elucidated with additional experience, suggestions for education of first-line providers are provided to accurately communicate results and compassionately counsel families regarding anxiety-provoking positive newborn screen results.

Keywords: Pompe disease; late-onset; infantile-onset; newborn screening; presymptomatic; c.-32-13T>G

---

1. Introduction

Pompe disease, caused by acid α-glucosidase enzyme deficiency (GAA; EC 3.2.1.20) due to pathogenic variants in *GAA*, is characterized by intralysosomal accumulation of glycogen throughout bodily tissues, most notably within cardiac and skeletal muscle.

Muscle lysosomal glycogen storage results in hypertrophic cardiomyopathy and skeletal muscle weakness varying in age of onset and severity according to residual GAA enzymatic activity. Skeletal myopathy is also augmented by spinal cord anterior horn and brain neuronal glycogen storage and dysfunction [1]. Infantile-onset Pompe disease (IOPD), caused by near-absence of lysosomal GAA enzyme, typically manifests in the first two months of life with progressive and severe hypertrophic cardiomyopathy, heart failure, marked hypotonia, respiratory failure; if untreated, death from cardiopulmonary complications typically occurs within the first 14 months of life [2].

Late-onset Pompe disease (LOPD) patients have pathogenic *GAA* variants that reduce, but do not completely abolish, acid α-glucosidase enzyme activity. The residual enzyme attenuates the disease course; prior to initiation of newborn screening programs for Pompe disease, LOPD patients were often diagnosed in adulthood following decades of proximal myopathic symptoms. Without treatment, LOPD patients experience deterioration of skeletal muscle strength, becoming nonambulatory and dependent upon artificial ventilation (non-invasive positive airway pressure, or invasive mechanical ventilation) [3].

Pompe disease patients typically have elevations of serum creatine phosphokinase and transaminases secondary to myopathic injury. However, these tests are neither sensitive nor specific for Pompe disease, nor is urinary hexose tetrasaccharide, which is an excreted marker of glycogen accumulation. A diagnosis of Pompe disease relies upon identification of deficient white blood cell GAA enzymatic activity and biparentally inherited variants in *GAA* [4].

Development of intravenous enzyme replacement therapy (ERT) in the form of recombinant human GAA (rhGAA) enzyme, has radically transformed the natural history of Pompe disease. The efficacy of rhGAA ERT is well documented for both IOPD and LOPD. IOPD patients' overall survival and ventilation-free survival are drastically prolonged; early initiation of rhGAA therapy is associated with better developmental and survival outcomes [5]. Since immune response and cross-reactive immunologic material (CRIM) status play a significant role in outcomes, pre-rhGAA immunomodulation is also indicated to mitigate the neutralizing effect of the anti-rhGAA immune response [6]. LOPD patients also demonstrate improvement in ambulatory and pulmonary function, with delayed onset of declines in six-minute walk and pulmonary function testing [7].

Given the significant improvement in survival, hypertrophic cardiomyopathy, and pulmonary outcomes in infantile-onset patients, Pompe disease was included in newborn screening (NBS) programs around the world. Taiwan, which has been screening for Pompe disease since 2005 due to a founder effect for IOPD [8], reported 28 newborns affected with either form of Pompe disease out of 473,738 screened (1 case per 16,919 newborns) [9]. Surprisingly, prevalences from NBS programs without known Pompe disease founder effects have also been much higher than expected. The Austrian program identified 4 Pompe disease infants out of 34,736 screened (1 case per 8,684 newborns) [10]. Pilot NBS programs in the United States also identified a high prevalence of Pompe disease; the state of Missouri identified 8 affected out of 43,701 screened (1 case per 5463 newborns) [11], while the state of Illinois identified 10 affected out of 219,973 screened (1 case per 21,979 newborns) [12].

Favorable outcomes of NBS-identified IOPD infants in these programs led to the eventual inclusion of Pompe disease to the United States Health and Human Services "Recommended Uniform Screening Panel" in 2013, leading to the implementation of universal newborn screening for Pompe disease in the United States. NBS for Pompe disease began in the state of California in July of 2018.

New challenges emerge with the implementation of every newborn screening program. Quantification of GAA enzymatic activity in NBS samples cannot distinguish between IOPD and LOPD patients. Consequently, for each IOPD case identified, there are anywhere from 1 to 4 LOPD cases identified. If GAA enzymatic activity alone is utilized as the first-tier analyte, heterozygous and pseudodeficiency-carrying infants are also identified. Though rapid initiation of rhGAA ERT is clearly beneficial for IOPD babies, the management—including potential decisions regarding ERT—of NBS-identified, presymptomatic LOPD infants is not clearly defined [13].

Because NBS for Pompe disease was recently introduced in the United States, a clearer understanding of early childhood LOPD phenotypes and natural history will require more time for additional cases to be identified and followed longitudinally. Only then can clear guidelines for clinical follow-up and potential initiation of ERT be issued.

These early uncertainties present difficulties for the clinicians who are the initial evaluators of NBS-identified LOPD infants, and create anxiety and distress for the infants' parents. This scenario is not novel to the practice of newborn screening: Following implementation of universal screening for phenylketonuria, another inborn error of metabolism for which early institution of treatment significantly impacts outcome, parents of infants ultimately found to be false positives for the disorder demonstrated long-lasting anxiety about their baby's health [14]. In the era of tandem mass spectrometry-based NBS for multiple inborn errors of metabolism, infants with NBS false positives were hospitalized twice as often as infants with normal NBS [15] due to higher parental stress levels, dysfunction, and perceptions of fragility. If such a possibility for psychological harm exists for parents of infants with false positives, it is undoubtedly present for parents of infants with attenuated conditions for which no clear standard of care yet exists.

The purpose of this report is to highlight one case of LOPD identified through the California Newborn Screening program. More importantly, this report aims to gain insight into how the infant's parents initially responded to the revelation of their child's condition, and how they processed and coped with the realization that their child had LOPD. Their goal in sharing their experience and suggestions, which have been curated, is to help all medical staff involved in the newborn screening process—not only medical geneticists, but also the primary care pediatricians' offices and neonatal intensive care units—better understand the complexities of screening for a heterogeneous disorder and how to effectively counsel and communicate with families whose infants have been identified by NBS.

2. Case Report

Parents of the proposita have provided consent for publication of clinical data. The proposita is a second twin, born at 31 5/7 weeks' gestational age with a birth weight of 1550 g. Her mother was a 36-year-old gravida 2/para 1-2-0-3 woman whose twin pregnancy was monitored closely due to anti-protein S antibodies; she experienced prolonged premature rupture of membranes leading to the proposita's delivery via repeat Cesarean section. Prenatal screening included normal prenatal nuchal translucency, first trimester laboratory testing, and monitoring ultrasounds.

Initial Apgar scores were 7 at 1 min and 8 at 5 min. She experienced an uncomplicated neonatal course; in the perinatal period, she received empiric antibiotics, phototherapy, and was placed on nasal continuous positive airway pressure. She did not require intubation or supplemental oxygen, and was hospitalized for a total of four weeks in the neonatal intensive care unit advancing oral feedings.

Her newborn screening was flagged for potential Pompe disease as blood spot GAA enzymatic activity was low at 2.7 nmol/mg protein/h (reference range 20.9–140.7). Control β-galactosidase enzyme was within normal range. Blood creatine phosphokinase level was 134 units/liter (reference range <235 units/liter). While urinary hexose tetrasaccharide (uHex4) and *GAA* molecular sequencing were pending, an echocardiogram was performed which documented normal atrial and ventricular dimensions, normal left ventricular wall thickness without evidence of cardiomyopathy, and a normal left ventricular ejection fraction of 72.4%.

Initial uHex4 level was elevated at 25.2 mmol/mol creatinine (reference range <17.6 mmol/mol creatinine); because this was obtained when she was 32 5/7 weeks' adjusted gestational age, when low urinary creatinine excretion of a premature infant could interfere with accurate measurement, it was repeated five weeks later which was normal at 4.1 mmol/mol creatinine. *GAA* sequencing identified two pathogenic variants: the paternally inherited "common" late-infantile onset c.-32-13T>G variant, and the maternally inherited c.29delA (p.His10Profs*33) variant.

Subsequent measurements of creatine phosphokinase continued to be normal at 215 units/L (23 days of life) and 212 units/L (2.5 months of life). An echocardiogram performed at two months of life continued to show normal ventricular dimensions and function without left ventricular hypertrophy. She had retinopathy of prematurity, which subsequently resolved. She also had apnea of prematurity, for which she was initially placed on caffeine citrate while hospitalized, and subsequently monitored with an apnea monitor after two episodes of apnea following discharge.

Prior to her first evaluation with the author, she was rehospitalized twice for respiratory issues. The first, occurring at 6 weeks of age, was due to respiratory distress caused by rhinovirus bronchiolitis, for which she was placed on nasal continuous positive airway pressure with supplemental oxygen. The second, occurring at 8 weeks of age, took place because she experienced apnea at home requiring cardiopulmonary resuscitation. She was hospitalized for intravenous antibiotics for treatment of presumptive pneumonia and for observation.

Following her hospitalizations, she experienced good subsequent weight gain without any feeding difficulties. At approximately four months of age (two months adjusted for prematurity), her weight was 5.13 kg (50th percentile), length was 54.6 cm (15th percentile), and head circumference 39.5 cm (75th percentile). Examination identified head lag, absence of calf pseudohypertrophy, normal patellar/biceps/triceps/brachioradialis deep tendon reflexes, and reduced truncal and appendicular muscle tone.

3. Parental Perspective

We had finally escaped the fluorescent lighting and beeps of the machines in the NICU for a brief moment to take our older son and my mother out for a well-needed frozen yogurt. The phone rang—with the number of the hospital on the screen—sending chills down my spine. The doctor informed us that one of our twins, who were born two months prematurely, had an abnormality on the newborn screening test. "What disease and what baby?" I asked.

"Pompeii disease in baby B" he seemed to have said. Images of an entire civilization frozen in molten lava came flooding through my mind. "It's a metabolic disease. It's most likely a false positive. We see this a lot. Once the baby eats and the metabolism stabilizes, the test will most likely be normal. We will confirm with a genetic test and a few other tests. Just don't look it up online." So, of course, immediately, my husband and I looked it up. Autocorrect changed "Pompeii" to "Pompe." From the (now I understand outdated) catastrophic and deadly description of the disease online, I would have preferred a Roman volcanic eruption.

We would later learn that this description was for IOPD before the current enzyme replacement therapy treatments, which have dramatically improved the outcome for Pompe disease patients. We would also later learn that there are at least two very distinct types of Pompe disease, infantile, and late-onset, and that doctors, researchers, and biotech companies have made tremendous strides in understanding, treating, and halting the progression of the disease. Some born with IOPD can walk, dance, sing, and even attend college. Late-onset patients are now identified more quickly due to newborn screening, and can be treated before muscular deterioration occurs. I have since met a successful scientist, a neurologist, and the head of a foundation who all have LOPD, and you would most likely never know they had it. Furthermore, with gene therapy clinical trials already accepting applicants and gene editing on the horizon, there is even the prospect of the eliminating the disease entirely.

However, at this point, we were only seeing what was online. "It's a lysosomal storage disease", I said to my mother while driving back in the car. She stopped the car, paralyzed. "That's what your brother had. It's a different gene but the same category of disease." How could this be? My brother had died of Batten Disease, and my husband and I underwent extensive genetic counseling to help insure that none of our children would have a rare genetic disease.

What I found out later about prenatal carrier testing was that I was only tested for the common variant of Pompe disease (c.-32-13T>G), which I do not carry, but my husband does. I later discovered that I carry a previously unrecorded, but most likely very severe, mutation that contains a deletion. In our prenatal counseling, my husband was not tested as a carrier for Pompe disease at all. One counselor had told me I had the same risk as the general population. Another doctor said it would be unlikely that I would carry Pompe disease because I was not of Dutch descent.

When we did receive the genetic confirmation that our baby did indeed have the disease, the genotype–phenotype correlation baffled the NICU doctors and the consulting geneticist. She had the common variant (predicting late-onset Pompe disease) and this unrecorded severe mutation (predicting infantile Pompe disease). Whereas classic IOPD, defined by cardiomyopathy as well as low GAA enzymatic levels in an infant younger than one year of age, is very severe, LOPD can be potentially mild with a later multi-symptom disease progression. Cardiac involvement is rarely involved in the c.-32-13T>G mutation [16]. In one study, ERT was initiated early with some LOPD infants exhibiting very mild early signs of muscle weakness [17].

However, because one of our child's confirmatory tests were abnormal with elevated uHex4 levels, which could indicate glycogen storage, the doctors did not know whether the baby had infantile or late-onset Pompe disease. Although infantile Pompe disease is sometimes known as "floppy baby syndrome," she was not floppy at all but had excellent muscle tone. Her treatment depended upon a correct diagnosis: infantile-onset Pompe disease needed enzyme replacement therapy treatment right away, while for late-onset Pompe disease, enzyme replacement therapy was less urgent. The laboratory performing the uHex4 test informed us that this elevation was due to prematurity; thankfully, in the next test, the uHex4 levels were normal.

There was quite a learning curve with terms like "uHex4," "ERT (enzyme replacement therapy)", "leaky splice site," "c.-32-13T>G," "GAA-levels", "CK levels," "exon," "del (deletion)," and "dup (duplication)", but after a few months of research, we found ourselves able to understand much of the genetic lingo and code. I found it most helpful to start with the articles referencing the specific alleles (if previously reported), which were cited in the genetic confirmation of the disease. This evolved to understanding broader issues and concepts in the Pompe community by attending conferences focusing on Pompe or rare disease and by making contact with leading researchers, doctors, and biotech companies interested in Pompe as well as parents of kids with Pompe and patients with Pompe.

We also researched observational studies and clinical trials. There are many groups on social media to connect people as well. In the rare disease community, we discovered, as one patient put it, "patients and parents are treated as collaborators." There is so much hope in this field, and no parent needs to be devastated by the newborn screening results. In fact, we are also filled with gratitude that this disease was caught early and can be treated and eventually eliminated.

4. Suggestions from Parents, to Medical Staff Counseling or Seeing Families Screening Positive for Pompe NBS

4.1. Screening and Genetic Counseling

Do not minimize the initial results for the parents by telling them that chances are the test is a false positive. The follow up testing may in fact demonstrate that the initial result was in fact a true positive.

Do not tell parents that infantile Pompe disease means that the child will die as an infant.

Do not tell parents not to look up the disease online. Instead, give them suggestions of what to look up and what to ignore.

A person does not have to be Dutch to carry a Pompe disease gene mutation.

A baby that "looks healthy" can still have a genetic disease.

The common c.-32-13T>G variant of Pompe, even when present on one allele with a normal echo, does not result in IOPD. It predicts later onset Pompe disease.

4.2. Pompe Disease Management and Treatment

Do not early discharge premature infants from the NICU if Pompe disease, or any other serious metabolic disorder, is suspected. The geneticist should perform a clinical evaluation and examination of the child. Prematurity should also be closely monitored.

Teach other health care staff about the difference between infantile and late-onset Pompe disease.

Learn about enzyme replacement therapy and inform the parents about it.

IOPD babies must be treated with enzyme replacement therapy as soon as possible once CRIM status has been confirmed and immunomodulation potentially initiated [6].

Give a referral to a dietician versed in Pompe disease. Diets should be high in protein but low in simple carbohydrates [18].

Give a referral to physical therapy if possible and if necessary. We have found that physical therapy can help build up muscle strength even without ERT yet.

4.3. Family Advocacy

Tell the parents about all the incredible resources there are for Pompe patients, which will inform parents of gene therapy studies, observational newborn studies, clinical trials, next generation ERT therapies, pharmacological chaperones and put them in touch with the Pompe community.

Tell parents to research and contact the leading Pompe doctors, researchers, and biotech companies in the country.

Inform the parents about registries.

Tell the parents to have hope! Pompe disease has been thoroughly researched. It is precisely because there is treatment that it is on the NBS, and the one word that continuously circulates in discussions of upcoming and eventual gene therapies for Pompe disease is "cure."

5. Discussion

This report highlights a case of a neonate in the State of California screening positive for Pompe disease. Reported herein are findings of clinical, biochemical, and molecular confirmatory testing that ultimately identified a diagnosis of late-onset Pompe disease. Additionally reported are the reactions and emotional journey taken by the infant's parents from initial notification, to definitive diagnosis, and subsequent follow-up.

The child's neonatal course was complicated by prematurity, not only due to premature physiology resulting in increased excretion of urinary hexose tetrasaccharide, but also due to apnea of prematurity episodes/intercurrent illness in which she required supplemental oxygen or cardiopulmonary resuscitation. She has hypotonia on physical examination, and it is too early to tell if the hypotonia is a result of her prematurity, potential neurologic sequelae from hypoxia, or due to early symptoms of LOPD.

Review of clinically-diagnosed (not NBS-identified) Pompe disease patients indicates that patients with the common c.-32-13T>G intronic splice site *GAA* variant uniformly develop LOPD are very rarely develop childhood-onset cardiac disease [16]. While most of these patients develop myopathic symptoms and are at risk of dysrhythmias and left ventricular hypertrophy in adulthood, a small subset may manifest gross motor delay and proximal muscle weakness during their first years of life. A retrospective review of 84 symptomatically-identified LOPD patients with at least one c.-32-13T>G variant identified four patients presenting with symptoms prior to 20 months of age; of these patients, three had elevated creatine phosphokinase and two had elevated uHex4 levels [19]. An examination of 7 NBS-identified LOPD patients with the c.-32-13T>G variant demonstrated that while all infants had some degree of muscle weakness, the four patients with the most notable weakness had elevations in creatine phosphokinase. All NBS-identified infants had normal uHex4 levels [17].

For the infant in this report, physical therapy was recommended due to her hypotonia, prematurity, apnea of prematurity, and LOPD diagnosis. Quarterly monitoring for signs and symptoms of spinal and pelvic girdle muscle weakness, calf pseudohypertrophy, as well as laboratory quantification of transaminases, creatine phosphokinase, and uHex4 was instituted. Given the difficulties of secure intravenous access, potential for infusion-associated reactions, and absence of creatine phosphokinase/uHex4 elevation at assessment, ERT was deferred. The infant is now considered a "patient-in-waiting", with her parents and her metabolic physician placing her under surveillance for development of symptoms, "living between health and disease" and unable to determine when treatment should be instituted [20].

Pompe disease was added to newborn screening panels in order to rapidly identify and initiate treatment for neonates with the severe, infantile-onset form of the disease. Cardiac, motor, and overall survival outcomes in early-treated IOPD babies is superior to outcomes in IOPD babies initiated with ERT after symptomatic presentation [13]. However, since NBS identifies neonates with LOPD as well as those bearing pseudodeficiency variants and *GAA* variant heterozygotes, the implementation of NBS for Pompe disease has created considerable uncertainty. First, for parents of NBS-flagged infants, who must wait for results of confirmatory testing and undoubtedly experience some degree of anxiety after reading about the morbidity and mortality associated with Pompe disease; second, for medical providers—especially primary care practitioners and non-physician staff—who are often tasked with notifying parents about NBS results, but may feel their knowledge about Pompe disease is inadequate and subsequently either minimize the significance of the NBS or transmit their apprehension to the parents. Finally, after confirmation of LOPD, uncertainty exists for parents and specialty caregivers as there is currently no established management guideline for presymptomatically-identified LOPD infants. Our family's experience mirrors closely those of other families receiving Pompe disease NBS results [21]. As additional LOPD cases are identified and followed longitudinally with existing NBS-identified LOPD cases, a clearer natural history, prognosis, and recommendations for timing of treatment initiation will arise. Increased knowledge will help allay some of the anxieties and uncertainties faced by families of NBS-identified LOPD babies.

It is our parents' hope that their suggestions, which we are in agreement with, and the experience of other families will enhance health care practitioners' abilities to accurately communicate results and compassionately counsel families regarding anxiety-provoking positive newborn screen results.

Acknowledgments: The author is grateful to the patient and her family, for sharing their experiences.

References

1. Fuller, D.D.; ElMallah, M.K.; Smith, B.K.; Corti, M.; Lawson, L.A.; Falk, D.J.; Byrne, B.J. The respiratory neuromuscular system in Pompe disease. *Respir. Physiol. Neurobiol.* **2013**, *189*, 241–249. [CrossRef] [PubMed]
2. Kishnani, P.S.; Goldenberg, P.C.; DeArmey, S.L.; Heller, J.; Benjamin, D.; Young, S.; Bali, D.; Smith, S.A.; Li, J.S.; Mandel, H.; et al. Cross-reactive immunologic material status affects treatment outcomes in Pompe disease infants. *Mol. Genet. Metab.* **2010**, *99*, 26–33. [CrossRef] [PubMed]
3. Hagemans, M.L.; Winkel, L.P.; Van Doorn, P.A.; Hop, W.J.; Loonen, M.C.; Reuser, A.J.; Van der Ploeg, A.T. Clinical manifestation and natural course of late-onset Pompe's disease in 54 Dutch patients. *Brain* **2005**, *128*, 671–677. [CrossRef]
4. Bali, D.S.; Goldstein, J.L.; Banugaria, S.; Dai, J.; Mackey, J.; Rehder, C.; Kishnani, P.S. Predicting cross-reactive immunological material (CRIM) status in Pompe disease using, G.A.A mutations: Lessons learned from 10 years of clinical laboratory testing experience. *Am. J. Med. Genet. C Semin. Med. Genet.* **2012**, *160*, 40–49. [CrossRef] [PubMed]
5. Chien, Y.H.; Lee, N.C.; Chen, C.A.; Tsai, F.J.; Tsai, W.H.; Shieh, J.Y.; Huang, H.J.; Hsu, W.C.; Tsai, T.H.; Hwu, W.L. Long-term prognosis of patients with infantile-onset Pompe disease diagnosed by newborn screening and treated since birth. *J. Pediatr.* **2015**, *166*, 985–991. [CrossRef] [PubMed]
6. Desai, A.K.; Li, C.; Rosenberg, A.S.; Kishnani, P.S. Immunological challenges and approaches to immunomodulation in Pompe disease: A literature review. *Ann. Transl. Med.* **2019**, *7*, 285. [CrossRef]
7. Schoser, B.; Stewart, A.; Kanters, S.; Hamed, A.; Jansen, J.; Chan, K.; Karamouzian, M.; Toscano, A. Survival and long-term outcomes in late-onset Pompe disease following alglucosidase alfa treatment: A systematic review and meta-analysis. *J. Neurol.* **2017**, *264*, 621–630. [CrossRef]
8. Chien, Y.H.; Lee, N.C.; Huang, H.J.; Thurberg, B.L.; Tsai, F.J.; Hwu, W.L. Later-onset Pompe disease: Early detection and early treatment initiation enabled by newborn screening. *J. Pediatr.* **2011**, *158*, 1023–1027. [CrossRef]
9. Chiang, S.C.; Hwu, W.L.; Lee, N.C.; Hsu, L.W.; Chien, Y.H. Algorithm for Pompe disease newborn screening: Results from the Taiwan screening program. *Mol. Genet. Metab.* **2012**, *106*, 281–286. [CrossRef]
10. Mechtler, T.P.; Metz, T.F.; Müller, H.G.; Ostermann, K.; Ratschmann, R.; de Jesus, V.R.; Shushan, B.; Di Bussolo, J.M.; Herman, J.L.; Herkner, K.R.; et al. Short-incubation mass spectrometry assay for lysosomal storage disorders in newborn and high-risk population screening. *J. Chromatogr. B Anal. Technol. Biomed. Life Sci.* **2012**, *908*, 9–17. [CrossRef]
11. Hopkins, P.V.; Campbell, C.; Klug, T.; Rogers, S.; Raburn-Miller, J.; Kiesling, J. Lysosomal storage disorder

screening implementation: Findings from the first six months of full population pilot testing in Missouri. *J. Pediatr.* **2015**, *166*, 172–177. [CrossRef] [PubMed]
12. Burton, B.K.; Charrow, J.; Hoganson, G.E.; Waggoner, D.; Tinkle, B.; Braddock, S.R.; Schneider, M.; Grange, D.K.; Nash, C.; Shryock, H.; et al. Newborn Screening for Lysosomal Storage Disorders in Illinois: The Initial 15-Month Experience. *J. Pediatr.* **2017**, *190*, 130–135. [CrossRef] [PubMed]
13. Kronn, D.F.; Day-Salvatore, D.; Hwu, W.L.; Jones, S.A.; Nakamura, K.; Okuyama, T.; Swoboda, K.J.; Kishnani, P.S. Pompe Disease Newborn Screening Working Group. Management of Confirmed Newborn-Screened Patients with Pompe Disease across the Disease Spectrum. *Pediatrics* **2017**, *140*, S24–S45. [CrossRef] [PubMed]
14. DeLuca, J.M.; Kearney, M.H.; Norton, S.A.; Arnold, G.L. Parents' experiences of expanded newborn screening evaluations. *Pediatrics* **2011**, *128*, 53–61. [CrossRef] [PubMed]
15. Waisbren, S.E.; Albers, S.; Amato, S.; Ampola, M.; Brewster, T.G.; Demmer, L.; Eaton, R.B.; Greenstein, R.; Korson, M.; Larson, C.; et al. Effect of expanded newborn screening for biochemical genetic disorders on child outcomes and parental stress. *JAMA* **2003**, *290*, 2564–2572. [CrossRef]
16. Herbert, M.; Cope, H.; Li, J.S.; Kishnani, P.S. Severe Cardiac Involvement Is Rare in Patients with Late-Onset Pompe Disease and the Common c.-32-13T>G Variant: Implications for Newborn Screening. *J. Pediatr.* **2018**, *198*, 308–312. [CrossRef]
17. Rairikar, M.V.; Case, L.E.; Bailey, L.A.; Kazi, Z.B.; Desai, A.K.; Berrier, K.L.; Coats, J.; Gandy, R.; Quinones, R.; Kishnani, P.S. Insight into the phenotype of infants with Pompe disease identified by newborn screening with the common c.-32-13T>G "late-onset" GAA variant. *Mol. Genet. Metab.* **2017**, *122*, 99–107. [CrossRef]
18. Tarnopolsky, M.A.; Nilsson, M.I. Nutrition and exercise in Pompe disease. *Ann. Transl. Med.* **2019**, *7*, 282. [CrossRef]
19. Herbert, M.; Case, L.E.; Rairikar, M.; Cope, H.; Bailey, L.; Austin, S.L.; Kishnani, P.S. Early-onset of symptoms and clinical course of Pompe disease associated with the c.-32-13 T > G variant. *Mol. Genet. Metab.* **2019**, *126*, 106–116. [CrossRef]
20. Timmermans, S.; Buchbinder, M. Patients-in-waiting: Living between sickness and health in the genomics era. *J. Health Soc. Behav.* **2010**, *51*, 408–423. [CrossRef]
21. Pruniski, B.; Lisi, E.; Ali, N. Newborn screening for Pompe disease: Impact on families. *J. Inherit. Metab. Dis.* **2018**, *41*, 1189–1203. [CrossRef] [PubMed]

10

Newborn Screening for Sickle Cell Disease and Other Hemoglobinopathies: A Short Review on Classical Laboratory Methods—Isoelectric Focusing, HPLC and Capillary Electrophoresis

Claudia Frömmel [1,2]

1 MVZ Alexianer Labor GmbH, Groβe Hamburger Str. 5–11, 10115 Berlin, Germany; c.froemmel@alexianer.de;

2 Newborn Screening Laboratory, Charité-Universitätsmedizin Berlin, Augustenburger Platz 1, 13353 Berlin, Germany

Abstract: Sickle cell disease (SCD) and other hemoglobinopathies are a major health concern with a high burden of disease worldwide. Since the implementation of newborn screening (NBS) for SCD and other hemoglobinopathies in several regions of the world, technical progress of laboratory methods was achieved. This short review aims to summarize the current practice of classical laboratory methods for the detection of SCD and other hemoglobinopathies. This includes the newborn screening technologies of high-performance liquid chromatography (HPLC), capillary electrophoresis (CE), and isoelectric focusing (IEF).

Keywords: newborn screening; sickle cell disease; hemoglobinopathy; laboratory methods; neonatal screening; hemoglobin pattern; HPLC; IEF; capillary electrophoresis

---

1. Introduction

Newborn screening (NBS) for sickle cell disease (SCD) as one element of prevention programs for hemoglobinopathies has been in place in several regions in the world for more than 40 years now. First attempts were made in the United States of America (USA) and Jamaica, as well as in Great Britain in the 1970s [1,2]. Starting with alkaline electrophoresis, the development of faster and more precise methods permitted the development of extended and more sophisticated prevention programs of hemoglobinopathies. The aim of NBS for SCD is to prevent major health complications of SCD from early childhood onward. SCD in this context comprises all forms of relevant sickling disorders, originating from different genetic constellations (e.g., homozygous HbS (HbSS) and compound heterozygous forms as HbS/β^0 thalassemia, HbS/β^+ thalassemia, HbS/HbC, HbS/HbD^{Punjab}, HbS/HbE, HbS/HbO^{Arab}, HbS/Hb Lepore, and HbS/$\delta\beta$ thalassemia). As life-threatening events can occur in children with SCD from three months of age onward, early diagnosis is desirable to establish preventive measures. Patients with thalassemia and other major hemoglobin disorders do not benefit in the same way from early diagnosis. However, these disorders have important implications for family health, and the burden of disease is very high in several regions of the world, thus demanding preventive action. In this context, many newborn screening programs make use of the possibility to detect carriers of hemoglobin variants as a by-product to provide families with reproductive knowledge and informed decision-making regarding hemoglobinopathies.

Laboratory methods to detect disease states and carrier states (if included in the program) should be very sensitive and highly specific. To prevent harm, they should not miss patients and should not falsely identify patients. Psychosocial and logistic burdens to families from screening or diagnostic evaluation, an increased risk of unnecessary medical treatment, or a delayed diagnosis from false negative results, as well as psychosocial harm from false positive results and uncertainty of clinical diagnosis, should be minimized and be outweighed by the benefits [3].

While laboratories for newborn screening for endocrine and metabolic disorders mainly use tandem mass spectrometry (MS/MS) or photometric assays, technologies, which are commonly established for NBS for hemoglobinopathies include HPLC, isoelectric focusing (IEF), and capillary electrophoresis (CE). They were developed for larger sample sizes from routine hemoglobinopathy testing and permit the clear separation of hemoglobin variants of interest in an automated or semi-automated way. Recent developments of screening methods like tandem mass spectrometry (MS/MS) and Matrix-assisted laser desorption/ionization time-of-flight mass spectrometry (MALDI-TOF MS) or molecular genetic testing are explained elsewhere.

2. Technologies

Technologies are based on the separation of hemoglobin species (Hb) and the quantification of respective hemoglobin fractions from dried blood spot (DBS) or fresh cord blood samples. They should be able to detect HbS and HbC, and separate HbF and HbA, as well as being able to detect other hemoglobin variants of clinical relevance, such as HbD^{Punjab}, HbE, Hb Lepore, and HbO^{Arab}. The screening methods reviewed here provide provisional results and identify putative abnormal fractions of hemoglobin and have to be confirmed to give a definite diagnosis.

In contrast to the diagnosis of carriers and patients with hemoglobinopathies in clinical routine or carrier screening programs, where a complete blood count with erythrocyte indices and parameters of iron metabolism are included, newborn screening is only based on the separation of hemoglobin from DBS or cord blood. Additional tests such as the solubility test for HbS are not applicable. As symptoms usually do not occur before two months of age, results of screening should be provided within this period. An algorithm designed to clearly state when parents should be informed and a defined follow-up help avoid reduced effectiveness of the whole process.

2.1. HPLC

Automated cation-exchange high-performance liquid chromatography (HPLC) is a widely used method to screen for hemoglobinopathies with a clear separation and quantification of hemoglobin fractions [4–11]. The method is based on the elution of hemoglobin bound to a solid phase over time by buffers with a pH gradient. The time from the injection of the sample into the column to the elution of the hemoglobin fraction is called the retention time. Eluted hemoglobin is detected by a dual-wavelength detector and quantified by integrating the area under curve of the produced chromatogram, expressed as a percentage of the total area (Figure 1). A characteristic retention time (window of detection), together with the relative quantification, permits presumptive identification of all relevant hemoglobin species: HbF, HbA, HbA_2, HbS, HbC, HbD^{Punjab}, HbE, Hb Lepore, and HbO^{Arab}. Hb Bart's is also detected. HPLC analysis is very precise and reproducible with an inter-run coefficient of variation (CV) of <5%. The detection limit for HbA and HbS was shown to be around 1% of total hemoglobin [4,6,12]. Calibrators and material for internal quality assurance containing Hb FAES and FADC (where letters represent different Hb species) are available.

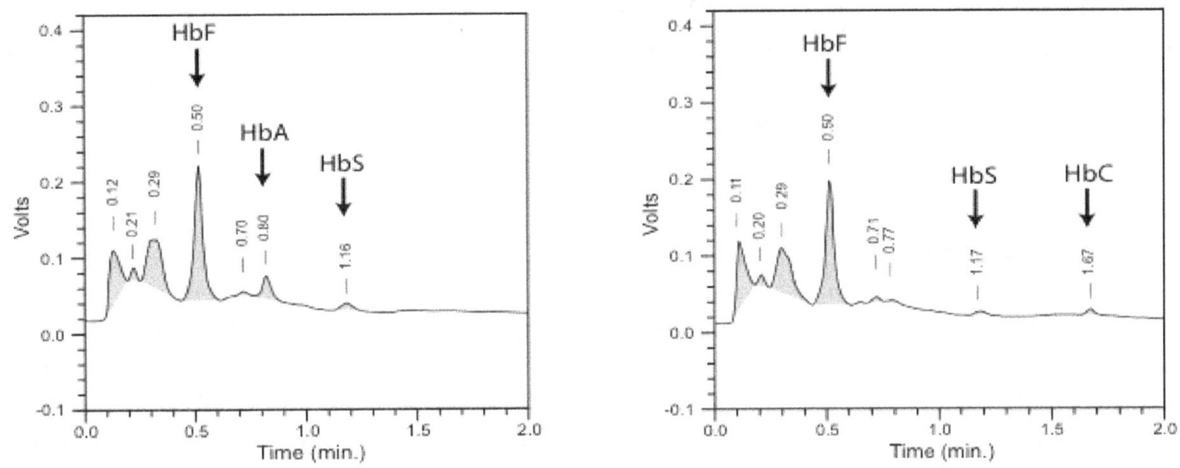

(a) (b)

Figure 1. Chromatogram of HPLC (Variant™ newborn screening (nbs), Bio-Rad laboratories, Europe): the x-axis represents the time in minutes, and the y-axis represents the response in volts; retention times of integrated peaks are shown above the peaks, and peaks of Hb variants included in the pattern are named and indicated with an arrow: (**a**) pattern of HbF/HbA/HbS (FAS); (**b**) pattern of HbF/HbS/HbC (FSC).

2.2. CE

Capillary electrophoresis (CE) combines two principles of separation of hemoglobins, the electrophoretic mobility in alkaline buffer and the electro-osmotic flow resulting in excellent separation. High voltage applied to an in silica glass capillary prompt hemoglobin molecules to migrate toward a detector of 415-nm wavelength. Detected hemoglobin fractions can be relatively quantified and produce a pherogram. HbF is centered in the neonatal system (note: it is HbA in the adult system), followed by the automated integration of peaks and defined migration zones (N1 to N13—specific to the neonatal system) which allow the easy interpretation of pherograms and help identify hemoglobin patterns (Figure 2).

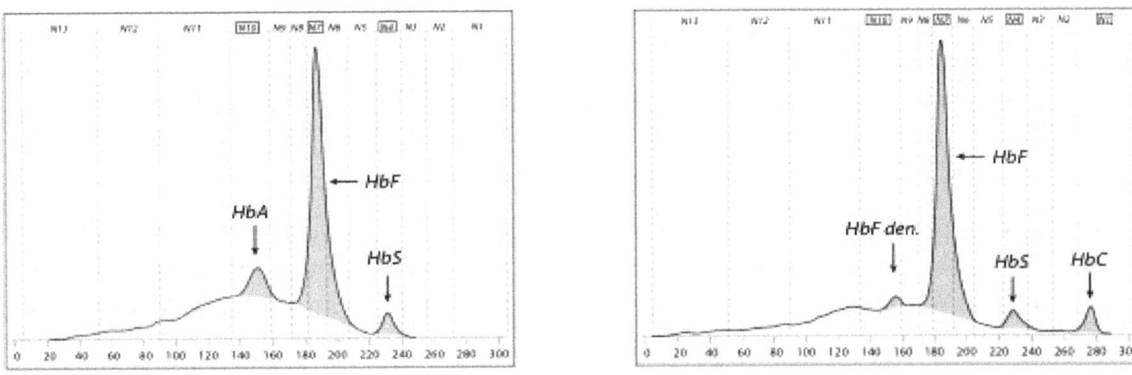

(a) (b)

Figure 2. Pherogram of capillary electrophoresis (CE; Capillarys™ neonat fast, Sebia, France); zone from left to right: N13–N1. Peaks of Hb variants included in the pattern are named: (**a**) pattern of FAS; (**b**) pattern of FSC.

CE is able to detect and relatively quantify HbF, HbA, HbA_2, HbS, HbC, HbD^{Punjab}, HbO^{Arab}, HbE, and Hb Lepore. Hb Bart's is also detected. Many other Hb variants may be detected including γ- and α-chain abnormalities with an overlap in the zones of the more common hemoglobins, e.g.,

HbD^{Punjab} and Hb Korle Bu in zone N5 [13]. Interpretation has to be diligent with regards to reporting named hemoglobin variants following the presumptive identification of the system. Controls for internal quality assurance are provided containing HbF, HbA, HbS and HbC. The detection limit for HbA and HbS was found to be around 1% of total hemoglobin.

2.3. IEF

IEF is a very sensitive method and is widely used at relatively low costs. IEF separates hemoglobin species according to their isoelectric point on a gel medium with very high resolution. Hb variants migrate in a pH gradient to the point where their net charge becomes zero. Bands are narrow compared to classical electrophoresis and give a precise picture (Figure 3). HbF and HbA, as well as relevant hemoglobins HbS, HbC, HbD^{Punjab}, HbE, and HbO^{Arab}, can be separated. Hb Bart's can also be detected. IEF separates post-translationally modified variants, which sometimes makes interpretation difficult; thus, an experienced staff is needed to read results.

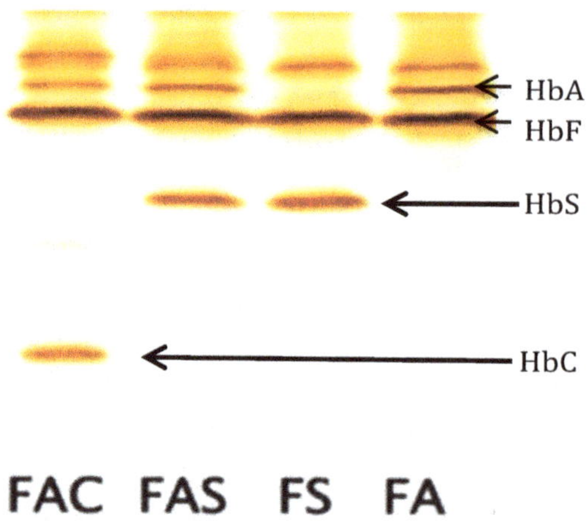

Figure 3. Isoelectric focusing gel picture (RESOLVE™, Perkin Elmer, Finland); from left to right: patterns of FAC, FAS, FS, and FA, adopted from Reference [14].

IEF is a semi-automated system, which allows the parallel run of several gels entailing some labor-intensive steps. Easier work-up and documentation of gels are achieved using a scanning software. Controls for internal quality assurance contain HbF, HbA, HbS and HbC.

3. Interpretation of Newborn Screening Results and Hemoglobin Patterns

Normal newborn samples mainly contain HbF ($\alpha 2/\gamma 2$) and a smaller amount of HbA ($\alpha 2/\beta 2$). HbA levels range from 6 to 40% with an average of 19%, showing inter-individual variations. HbA levels in newborns are dependent on gestational age and date of sampling, reflecting the stage of hemoglobin switch [6,12]. In Table 1, patterns of the detected hemoglobins are listed in the order of highest percentage to the lowest. One has to be aware that relevant Hb variants may present an abnormal pattern similar to those consistent with a target disease. Today, there are more than 1000 variants of hemoglobin known. Software solutions for HPLC and CE suggest a pattern, which has to be verified by the technician reviewing the chromatogram or pherogram. In IEF, an experienced staff reviews the gel, and densitometry helps quantify hemoglobin variants to determine the pattern. Guidelines and lab handbooks can be used to interpret hemoglobin patterns, specifying the significance of a found pattern and the possible pitfalls according to the methods applied. An abnormal result with the screening method (first line) is repeated from the sample using a secondary method (second line), or using the same method if another is not available.

Table 1. Hemoglobinopathies relevant in newborn screening (NBS) and their respective patterns.

Target Disease	Pattern
Sickle cell disease Primary target	
HbSS, HbS/β^0 thalassemia, HbS/$\delta\beta$ thalassemia, HbS/HPFH	FS [1]
HbS/C	FSC
HbS/β^+ thalassemia	FSA
HbS/D^{Punjab}	FSD [2]
HbS/E	FSE
HbS/other variant [3]	FSX
Thalassemia syndromes and other hemoglobinopathies	Secondary target
β^0 thalassemia	F only
β^+ thalassemia	FA [4]
HbEE, HbE/β^0 thalassemia	FE
HbE/β^+ thalassemia	FEA
HbCC or HbC/β^0 thalassemia	FC
HbC/β^+ thalassemia	FCA
$HbDD^{Punjab}$ or HbD^{Punjab}/β^0 thalassemia	FD
HbD^{Punjab}/β^+ thalassemia	FDA
Hb variant not specified homozygous	FX
Hb variant/β^0 or β^+ thalassemia	FXA
Severe α thalassemia, HbH disease	FABart's [5]
Severe α thalassemia, HbH disease with other variants [6]	FE Bart's (e.g) FAX Bart's
Traits Secondary target	
HbS	FAS
HbD^{Punjab}	FAD
HbC	FAC
HbE	FAE
Other Hb variant [7]	FAX
Normal	FA

[1] Hb variants migrating similarly to HbS may be hidden; [2] HbD has to be verified as HbD^{Punjab}, as many other variants run like HbD^{Punjab}; [3] Hb variants not specified during screening, or specified with second-line methods, e.g., Hb Lepore, or HbO^{Arab} if included in the program; [4] HbA <5% or <1.5% (overlap of premature newborns and normal newborns) depend on cut-off used; [5] detected Hb Bart's (over cut-off or qualitative); [6] includes detected Hb Bart's with combined α- or β-variants and, e.g., HbE with Hb Bart's; [7] Hb variants not specified during screening or specified with second-line methods, e.g., Hb Lepore, or HbO^{Arab} if included in the program.

3.1. Target Diseases

Patients with sickle cell disease and non-sickling disorders, as well as carriers of abnormal hemoglobin variants, can be detected by NBS. Choosing primary and secondary target diseases influences false negative and false positive results of the overall screening program and, therefore, are important to the evaluation of the screening process. NBS for hemoglobinopathies has sensitivity and specificity close to 100% for SCD with regards to the different genetic forms defined as target diseases (see below); however, it loses sensitivity and specificity when non-sickling disorders are included. Furthermore, pre-analytic factors like prematurity and blood transfusions prior to sampling influence the sensitivity. The positive and negative predictive values vary with prevalence of the abnormal variants and thalassemia syndromes.

3.2. Sickle Cell Disease

Sickle cell disease is a severe hematological disorder with acute and chronic manifestations caused by a complex pathomechanism of hemolysis and recurrent vaso-occlusive events. Life-threatening early complications can be largely avoided by initiating simple and effective prophylactic measures such as penicillin, vaccination, and parent education. Primary target diseases are all common and are generally severe sickling disorders (see Table 1).

HbS/hereditary persistence of fetal hemoglobin (HPFH) is included as a very mild disorder, as it cannot be distinguished from homozygous HbS and β^0 thalassemia/HbS. This is accepted, as the disorder seems relatively rare. The definite diagnosis should be ruled out by confirmatory diagnostics for appropriate counseling and treatment [15].

For the distinction between the disease states of HbS/β^+ thalassemia or HbS/β^{++} thalassemia and a simple carrier state for HbS, the relative quantification of HbA and HbS and the ratio between HbA/HbS is used (mainly a cut-off of <1). This approach bears the risk of false positive and false negative results, as there is an overlap between HbS/β^+ thalassemia or HbS/β^{++} thalassemia and a simple carrier state for HbS, especially in premature babies. In these cases, HbA is present, but at different levels depending on gestational age. Additionally, precise quantification is a problem close to the detection limit of a variant for HPLC and CE [5,7]. To standardize quantitative interpretation of screening results, cut-offs and ratios can be expressed as multiples of median (MoM) [12]. IEF is a method with a very high resolution, but it sometimes hampers precise quantification and correct classification of bands, and there is a slight tendency to over-detect variants of no significance, e.g., modified HbA or γ-variants [5,16].

For all described methods, there are difficulties due to the fact that, with over 1000 known abnormal Hb variants, some of them will migrate, differently from HbA, but together with HbS or other common variants (HbC, HbD, and HbE). Genetic constellations like Hb Hope and HbS can lead to false positive screening results for SCD, which can then be excluded by a second-line method or by confirmatory testing [17]. Unusual analytical pictures may occur, depending on whether these rare abnormal variants with migration properties similar to HbS (or other common variants) derive from γ-, α-, or β-globin chain mutations. Heterozygous α-globin chain variants produce additional peaks or bands and comprise about one-fourth of HbF and HbA (or HbS if an additional β-mutation is present) if all four α-genes are functional, or about one-third if one α-gene is missing, or one-half if two α-genes are missing, provided the α-variant is stable. From all possible genotypes for SCD, the suitable target diseases should be defined according to the whole screening process, in both the screening laboratory and the confirmatory laboratory. With regards to this definition, cases of SCD caused by very rare genotypes, such as dominant HbS with a double mutation, are missed by classical NBS [17]; moreover, milder disorders such as HbS/β^{++} thalassemia or HbS/HPFH might be detected.

3.3. Non-Sickling Disorders

Other hemoglobinopathies with clinical relevance, including severe disorders such as β-thalassemia major and severe α-thalassemia (HbH disease), are often also included in NBS for SCD as secondary target diseases.

3.3.1. β-Thalassemia Major and Intermedia

β-thalassemia major or intermedia results from homozygous or compound heterozygous β^0 or β^+ mutations. Patients suffer from severe anemia, which requires regular or irregular blood transfusion and chelation therapy to prevent iron overload. Early detection is wanted to prevent babies from becoming severely anemic and to support family health in social and medical aspects by giving the possibility of informed choice for future pregnancies and by including the affected child in a comprehensive care program for thalassemia. β-thalassemia major can be expected in samples with a hemoglobin pattern of HbF only, or HbF and HbA below a certain cut-off from 0–5% (<1.5% in the United Kingdom (UK)) [18,19].

3.3.2. Severe α-Thalassemia, HbH Disease

HbH disease has a variable phenotype ranging from mild microcytic anemia to severe transfusion-dependent anemia. HbH disease is caused by deletion or inactivation of three α-globin genes with an imbalance of chain synthesis, leading to the association of β-chains in adults (β2/β2), known as HbH, and of γ-chains in newborns, known as Hb Bart's (γ2/γ2). Clinically significant hemolytic anemia, which possibly necessitates blood transfusion, can occur during fever, infections, and pregnancy. Severe aplastic crises after infection with parvovirus B19 or growth retardation during childhood, as well as iron overload in adults with or without previous transfusion, are possible complications in a minority of patients. In regions with high prevalence and also in some low prevalence areas for α-thalassemia, HbH disease is included in the newborn screening program as a target disease. Technologies such as IEF, HPLC, and CE are able to detect Hb Bart's [20–24]. Several cut-offs were evaluated for HPLC or a qualitative detection of Hb Bart's in the fraction of fast-eluting hemoglobins (≥15% or ≥20% or ≥25% for the FAST fraction on the Bio-Rad™ nbs System, evaluated on different integration principles). IEF and CE represent a qualitative analysis of Hb Bart's. Detection of Hb Bart's shows considerable overlap between HbH disease and heterozygous α^0 thalassemia. Literature about the sensitivity and the specificity for Hb Bart's is scarce. Specificity seems lower than that for β-thalassemia and positive predictive values in a low-prevalence region will be unsatisfactory. Screening policy should decide on whether false negative results outweigh false positive results or vice versa. As Hb Bart's is unstable, sensitivity also depends on material (DBS vs. fresh-cord blood), the day of sampling, and the storage of samples until measurement.

Including HbH disease in a neonatal screening setting is still controversial, as over-diagnosis is probable [20]. It seems more acceptable in high-prevalence areas and if the definite diagnosis by verifying deletional and/or non-deletional α-thalassemia through DNA analysis is done in the screening center [10,23]. Asian publications show a higher detection rate using DNA analysis in the first line [25].

3.4. Carrier Detection

With IEF, CE, and HPLC, carriers of relevant Hb variants can be incidentally detected. HPLC and CE provide presumptive identification of a variant. Variant peaks occur in their respective windows or zones and, together with the percentages of HbA and the variant peak, a presumptive result can be reported. All screening programs which include carrier detection recommend two independent methods as first- and second-line laboratory methods (e.g., IEF and HPLC or HPLC and CE). Whereas carriers of heterozygous β-thalassemia are not detectable in newborns by measurement of HbA_2, the measurement of HbA and a cut-off <15% may be indicative for the β-thalassemia trait in newborns [19]. Confirmatory diagnostic follow-ups using a new sample with blood count, hemoglobin separation analysis, and, if necessary, DNA analysis then provide a definite result. These inexpensive methods can be used for carrier detection to improve family health, as well as in states where no antenatal screening program is in place; however, they can also lead to stigmatization and counterproductive effects [26–28].

4. Pre-Analytics

Limitations of the aforementioned methods lie often in the pre-analytical phase. The used material can be fresh cord blood or dried blood spot from a heel prick. Storage of cord blood should not exceed seven days at 4 °C and that of dried blood spots should not exceed 1 month. Older samples show lower elution of samples from the DBS and, often, the degradation of hemoglobin, resulting in a high baseline, increased noise, and unclear peaks with difficulties in zone adjustment and quantification, especially in Hb species present at low percentage.

Blood from premature babies contains lower percentages of HbA or other β-chain variants, which may lead to false negative results in screening for SCD. Although an exact gestational age for requesting a second sample is not defined, premature babies under 33 weeks of gestational age should receive repeated testing.

Babies who received blood transfusions show increased percentages of adult hemoglobin HbA and HbA_2 and the presence of a severe hemoglobinopathy may be masked. Therefore, it seems essential that transfused babies can be identified using either HbA levels above the 2.5 multiples of median (MoM) dependent on gestational age or ratios of HbF/HbA [12].

5. Conclusions

HPLC, CE, and IEF have proven to be suitable methods for NBS for sickle cell disease and other hemoglobinopathies in several different states and regions with specific legal and economic conditions. They have very high sensitivity and high specificity regarding SCD with patterns of FS, FSC, and FSE, and just slightly lower for patterns of FSA and FSD. Other non-sickling hemoglobinopathies were successfully included in newborn screening programs, and future developments must match the achievements of this recent era of hemoglobin analysis systems and will add new flexibility.

Acknowledgments: I would like to thank Stephan Lobitz and Jeanette Klein for their constant support, Cornelius Frömmel, Bryony Fox, and Daniel Wiesenfeld for their help with the manuscript, Barbara Wild for providing the gel picture and Thomas Burmeister for assistance refining the figures. Cornelis Harteveld and Bichr Allaf for helpful discussions, and Annemarie Brose for technical advice.

References

1. Serjeant, B.E.; Forbes, M.; Williams, L.L.; Serjeant, G.R. Screening cord bloods for detection of sickle cell disease in Jamaica. *Clin. Chem.* **1974**, *20*, 666–669. [PubMed]
2. Pearson, H.A.; O'Brien, R.T.; McLntosh, S.; Aspnes, G.T.; Yang, M. Routine screening of umbilical cord blood for sickle cell diseases. *JAMA* **1974**, *227*, 420–421. [CrossRef] [PubMed]
3. Goldenberg, A.J.; Comeau, A.M.; Grosse, S.D.; Tanksley, S.; Prosser, L.A.; Ojodu, J.; Botkin, J.R.; Kemper, A.R.; Green, N.S. Evaluating Harms in the Assessment of Net Benefit: A Framework for Newborn Screening Condition Review. *Matern. Child Health J.* **2016**, *20*, 693–700. [CrossRef] [PubMed]
4. Eastman, J.W.; Wong, R.; Liao, C.L.; Morales, D.R. Automated HPLC screening of newborns for sickle cell anemia and other hemoglobinopathies. *Clin. Chem.* **1996**, *42*, 704–710. [CrossRef]
5. Campbell, M.; Henthorn, J.S.; Davies, S.C. Evaluation of cation-exchange HPLC compared with isoelectric focusing for neonatal hemoglobinopathy screening. *Clin. Chem.* **1999**, *45*, 969–975.
6. Bouva, M.J.; Mohrmann, K.; Brinkman, H.B.; Kemper-Proper, E.A.; Elvers, B.; Loeber, J.G.; Verheul, F.E.; Giordano, P.C. Implementing neonatal screening for haemoglobinopathies in the Netherlands. *J. Med. Screen.* **2010**, *17*, 58–65. [CrossRef] [PubMed]
7. Frommel, C.; Brose, A.; Klein, J.; Blankenstein, O.; Lobitz, S. Newborn screening for sickle cell disease: Technical and legal aspects of a German pilot study with 38,220 participants. *BioMed Res. Int.* **2014**, *2014*, 695828–695838. [CrossRef] [PubMed]
8. Greene, D.N.; Pyle, A.L.; Chang, J.S.; Hoke, C.; Lorey, T. Comparison of Sebia Capillarys Flex capillary electrophoresis with the BioRad Variant II high pressure liquid chromatography in the evaluation of hemoglobinopathies. *Clin. Chim. Acta* **2012**, *413*, 1232–1238. [CrossRef] [PubMed]
9. Lorey, F.; Cunningham, G.; Shafer, F.; Lubin, B.; Vichinsky, E. Universal screening for hemoglobinopathies using high-performance liquid chromatography: Clinical results of 2.2 million screens. *Eur. J. Hum. Genet.* **1994**, *2*, 262–271. [CrossRef] [PubMed]
10. Hoppe, C.C. Newborn screening for hemoglobin disorders. *Hemoglobin* **2011**, *35*, 556–564. [CrossRef] [PubMed]
11. Upadhye, D.S.; Jain, D.L.; Trivedi, Y.L.; Nadkarni, A.H.; Ghosh, K.; Colah, R.B. Newborn screening for haemoglobinopathies by high performance liquid chromatography (HPLC): Diagnostic utility of different approaches in resource-poor settings. *Clin. Chem. Lab. Med.* **2014**, *52*, 1791–1796. [CrossRef] [PubMed]

12. Allaf, B.; Patin, F.; Elion, J.; Couque, N. New approach to accurate interpretation of sickle cell disease newborn screening by applying multiple of median cutoffs and ratios. *Pediatr. Blood Cancer* **2018**, *65*, e27230. [CrossRef] [PubMed]
13. Renom, G.; Mereau, C.; Maboudou, P.; Perini, J.M. Potential of the Sebia Capillarys neonat fast automated system for neonatal screening of sickle cell disease. *Clin. Chem. Lab. Med.* **2009**, *47*, 1423–1432. [CrossRef] [PubMed]
14. Wild, B. The Haemoglobinopathies: Learning from EQA, UK NEQAS. Available online: https://www.ukneqash.org/documents.php (accessed on 29 September 2018).
15. Serjeant, G.R.; Serjeant, B.E.; Hambleton, I.R.; Oakley, M.; Thein, S.L.; Clark, B. A Plea for the Newborn Diagnosis of Hb S-Hereditary Persistence of Fetal Hemoglobin. *Hemoglobin* **2017**, *41*, 216–217. [CrossRef] [PubMed]
16. Hustace, T.; Fleisher, J.M.; Sanchez Varela, A.M.; Podda, A.; Alvarez, O. Increased prevalence of false positive hemoglobinopathy newborn screening in premature infants. *Pediatr. Blood Cancer* **2011**, *57*, 1039–1043. [CrossRef] [PubMed]
17. Moradkhani, K.; Riou, J.; Wajcman, H. Pitfalls in the genetic diagnosis of Hb S. *Clin. Biochem.* **2013**, *46*, 291–299. [CrossRef] [PubMed]
18. Ryan, K.; Bain, B.J.; Worthington, D.; James, J.; Plews, D.; Mason, A.; Roper, D.; Rees, D.C.; de la Salle, B.; Streetly, A. Significant haemoglobinopathies: Guidelines for screening and diagnosis. *Br. J. Haematol.* **2010**, *149*, 35–49. [CrossRef]
19. Mantikou, E.; Arkesteijn, S.G.; Beckhoven van, J.M.; Kerkhoffs, J.L.; Harteveld, C.L.; Giordano, P.C. A brief review on newborn screening methods for hemoglobinopathies and preliminary results selecting beta thalassemia carriers at birth by quantitative estimation of the HbA fraction. *Clin. Biochem.* **2009**, *42*, 1780–1785. [CrossRef] [PubMed]
20. Bouva, M.J.; Sollaino, C.; Perseu, L.; Galanello, R.; Giordano, P.C.; Harteveld, C.L.; Cnossen, M.H.; Schielen, P.C.; Elvers, L.H.; Peters, M. Relationship between neonatal screening results by HPLC and the number of alpha-thalassaemia gene mutations; consequences for the cut-off value. *J. Med. Screen.* **2011**, *18*, 182–186. [CrossRef] [PubMed]
21. Jindatanmanusan, P.; Riolueang, S.; Glomglao, W.; Sukontharangsri, Y.; Chamnanvanakij, S.; Torcharus, K.; Viprakasit, V. Diagnostic applications of newborn screening for alpha-thalassaemias, haemoglobins E and H disorders using isoelectric focusing on dry blood spots. *Ann. Clin. Biochem.* **2014**, *51*, 237–247. [CrossRef]
22. Liao, C.; Zhou, J.Y.; Xie, X.M.; Tang, H.S.; Li, R.; Li, D.Z. Newborn screening for Hb H disease by determination of Hb Bart's using the Sebia capillary electrophoresis system in southern China. *Hemoglobin* **2014**, *38*, 73–75. [CrossRef] [PubMed]
23. Uaprasert, N.; Settapiboon, R.; Amornsiriwat, S.; Sarnthammakul, P.; Thanapat, T.; Rojnuckarin, P.; Sutcharitchan, P. Diagnostic utility of isoelectric focusing and high performance liquid chromatography in neonatal cord blood screening for thalassemia and non-sickling hemoglobinopathies. *Clin. Chim. Acta* **2014**, *427*, 23–26. [CrossRef] [PubMed]
24. Rugless, M.J.; Fisher, C.A.; Stephens, A.D.; Amos, R.J.; Mohammed, T.; Old, J.M. Hb Bart's in cord blood: An accurate indicator of alpha-thalassemia. *Hemoglobin* **2006**, *30*, 57–62. [CrossRef]
25. Wu, M.Y.; Xie, X.M.; Li, J.; Li, D.Z. Neonatal screening for alpha-thalassemia by cord hemoglobin Barts: How effective is it? *Int. J. Lab. Hematol.* **2015**, *37*, 649–653. [CrossRef] [PubMed]
26. Bain, B.J. Haemoglobinopathy diagnosis: Algorithms, lessons and pitfalls. *Blood Rev.* **2011**, *25*, 205–213. [CrossRef] [PubMed]
27. Bombard, Y.; Miller, F.A.; Hayeems, R.Z.; Wilson, B.J.; Carroll, J.C.; Paynter, M.; Little, J.; Allanson, J.; Bytautas, J.P.; Chakraborty, P. Health-care providers' views on pursuing reproductive benefit through newborn screening: The case of sickle cell disorders. *Eur. J. Hum. Genet.* **2012**, *20*, 498–504. [CrossRef] [PubMed]
28. Ross, L.F. Newborn screening for sickle cell disease: Whose reproductive benefit? *Eur. J. Hum. Genet.* **2012**, *20*, 484–485. [CrossRef]

11

Constructing a Bioethical Framework to Evaluate and Optimise Newborn Bloodspot Screening for Cystic Fibrosis

Rachael E. Armstrong [1], Lucy Frith [2], Fiona M. Ulph [3] and Kevin W. Southern [1,*]

[1] Department of Women's and Children's Health, University of Liverpool, Liverpool L12 2AP, UK; r.armstrong3@doctors.org.uk
[2] Institute of Population Health, University of Liverpool, Liverpool L69 3GL, UK; frith@liverpool.ac.uk
[3] Division of Psychology & Mental Health, School of Health Sciences, Faculty of Biology, Medicine and Health, University of Manchester, Manchester Academic Health Science Centre, Manchester M13 9PL, UK; Fiona.Ulph@manchester.ac.uk
* Correspondence: kwsouth@liv.ac.uk;

Abstract: Newborn bloodspot screening for cystic fibrosis is a valid public health strategy for populations with a high incidence of this inherited condition. There are a wide variety of approaches to screening and in this paper, we propose that a bioethical framework is required to determine the most appropriate screening protocol for a population. This framework depends on the detailed evaluation of the ethical consequences of all screening outcomes and placing these in the context of the genetic profile of the population screened, the geography of the region and the healthcare resources available.

Keywords: cystic fibrosis; newborn bloodspot screening; cystic fibrosis screen positive; inconclusive diagnosis (CFSPID); bioethics

---

1. Introduction

In this paper, we develop a bioethical framework that can be used to assess newborn bloodspot screening (NBS) for cystic fibrosis (CF) protocols [1,2]. This approach provides a means to appraise the impact of the evolving technologies that are increasingly being used as part of screening protocols, for example more extensive DNA analyses [3]. An ethical consideration is essential for all screening strategies but particularly pertinent for NBS for CF for three main reasons: (1) NBS for CF protocols are complex and varied, (2) expanded DNA analysis including sequencing is increasingly common and (3) outcomes are complicated and not comprehensively recognised or characterised.

The measurement of immuno-reactive trypsinogen (IRT) from a dried bloodspot (DBS) sample enabled screening for CF by providing a simple and inexpensive test, as per the criteria outlined by the World Health Organisation (WHO) [4]. However, other criteria outlined by Wilson and Jungner were more challenging to fulfil, namely that an early diagnosis following a positive NBS resulted in improved outcomes for children with CF. This felt at odds with the lived experience of regions in which NBS for CF was established, when qualitatively the impact of an earlier diagnosis seemed considerable [5].

In an important study undertaken in Wisconsin (USA), over 650,000 DBS samples were analysed for IRT (and in some cases DNA analysis), but only results from alternative samples were reported [6]. In 54 of the samples reported, a positive NBS result was associated with an early diagnosis and significantly improved nutritional outcomes, compared to 67 infants diagnosed clinically. These early differences in nutritional well-being were transient, reflecting the capacity of standard care to address the early challenges of growth delay in clinically diagnosed children [7]. There were no clinically significant differences in respiratory outcomes, and this was consistent with a study undertaken in the United Kingdom [8,9].

For those who work in the field, there was a disconnection between the apparent positive impact of NBS in the clinical environment and the relative lack of evidence for improved outcomes for people with CF after NBS. To some degree, this reflects the ability of CF teams and parents to provide high quality CF care following a clinical diagnosis, even if delayed [9]. However, evidence is increasing that small differences in clinical outcomes in the early months of life can lead to significant and sometimes dramatic differences in outcomes later in life. This is supported by the historical cohort study undertaken in Australia that compared two groups of children with CF before and after the implementation of NBS for CF [10]. Over the first two decades, differences between the two cohorts were minimal, but a distinct and large difference in survival became apparent as the cohorts entered their adult years, with the clinically diagnosed group faring much less well. These data are supported by data from other programmes, including an Italian group reinforcing the view that early recognition and treatment through NBS may have a more profound impact on clinical outcomes later in life [11,12] (Figure 1).

a) Severe

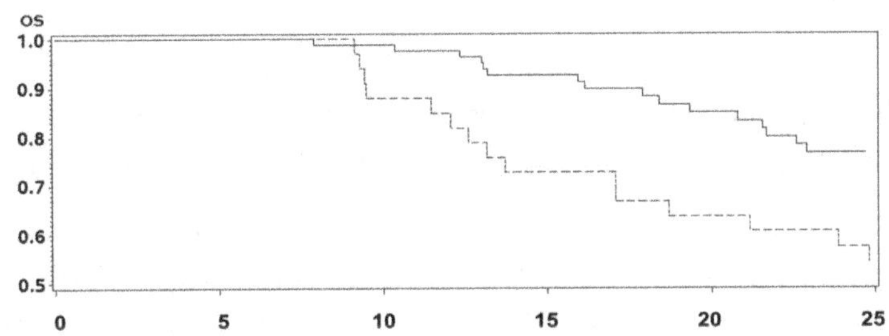

Age (years)		0	5	10	15	20	25
Screening	———	95	87	82	69	52	43
Symptoms	- - - - - - -	34	34	29	24	21	17

Diagnosis	Pts	Events	HR (95% C.I.)	20 years OS (95% C.I.)	p
NBS	95	23	1.00	84.93 (74.29, 91.41)	0.007
Symptoms	34	21	2.23 (1.23-4.03)	63.64 (44.95, 77.46)	

b) Moderate

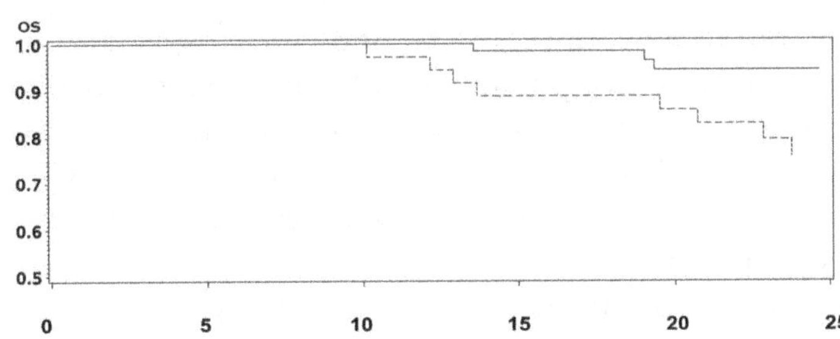

Age (years)		0	5	10	15	20	25
Screening	———	80	78	71	61	45	33
Symptoms	- - - - - - -	40	39	36	32	29	21

Diagnosis	Pts	Events	HR (95% C.I.)	20 years OS (95% C.I.)	p
NBS	80	4	1.00	94.48 (83.72, 98.20)	0.016
Symptoms	40	12	3.86 (1.21-12.38)	85.93 (69.41, 93.89)	

Figure 1. *Cont.*

c) Mild

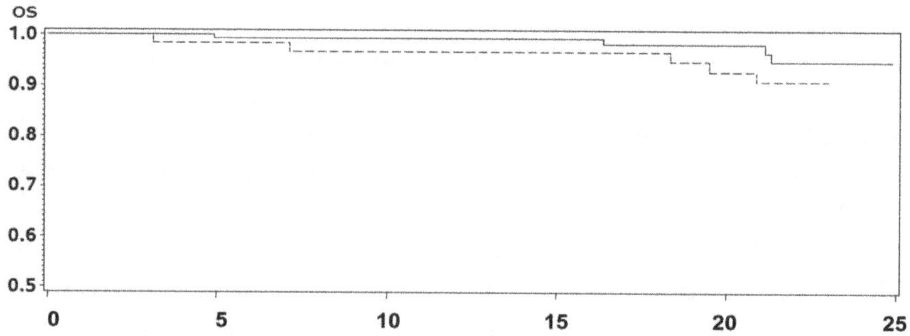

Age (years)		0	5	10	15	20	25
Screening	———	149	139	114	96	69	25
Symptoms	- - - - - - -	58	57	55	53	49	46

Diagnosis	Pts	Events	HR (95% C.I.)	20 years OS (95% C.I.)	p
NBS	149	6	1.00	98.21 (92.83, 99.56)	0.6
Symptoms	58	12	1.35 (0.44-4.15)	92.80 (81.92, 97.24)	

Figure 1. Results from an Italian study that illustrates the impact of early diagnosis through NBS on survival. The impact on survival is most apparent in infants with severe (**a**) or moderate disease (**b**) after diagnosis, highlighting the reduced impact of early diagnosis on people with mild or less typical CF (**c**) [12].

There are other important but "softer" outcomes that support the rationale of NBS for CF—namely, preventing the diagnostic odyssey that many families have to endure, providing families with information to inform future reproductive decisions and providing a framework for improved and more systematic CF services to be established across a region [1].

On the basis of these data, there is a compelling rationale to support NBS for CF, but also a responsibility to ensure that protocols are designed to minimise negative outcomes [1]. It is clear that the WHO screening criteria alone are not sufficient to critically judge the validity of a programme. Petros suggests an expanded list of criteria which provides a more comprehensive picture of the worth of an NBS programme [13]. Using these criteria, he argues that NBS for CF is a valid and worthwhile undertaking. These additional criteria are helpful, but still not adequate to rigorously evaluate a programme in the era of new emerging technologies, especially the ability to undertake extensive DNA testing in a cheap and timely manner. Advances in the capability to undertake extensive genetic testing have outpaced the capacity of most to assimilate this knowledge, and for many it is a potential cause of significant anxiety [14]. In such a climate, we propose that a bioethical approach is required to provide a framework to assess and optimise NBS for CF to ensure that the most appropriate protocol is used for a given population.

To work towards a bioethical framework, it is important to consider the impact of all possible outcomes from NBS for CF both in isolation and collectively, weighing up the relative importance to society and individuals. To establish a framework, we examined all potential outcomes for NBS for CF and related these to ethical considerations.

This work was undertaken in a series of small group meetings between the author team, with subsequent email correspondence and a literature review.

2. Outcomes from Newborn Bloodspot Screening for CF

Below, we list the potential outcomes from NBS for CF and the bioethical issues raised by each.

2.1. *True Negative: An Infant with a Negative NBS Result, Not Affected by CF*

An effective outcome of the screening programme is the accurate exclusion of cystic fibrosis. The accurate identification of infants who do not have CF is a positive outcome with no associated adverse consequences. As with all screening, this societal benefit is accepted and often underappreciated by the general population.

2.2. *True Positive: An Infant with CF Detected by NBS*

Early diagnosis provides a window of opportunity for proactive nutritional intervention. The impact on well-being later in life is now becoming apparent, as outlined in the introduction.

The beneficial implications of a true positive NBS result are:

- Proactive treatment.
- An earlier diagnostic period provides an opportunity to initiate an earlier referral into specialist tertiary care centres and to start positive intervention at the earliest opportunity.
- Preventing a potentially protracted and painful diagnostic journey.
- Diagnostic delays for children affected by cystic fibrosis have been shown to be associated with negative psychosocial consequences [15]. The journey to a clinical diagnosis may be protracted and more complicated, with higher levels of psychological distress for the individual and family. The early detection of CF in a newborn prevents this by providing a timely diagnosis and access to the appropriate specialist CF team [16].
- Information for reproductive decision making.
- A positive NBS result, subsequently confirmed by diagnostic assessment, provides an opportunity for the parents (and other family members) to obtain further information about the implications of CF and to have the option to consider future reproductive decisions. The parents should be provided with genetic counselling to guide them through this process, mitigate unaddressed fears and uncertainty and enable them to make informed decisions.

A potential negative impact of a true positive NBS result is the possibility of revealing non-paternity (for example, an infant is recognised to be homozygous for F508del, but subsequent genetic testing of the parents demonstrates that the father is not a carrier). Although this is a rare negative compared to the considerable positive impact, it is important that appropriate follow up is in place for parents to seek genetic counselling and support following the NBS process, and this should be empathetic and sensitive.

Whilst a true positive result is of benefit to the infant and family, this needs to be balanced with the potential for harm. Parents/carers may consider that they have had time with a "normal" child diminished, and the initial processing of a positive result needs to be handled sensitively, with a particular focus on timeliness and clear information. It is important that this situation is not presented to families as a "good news story" that their child has been diagnosed early, and neither should it be presented dramatically. Rather, it should be presented as the start of a journey to a hopefully full and active life. The communication of the result and the subsequent diagnostic assessment is a task requiring experience and skill, and some parents are particularly vulnerable at this point. Healthcare professionals should be able to recognise this and address the parents' needs appropriately over time.

It is essential that a newly diagnosed infant with CF has access to high quality CF care which does not place them at risk (for example, from cross infection with airway pathogens). Health economic analysis demonstrates that whilst infants with CF recognised through NBS may have similar outcomes to those diagnosed clinically, this is at the expense of less treatment intervention (i.e., clinically diagnosed infants need more treatment to achieve similar outcomes) [17]. Hence, a societal benefit is achieved. It is clear that from a bioethical view, a true positive result achieves considerable individual and societal benefit but occasional harm; programmes must strive to minimise harm (non-maleficence).

This can be done through the effective and timely processing of the NBS result, effective communication and a clear pathway to high quality multi-disciplinary care.

2.3. Recognition of an Infant as a Carrier (Negative NBS Result)

For some programmes (for example, The Netherlands and UK), carrier reporting is a possible outcome. For most programmes using DNA analysis as a second tier of testing, carriers are only confirmed after clinical assessment and sweat testing. For these families, this result would be consistent with a false positive experience (see next section). Carrier reporting may leave the family with some anxiety around the possibility of an unrecognised second Cystic Fibrosis Transmembrane Conductance Regulator (CFTR) variant, and clear information is required to minimise this potential harm.

The detection of carrier status in a baby provides an opportunity for the parents to undergo genetic counselling and testing, which may impact on future reproductive decision making and cascade screening for other family members. There is a potential for negative impact arising from carrier recognition. There is evidence of increased parental anxiety about the child; in one study, a significant number of parents (18%) felt anxious about the health of their child four years after screening, suggesting a lack of assimilation of the "healthy carrier" concept [18]. The delivery and communication of carrier status are key factors, with most concern being caused by uncertainty or confusion regarding the use of negative terms such as "query" around the screening result [19]. A perceived negative style of communication from the healthcare professional can cause increased anxiety, and lead to family issues (stigma), depression and relationship difficulties [20]. Indeed, this study suggested that parents do not perceive the information that their child is a carrier as negative, rather, the distress arises from communication practices. Concerns for the family include anxiety about the status of their other children and how to communicate the result with other family members [21]. This work found that whilst some families could be very supportive, other families could find this communication very challenging and may effectively "shut down" conversations, blame the person starting the conversation, or increase existing family stress. Providing effective support for people could lead to families benefiting from the information rather than it becoming a disruptive factor.

As with a true positive result, carrier recognition is associated with the potential risk of recognising non-paternity. This needs to be considered in the processing of a carrier result, for example leaving further genetic counselling as an option to the parents rather than making it compulsory, as in some programmes.

An ethical issue raised by all newborn screening is the possibility of reducing autonomy, as those screened have no opportunity for consent or control over the data generated. Self-determination does not feature in these public health screening strategies. This is balanced against the rights of children to receive optimal healthcare. Carrier recognition throws this into sharp relief, and the ownership of this information requires careful consideration. It is imperative that young adults identified as carriers through NBS receive this information in a clear and sensitive manner. At present, there is no clear guidance for programmes on this issue on what information and in what format to pass on [22]. It is assumed to be the responsibility of the adults who receive the initial result (parent/carers and primary healthcare professionals), who may not appreciate or want to pass on the information. As there is no clear guidance on how to manage this situation, there is a potential for harm when the index case becomes aware of their carrier status or if they are denied information on which to make fully informed decisions about their reproductive options.

2.4. False Positive: An Infant with a Positive NBS Result, Who Does Not Have CF

False positive NBS results are associated with acute psychological distress for the parent/carers, and for some this may extend into longer-term psychological morbidity [23]. The period of time between a false positive NBS result and the subsequent diagnostic testing has been shown to be acutely stressful for the family [24]. Qualitative research has shown that parents experience feelings of guilt for having passed on a "faulty" gene, and that even following confirmative diagnostic testing to exclude

CF, they still harbour feelings of scepticism and fear that the test may be wrong, with subsequent anxiety for their child's health. This may affect how parents perceive and respond to healthcare services in the future, and may undermine their confidence in medical services [23,25].

A population-based cohort study reported higher maternal worry scores for mothers with an infant with a false positive NBS result and, even following adjustment for confounding variables, there was a higher proportion of parents using outpatient and accident and emergency services for infants with a false positive NBS result compared to matched controls [26]. Care should be taken to ensure parents are fully informed in the antenatal period about the screening process and subsequent diagnostic testing, in order to avoid misconceptions about the screening result and prevent psychosocial confusion and the over-medicalisation of healthy infants [19]. In one prospective study, 96% of parents expressed having been anxious at the time of being informed about the need for a diagnostic sweat test, and the anxiety increased proportionally to the waiting time for diagnostic testing; 86% felt entirely reassured three months after the test. This suggests that the distress associated with a false positive result is most likely to be temporary [27]. Participants in a qualitative study have commented that they would be willing to endure the acute psychosocial risks of a false positive result in acknowledgement of the potential value of a true positive result and the recognition of the health benefits of an early diagnosis [23,26].

Families who remained anxious 3 months after diagnostic testing described doubts regarding the test's reliability, a poor understanding of the screening and diagnostic process and fears of CF being transmitted to future generations [27]. To minimise undermining parental confidence in the healthcare system, it is important to counsel families about the screening process, particularly when the initial result requires further diagnostic confirmation; this is particularly important when the initial screening result is positive, as there is an increased potential for misconceptions and doubt about the reliability of further testing. This information and support needs to be provided antenatally and be reinforced throughout the pregnancy, birth and postnatal period.

A small subset of parents continued to have persisting concerns about the health implications for their child following a false positive NBS result; namely, concerns of the possibility of poor health and illness for the infant, the fear of CF affecting another child or a genetic mutation affecting another family member, with some cases leading to a 'finger pointing' culture of attempting to identify the source of a suspected mutation [23]. It is important that screening programmes incorporate a recognition of the importance of counselling families on the meaning of a false positive NBS result, and that parents have the opportunity to express and discuss their concerns, with access to appropriate genetic counselling services where required.

Although, in general, the distress associated with a false positive result is considered transient, it may be that there are subtle longer-term psychosocial issues that quantitative studies may not have been sensitive enough to identify. Regardless, there is good agreement that NBS for all conditions should aim to minimise false positives. The European CF Society (ECFS) standards of care document suggests that CF programmes should aim for a positive predictive value greater than 0.3 (i.e., for every 10 infants with a positive NBS result, more than three will have a confirmed diagnosis of CF) [28].

2.5. *Unresolved Cases*

In some cases, a positive NBS result may remain unresolved. For example, an extremely preterm infant may have a positive NBS result, with a raised IRT level and one CF-causing gene variant detected. The infant may die from complications of preterm birth before further diagnostic testing is possible. Although this is a rare event in screening programmes, the increased incidence of raised IRT measurements in sick infants and infants with profound chromosomal abnormalities makes this a situation that occurs more frequently than might be anticipated by chance [29].

An unresolved screening outcome may cause psychological morbidity for the affected parents. The significance of the screening result is unknown, potentially causing increased concerns for future reproductive decisions. In addition, this result is presented during a period of extreme distress for parents, who may be unable to assimilate the information correctly.

Unresolved anxieties and a lack of diagnostic certainty may contribute to longer-term psychological distress, particularly in the context of further reproductive decisions in the face of uncertain genetic information.

2.6. Cystic Fibrosis Screen Positive, Inconclusive Diagnosis (CFSPID)

A potential outcome from a positive NBS result is an inconclusive diagnosis [30,31]. The number of infants with an unclear diagnosis is dependent on the NBS approach taken, with increased recognition associated with increased DNA analysis [32]. For example, a protocol that employs extended gene sequencing will recognise more infants with an unclear diagnosis, and these infants will be more likely to remain well. Biochemical protocols with no DNA analysis will still recognise infants with an unclear diagnosis but at a much lower rate and with intermediate sweat test results (a sweat chloride concentration of between 30 and 59 mmol/L). Infants with an intermediate sweat chloride are more likely to develop clinical features consistent with CF and convert to a CF diagnosis [33].

A number of papers have considered the evaluation and management of these infants and this is covered in another chapter in this series, as are the issues around designation [34]. Recently, a global exercise resulted in the harmonisation of the definition and designation of these infants as Cystic Fibrosis Transmembrane Conductance Regulator (CFTR)-Related Metabolic Syndrome/Cystic Fibrosis Screen Positive, Inconclusive Diagnosis (CRMS/CFSPID) [30,31]. For this paper, we will use the term CFSPID.

Infants with a CFSPID designation are by definition healthy, and the majority will remain healthy through their childhood. There are three pathways that can lead to a conversion to a CF diagnosis:

1. A repeat sweat test becomes supportive of a CF diagnosis (sweat chloride >59 mmol/L).
2. New information emerges that the CFTR variant is CF-causing (two CF-causing variants equates to a CF diagnosis, regardless of the sweat chloride value).
3. The CFSPID infant develops symptoms consistent with a CF diagnosis (most commonly a chronic cough).

For a programme using extended gene sequencing, around 5% of the infants designated as CFSPID will convert to a CF diagnosis [25]. For programmes with limited or no DNA analysis, conversion is more common (between 25% and 40%), although total numbers will be less [33]. If a programme that employs extended gene sequencing only reports variants that are CF-causing, this will significantly reduce the recognition of infants with CFSPID.

The majority of infants who do not convert to a CF diagnosis face an increased risk of a CFTR-related disorder (CFTR-RD) later in their life. A CFTR-RD is defined as a condition (usually single organ) that is associated with abnormal CFTR function [35]. The most common example is the congenital bilateral absence of the vas deferens (CBAVD), which is a cause of male infertility. Other potential CFTR-RDs include pancreatitis and rhinosinusitis. The risk of developing these conditions is not currently quantifiable, and counselling families and CFSPID individuals about the long-term risk is challenging. Whilst possibly the information may represent some benefit to the family of an early diagnosis in some cases, overall the situation raises a number of ethical issues, not least those around autonomy and non-maleficence, with the risk of over-medicalisation and iatrogenic harm. Qualitative studies of parents in this situation have demonstrated the profound negative impact this designation has on health beliefs and behaviours and the undermining of trust in health professionals [36].

There is no evidence that recognition of CFSPID improves outcomes, although some argue that it empowers families to make health decisions. In light of this, the European Neonatal Screening Working Group suggested in their best practice document that NBS protocols should aim to minimise the recognition of CFSPID infants [37]. This may be achieved by only reporting CF-causing variants in larger DNA panels and not reporting carriers or variants of varying clinical consequence. This raises the issue of autonomy in not reporting a result, even if that result is unclear and screened out by a computer (algorithm independent of human awareness). There may be an ethical argument that such selective reporting improves the performance of the programme in other regards, for example positive predictive value (PPV) and therefore this is compensated by the reduction in false positives. Consensus documents provide evidence-based guidance on the management of CFSPID with advice that minimises the medicalisation of these families [34]. Despite this, CFSPID infants are at risk of iatrogenic harm through inappropriate investigation and treatment, counter to the ethical principle of non-maleficence.

It is too early to evaluate the impact of a CFSPID designation on the child as they grow, but there is certainly a risk of psychological morbidity if it is not handled sensitively. This will need research to characterise the impact and provide guidance.

2.7. False Negative: An Affected, Undetected Infant—An infant with CF Not Detected by NBS

The outcome of newborn screening with the most potential for harm is a false negative result. The number of affected but not detected infants is a key performance measure of a screening programme. For most programmes, the commonest cause of a false negative result is an initial IRT result that is below the cut-off for further testing [32]. This is dependent on the cut-off used and the age of the baby when the dried blood sample is taken (IRT levels fall over the first weeks of life). Decreasing the IRT cut-off may improve the sensitivity, but this will be at the expense of a potential reduction in specificity [32]. A balance needs to be achieved between the improved sensitivity from lowering the cut-off and the reduction in the positive predictive value. Deciding this requires the weighing of different ethical values. Other strategies can be utilised to improve PPV and these include more extended DNA analysis, but again this can impact on the performance of other aspects of the NBS. For example, in a region with an ethnically diverse population, unusual CFTR variants may be missed and the sensitivity reduced. An approach to counter this has been the use of a "safety net", where extremely high IRT values result in further diagnostic testing even if no CFTR mutations are recognized [1]. Whilst this strategy is employed by many programmes, again it can result in a reduction in PPV. It can be seen, therefore, that different approaches can have positive and negative impacts on sensitivity and these need to be carefully considered in the bioethical framework.

The potential negative impacts of a false negative NBS result:

- The infant may have nutritional compromise or an airway infection that may have been avoided with early recognition.
- In a region with established NBS for CF, physicians may be less likely to consider a CF diagnosis and the family may have a prolonged diagnostic journey.
- Non-Caucasian populations may be disadvantaged by the use of DNA panels designed for populations from a North European background [1].
- Parents are denied knowledge (that their child has CF) that may inform future reproductive decision making.
- A false negative result may undermine confidence in the healthcare service.

Programmes should establish robust mechanisms to collect false negative data in order to usefully evaluate the impact on the population. However, it is important that false negative results are considered in the context of other aspects of the programme and not over emphasised at the expense of other performance metrics.

3. The Importance of Clear Communication

Research has shown the importance of effective and open communication with relatives during the newborn screening process; for example, the reasons for persisting anxieties experienced by parents affected by a false positive result were given as uncertainty about the reliability of tests and a poor understanding of the screening and diagnostic process, showing the importance of clear and accurate communication. A study on false positive results showed that there was almost a universal perception of the newborn screening test as an "indispensable tool"; admittedly, this is for parents affected by a false positive result and therefore cannot be generalised to those affected by a false negative result, but this finding does demonstrate the importance of educating and informing relatives about the screening process [27]. Certainly, consensus guidelines highlight the importance of ensuring positive and effective communication with families, and this is seen as an imperative component of all newborn screening programmes for CF.

4. Achieving an Ethical Balance

There are elements of the NBS protocol that will impact on the performance of the screening programme (Table 1). These need to be considered when developing a programme in light of four main factors:

1. What is the geographical spread of the population?
2. What healthcare provision is accessible for the population?
3. What is the CFTR genetic profile of the population?
4. What is the capacity of a health system to provide clear information to parents/carers (antenatally, postnatally) and for the child as they grow into adult life?

Table 1. Factors to consider when designing a protocol for cystic fibrosis (CF) newborn bloodspot screening (NBS).

Factors that will improve the sensitivity of a CF NBS programme
• A lower threshold for the first IRT value • An extensive DNA panel targeted for the population screened • A safety net, when a very high IRT-1 sample triggers further testing even if second tier testing (DNA or pancreatitis-associated-protein (PAP)) is negative
Factors that will improve the positive predictive value of a CF NBS programme
• A higher IRT-1 threshold • Obtaining the first DBS sample later • A second IRT measurement (at day 14-21) • Extended gene sequencing • A second biochemical test like PAP • Not screening pre-term infants • Not using a safety net
Factors that will reduce carrier recognition
• A higher IRT-1 threshold (and a later DBS sample) • No DNA analysis • Reduced DNA panel as a first line • A second IRT sample (day 14-21) • An algorithm with extended sequencing where carriers are not reported
Factors that will reduce CFSPID recognition
• A higher IRT-1 threshold (and later sampling) • A second biochemical test (PAP) • Reduced DNA analysis • Limiting reporting to CF causing variants after extended gene sequencing • A second IRT sample (day 14-21)

The first question to address is: is it ethically justified to screen this population for CF? The incidence of CF in a population correlates well with the prevalence of the F508del variant. In populations with a low F508del prevalence, the incidence of CF will be low, and the ethical balance will be tilted towards not screening, as screening will result in more negative impacts (for example, a poor PPV) than positive (actual cases of CF identified). An example to consider is screening in populations from sub-Saharan Africa. Studies in the US have demonstrated higher IRT levels in black infants compared to other ethnic populations, and it is reasonable to translate those data to the majority of infants born in sub-Saharan Africa [38]. This population also has a low F508del prevalence, consistent with a low overall prevalence of CF. Screening newborns from this population will result in a disproportionate number of false positive results (poor PPV) and an increased CFSPID recognition, especially if a DNA-based protocol is used. Our ethical framework clearly does not support NBS for CF in this population at present, as the balance of limited benefit is outweighed by the significant negative impact of diagnostic uncertainty and false positive tests for many families.

The decision to screen or not to screen is also influenced by the factors above; for example, if the family are geographically accessible and the healthcare infrastructure means the family can be visited to obtain a second DBS, then it may be possible to design a programme with improved PPV that is ethically acceptable. The "standards of care" published by the ECFS suggest that with an incidence of above 1 in 7000 births, the appropriateness of NBS for CF should be considered [28].

The geographical location and the framework of healthcare provision both impact on the capability to undertake a second DBS and high-quality sweat testing. These are important considerations when determining the ethical balance of a programme (Table 1). For example, if the programme is screening a geographically dispersed population with limited access to diagnostic testing, a protocol with good PPV, ideally from a single DBS sample, would be preferred from an ethical perspective, even at the expense of reduced sensitivity. In Turkey, because of the low F508del prevalence in the population, it was decided to implement a two stage IRT-IRT protocol. In most areas of the country, this required the family to travel to a local health centre for the collection of the second DBS sample, as it was not universally possible for a healthcare professional to travel to the family home. This subsequently resulted in a number of families not attending and incomplete testing. Establishing an IRT-IRT protocol reduced some of the harms associated with the recognition of CFSPID, but the inability to complete the protocol in some cases, together with a low PPV, raises an ethical discussion to consider the balance of this approach [39].

It is important that a country has an adequate health infra-structure to provide a good standard of care for infants with a positive NBS result and diagnosis of CF, although there should be a recognition that, in some countries, the implementation of NBS for CF may result in the development of better services to care for children with CF. The NBS process facilitates the regional concentration of positive results and improved utilisation of resources. Finally, it is important that NBS for CF is sensitive to the cultural and religious composition of a region.

5. Discussion

Newborn bloodspot screening for CF is complex, and there are numerous options for the screening protocol design. Surveys by the ECFS Neonatal Screening Working Group have identified over 50 different protocols in Europe [32]. It is clear that NBS for CF fulfils the traditional and more recent criteria that are used to determine the appropriateness of screening [13]. However, in this paper we have outlined the need for a bioethical consideration of this public health intervention to better determine the most appropriate protocol for a given population. Protocols should be assessed by considering the balance between beneficence (achieving a positive impact), non-maleficence (restricting the negative impacts) and the justice and autonomy of the parents, child and wider family. It is important to characterise and acknowledge the negative outcomes recorded in this paper in order to design the most appropriate programme for a population.

To design an ethical framework for screening is a multifaceted conceptual process, one which requires consideration of the impact of an intervention on the individual, family and society, and with perspectives that encompass the biological, psychological and social facets of the intervention. The consideration of beneficence and non-maleficence must be balanced against societal justice and the rights of the individual to benefit from early recognition and treatment of their condition, as well as self-determination.

This framework begins by addressing the ethical implications of each screening outcome, as outlined in the body of this article. This provides a guideline for those involved in the design or evaluation of newborn screening for CF and outlines the implications that ought to be considered and evaluated. The next step is to consider how to weigh the different outcomes and what ethical values should guide this, how to determine which factors should be given more significance, and how this impacts the overall outcome of the evaluation. Achieving this practice requires wide stakeholder engagement and discussion. This will allow a flexible, reflective evaluation that can be applied to programmes designed for varying populations. Once the relative ethical acceptability of the different outcomes has been determined, the next phase of the project will be using the framework to evaluate the active current screening programmes in order to determine the validity and effectiveness of the proposed framework. It is important that programmes critically review performance and adjust accordingly if they are not achieving the anticipated outcomes. Many programmes are resistant to change, but there are good examples of programmes that have adjusted cut-offs and DNA panels in light of sub-optimal performances. The national programme in France is an excellent example of a well performing programme that improved its "ethical balance" through a critical appraisal of its performance [40].

6. Conclusions

The complexities of newborn screening need to be considered and discussed in order to ensure the process of screening is ethical, fair, acceptable and just. The variety of potential approaches to screening introduces further complexity, and the ethical acceptability of the different outcomes will differ depending on the population screened. It is important to evaluate the process of NBS for CF and pay particular attention to the unintended consequences, including false negative results, carrier recognition and unresolved or inconclusive cases. We propose a framework for ethically evaluating NBS programmes that considers all the possible outcomes and evaluates their significance. The next step requires determining the relative acceptability of these outcomes, which will vary depending on the population; these can only be established for each population through stakeholder engagement. The framework can then be used to guide the design and evaluation of screening programmes. This framework will help guide policymakers to determine the most ethically acceptable programme, and to help identify, acknowledge and ameliorate the consequences of each outcome.

References

1. Castellani, C.; Massie, J.; Sontag, M.; Southern, K.W. Newborn screening for cystic fibrosis. *Lancet Respir. Med.* **2016**, *4*, 653–661. [CrossRef]
2. Goldenberg, A.J.; Lloyd-Puryear, M.; Brosco, J.P.; Therrell, B.; Bush, L.; Berry, S.; Brower, A.; Bonhomme, N.; Bowdish, B.; Clarke, A.; et al. Including ELSI research questions in newborn screening pilot studies. *Genet. Med.* **2019**, *21*, 525–533. [CrossRef]
3. Bell, S.C.; Mall, M.A.; Gutierrez, H.; Macek, M.; Madge, S.; Davies, J.C.; Burgel, P.R.; Tullis, E.; Castaños, C.; Byrnes, C.A.; et al. The future of cystic fibrosis care: A global perspective. *Lancet Respir. Med.* **2020**, *8*, 65–124. [CrossRef]
4. Wilson, J.M.; Jungner, Y.G. Principles and practice of mass screening for disease. *Bol Oficina Sanit Panam* **1968**, *65*, 281–393. [PubMed]
5. Hammond, K.B.; Abman, S.H.; Sokol, R.J.; Accurso, F.J. Efficacy of statewide neonatal screening for cystic fibrosis by assay of trypsinogen concentrations. *N. Engl. J. Med.* **1991**, *325*, 769–774. [CrossRef] [PubMed]
6. Farrell, P.M.; Kosorok, M.R.; Laxova, A.; Shen, G.; Koscik, R.E.; Bruns, W.T.; Splaingard, M.; Mischler, E.H.; Wisconsin Cystic Fibrosis Neonatal Screening Study Group. Nutritional benefits of neonatal screening for cystic fibrosis. *N. Engl. J. Med.* **1997**, *337*, 963–969. [CrossRef] [PubMed]

7. Farrell, P.M.; Kosorok, M.R.; Rock, M.J.; Laxova, A.; Zeng, L.; Lai, H.C.; Hoffman, G.; Laessig, R.H.; Splaingard, M.L.; Wisconsin Cystic Fibrosis Neonatal Screening Study Group. Early diagnosis of cystic fibrosis through neonatal screening prevents severe malnutrition and improves long-term growth. *Pediatrics* **2001**, *107*, 1–13. [CrossRef]
8. Farrell, P.M.; Li, Z.; Kosorok, M.R.; Laxova, A.; Green, C.G.; Collins, J.; Lai, H.-C.; Rock, M.J.; Splaingard, M.L. Bronchopulmonary disease in children with cystic fibrosis after early or delayed diagnosis. *Am. J. Respir. Crit. Care Med.* **2003**, *168*, 1100–1108. [CrossRef] [PubMed]
9. Chatfield, S.; Owen, G.; Ryley, H.C.; Williams, J.; Alfaham, M.; Goodchild, M.C.; Weller, P. Neonatal screening for cystic fibrosis in Wales and the West Midlands: Clinical assessment after five years of screening. *Arch. Dis. Child.* **1991**, *66*, 29–33. [CrossRef]
10. Dijk, F.N.; McKay, K.; Barzi, F.; Gaskin, K.J.; Fitzgerald, D.A. Improved survival in cystic fibrosis patients diagnosed by newborn screening compared to a historical cohort from the same centre. *Arch. Dis. Child.* **2011**, *96*, 1118–1123. [CrossRef]
11. Sanders, D.B.; Zhang, Z.; Farrell, P.M.; Lai, H.J.; Wisconsin, C.F.N.S.G. Early life growth patterns persist for 12years and impact pulmonary outcomes in cystic fibrosis. *J. Cyst. Fibros.* **2018**, *17*, 528–535. [CrossRef] [PubMed]
12. Tridello, G.; Castellani, C.; Meneghelli, I.; Tamanini, A.; Assael, B.M. Early diagnosis from newborn screening maximises survival in severe cystic fibrosis. *ERJ Open Res.* **2018**, *4*. [CrossRef] [PubMed]
13. Petros, M. Revisiting the Wilson-Jungner criteria: How can supplemental criteria guide public health in the era of genetic screening? *Genet. Med.* **2012**, *14*, 129–134. [CrossRef] [PubMed]
14. Scott, I.A.; Attia, J.; Moynihan, R. Promises and perils of using genetic tests to predict risk of disease. *BMJ* **2020**, *368*, m14. [CrossRef]
15. Tluczek, A.; Laxova, A.; Grieve, A.; Heun, A.; Brown, R.L.; Rock, M.J.; Gershan, W.M.; Farrell, P.M. Long-term follow-up of cystic fibrosis newborn screening: Psychosocial functioning of adolescents and young adults. *J. Cyst. Fibros.* **2014**, *13*, 227–234. [CrossRef]
16. Farrell, M.H.; Farrell, P.M. Newborn screening for cystic fibrosis: Ensuring more good than harm. *J. Pediatr.* **2003**, *143*, 707–712. [CrossRef]
17. Sims, E.J.; Mugford, M.; Clark, A.; Aitken, D.; McCormick, J.; Mehta, G.; Mehta, A.; UK Cystic Fibrosis Database Steering Committee. Economic implications of newborn screening for cystic fibrosis: A cost of illness retrospective cohort study. *Lancet* **2007**, *369*, 1187–1195. [CrossRef]
18. Lewis, S.; Curnow, L.; Ross, M.; Massie, J. Parental attitudes to the identification of their infants as carriers of cystic fibrosis by newborn screening. *J. Paediatr. Child Health* **2006**, *42*, 533–537. [CrossRef]
19. Ulph, F.; Wright, S.; Dharni, N.; Payne, K.; Bennett, R.; Roberts, S.; Walshe, K.; Lavender, T. Provision of information about newborn screening antenatally: A sequential exploratory mixed-methods project. *Health Technol. Assess.* **2017**, *21*, 1–240. [CrossRef]
20. Ulph, F.; Cullinan, T.; Qureshi, N.; Kai, J. Parents' responses to receiving sickle cell or cystic fibrosis carrier results for their child following newborn screening. *Eur. J. Hum. Genet.* **2015**, *23*, 459–465. [CrossRef]
21. Ulph, F.; Cullinan, T.; Qureshi, N.; Kai, J. Informing children of their newborn screening carrier result for sickle cell or cystic fibrosis: Qualitative study of parents' intentions, views and support needs. *J. Genet. Couns.* **2014**, *23*, 409–420. [CrossRef] [PubMed]
22. Oliver, S.; Dezateux, C.; Kavanagh, J.; Lempert, T.; Stewart, R. Disclosing to parents newborn carrier status identified by routine blood spot screening. *Cochrane Database Syst. Rev.* **2004**, CD003859. [CrossRef] [PubMed]
23. Tluczek, A.; Orland, K.M.; Cavanagh, L. Psychosocial consequences of false-positive newborn screens for cystic fibrosis. *Qual. Health Res.* **2011**, *21*, 174–186. [CrossRef] [PubMed]
24. Tluczek, A.; Koscik, R.L.; Farrell, P.M.; Rock, M.J. Psychosocial risk associated with newborn screening for cystic fibrosis: Parents' experience while awaiting the sweat-test appointment. *Pediatrics* **2005**, *115*, 1692–1703. [CrossRef] [PubMed]
25. Kharrazi, M.; Yang, J.; Bishop, T.; Lessing, S.; Young, S.; Graham, S.; Pearl, M.; Chow, H.; Ho, T.; Gaffney, L.; et al. Newborn Screening for Cystic Fibrosis in California. *Pediatrics* **2015**, *136*, 1062–1072. [CrossRef]
26. Hayeems, R.Z.; Miller, F.A.; Vermeulen, M.; Potter, B.K.; Chakraborty, P.; Davies, C.; Carroll, J.C.; Ratjen, F.; Guttmann, A. False-positive newborn screening for cystic fibrosis and health care use. *Pediatrics* **2017**, *140*, e20170604. [CrossRef]

27. Beucher, J.; Leray, E.; Deneuville, E.; Roblin, M.; Pin, I.; Bremont, F.; Turck, D.; Giniès, J.-L.; Foucaud, P.; Derelle, J.; et al. Psychological effects of false-positive results in cystic fibrosis newborn screening: A two-year follow-up. *J. Pediatr.* **2010**, *156*, 771–776.e1. [CrossRef]
28. Castellani, C.; Duff, A.J.; Bell, S.C.; Heijerman, H.G.; Munck, A.; Ratjen, F.; Sermet-Gaudelus, I.; Southern, K.W.; Barben, J.; Hodková, P.; et al. ECFS best practice guidelines: The 2018 revision. *J. Cyst. Fibros.* **2018**, *17*, 153–178. [CrossRef]
29. Heeley, A.F.; Fagan, D.G. Trisomy 18, cystic fibrosis, and blood immunoreactive trypsin. *Lancet* **1984**, *1*, 169–170. [CrossRef]
30. Farrell, P.M.; White, T.B.; Ren, C.L.; Hempstead, S.E.; Accurso, F.; Derichs, N.; Howenstine, M.; McColley, S.A.; Rock, M.; Sermet-Gaudelus, I.; et al. Diagnosis of cystic fibrosis: Consensus guidelines from the cystic fibrosis foundation. *J. Pediatr.* **2017**, *181*, S4–S15.e1. [CrossRef]
31. Southern, K.W.; Barben, J.; Gartner, S.; Munck, A.; Castellani, C.; Mayell, S.J.; Davies, J.C.; Winters, V.; Murphy, J.; McColley, S.A.; et al. Inconclusive diagnosis after a positive newborn bloodspot screening result for cystic fibrosis; clarification of the harmonised international definition. *J. Cyst. Fibros.* **2019**, *18*, 778–780. [CrossRef] [PubMed]
32. Barben, J.; Castellani, C.; Dankert-Roelse, J.; Gartner, S.; Kashirskaya, N.; Linnane, B.; Mayell, S.; Munck, A.; Sands, D.; Pybus, S.; et al. The expansion and performance of national newborn screening programmes for cystic fibrosis in Europe. *J. Cyst. Fibros.* **2017**, *16*, 207–213. [CrossRef] [PubMed]
33. Munck, A.; Bourmaud, A.; Bellon, G.; Picq, P.; Farrell, P.M.; DPAM Study Group. Phenotype of children with inconclusive cystic fibrosis diagnosis after newborn screening. *Pediatr. Pulmonol.* **2020**. [CrossRef] [PubMed]
34. Munck, A.; Mayell, S.J.; Winters, V.; Shawcross, A.; Derichs, N.; Parad, R.; Barben, J.; Southern, K.W. Cystic Fibrosis Screen Positive, Inconclusive Diagnosis (CFSPID): A new designation and management recommendations for infants with an inconclusive diagnosis following newborn screening. *J. Cyst. Fibros.* **2015**, *14*, 706–713. [CrossRef] [PubMed]
35. Bombieri, C.; Claustres, M.; De Boeck, K.; Derichs, N.; Dodge, J.; Girodon, E.; Sermet, I.; Schwarz, M.; Tzetis, M.; Bareil, C.; et al. Recommendations for the classification of diseases as CFTR-related disorders. *J. Cyst. Fibros.* **2011**, *10* (Suppl. 2), S86–S102. [CrossRef]
36. Johnson, F.; Southern, K.W.; Ulph, F. Psychological impact on parents of an inconclusive diagnosis following newborn bloodspot screening for cystic fibrosis: A qualitative study. *Int. J. Neonat. Screen.* **2019**, *5*, 23. [CrossRef]
37. Castellani, C.; Southern, K.W.; Brownlee, K.; Roelse, J.D.; Duff, A.; Farrell, M.; Mehta, A.; Munck, A.; Pollitt, R.; Wilcken, B.; et al. European best practice guidelines for cystic fibrosis neonatal screening. *J. Cyst. Fibros.* **2009**, *8*, 153–173. [CrossRef]
38. Korzeniewski, S.J.; Young, W.I.; Hawkins, H.C.; Cavanagh, K.; Nasr, S.Z.; Langbo, C.; TenEyck, K.R.; Grosse, S.D.; Kleyn, M.; Grigorescu, V. Variation in immunoreactive trypsinogen concentrations among Michigan newborns and implications for cystic fibrosis newborn screening. *Pediatr. Pulmonol.* **2011**, *46*, 125–130. [CrossRef]
39. Bulent, K.; Memorial Ataşehir Hospital, İstanbul, Turkey; Refika, E.; Marmara University, Istanbul, Turkey. Personal Communication, 2020.
40. Munck, A.; Delmas, D.; Audrezet, M.P.; Lemonnier, L.; Cheillan, D.; Roussey, M. Optimization of the French cystic fibrosis newborn screening programme by a centralized tracking process. *J. Med. Screen.* **2018**, *25*, 6–12. [CrossRef]

12

Newborn Screening for Pompe Disease: Pennsylvania Experience

Can Ficicioglu [1,*], Rebecca C. Ahrens-Nicklas [1], Joshua Barch [2], Sanmati R. Cuddapah [1], Brenda S. DiBoscio [1], James C. DiPerna [3], Patricia L. Gordon [4], Nadene Henderson [2], Caitlin Menello [1], Nicole Luongo [1], Damara Ortiz [2] and Rui Xiao [5,6]

1 Division of Human Genetics/Metabolism, Children's Hospital of Philadelphia, Perelman School of Medicine at the University of Pennsylvania, Philadelphia, PA 19104, USA; ahrensNicklasR@email.chop.edu (R.C.A.-N.); cuddapahs@email.chop.edu (S.R.C.); dibosciob1@email.chop.edu (B.S.D.); menelloc@email.chop.edu (C.M.); Luongon@email.chop.edu (N.L.)

2 Department of Pediatrics, Division of Medical Genetics, UPMC Children's Hospital of Pittsburgh, Pittsburgh, PA 15224, USA; joshua.barch@chp.edu (J.B.); nadene.henderson@chp.edu (N.H.); damara.ortiz@chp.edu (D.O.)

3 PerkinElmer, Mass Spectroscopy Unit, Pittsburgh, PA 15275, USA; James.DiPerna@perkinelmer.com

4 Division of Human Genetics, Penn State Heath Children's Hospital, Penn State University College of Medicine, Hershey, PA 17033, USA; pgordon@pennstatehealth.psu.edu

5 Department of Pediatrics, Division of Biostatistics, Children's Hospital of Philadelphia, Philadelphia, PA 19104, USA; xiaor@email.chop.edu

6 Department of Biostatistics, Epidemiology & Informatics, Perelman School of Medicine at the University of Pennsylvania, Philadelphia, PA 19104, USA

* Correspondence: ficicioglu@email.chop.edu

Abstract: Pennsylvania started newborn screening for Pompe disease in February 2016. Between February 2016 and December 2019, 531,139 newborns were screened. Alpha-Glucosidase (GAA) enzyme activity is measured by flow-injection tandem mass spectrometry (FIA/MS/MS) and full sequencing of the GAA gene is performed as a second-tier test in all newborns with low GAA enzyme activity [<2.10 micromole/L/h]. A total of 115 newborns had low GAA enzyme activity and abnormal genetic testing and were referred to metabolic centers. Two newborns were diagnosed with Infantile Onset Pompe Disease (IOPD), and 31 newborns were confirmed to have Late Onset Pompe Disease (LOPD). The incidence of IOPD + LOPD was 1:16,095. A total of 30 patients were compound heterozygous for one pathogenic and one variant of unknown significance (VUS) mutation or two VUS mutations and were defined as suspected LOPD. The incidence of IOPD + LOPD + suspected LOPD was 1: 8431 in PA. We also found 35 carriers, 15 pseudodeficiency carriers, and 2 false positive newborns.

Keywords: Pompe disease; newborn screening; alpha glucosidase

1. Introduction

Pompe disease is an autosomal recessive inborn error of metabolism caused by mutations in the glucosidase alpha acid (*GAA*) gene located on the long arm of chromosome 17q25.2-q25.3. These genetic mutations cause deficient GAA enzyme activity [1]. Due to the deficiency of this enzyme, glycogen cannot be metabolized in lysosomes. This causes glycogen accumulation that damages cells throughout the body, especially muscle cells. Pathologic changes in muscle usually begin long before patients present with symptoms [2].

The previously estimated overall incidence of Pompe disease is 1 in 40,000 [1 in 138,000 for Infantile Onset Pompe Disease (IOPD) and 1 in 57,000 for Late Onset Pompe Disease (LOPD)]

in the Netherlands [3]. This roughly corresponds to the incidence of clinically identified cases in New York state [4]. The frequency appears to vary significantly in different ethnic groups from 1 in 14,000 to 1 in 600,000 [1,3–7]. Recorded incidence is highest in African Americans and lowest in Portuguese populations.

Patients with IOPD present with hypertrophic cardiomyopathy, hypotonia, macroglossia, feeding difficulties, and failure to thrive at around 2 months of age [8]. Some cases develop hypertrophic cardiomyopathy in utero. IOPD is rapidly progressive, and if left untreated, patients usually die in the first year of life. IOPD patients, diagnosed clinically or by newborn screening, always have elevated CK levels as a marker of muscle damage, and elevated urinary glucose tetrasaccharide (Glc4 or Hex4). Hex4 was shown to correlate with glycogen content in quadriceps biopsies in patients with IOPD [9]. Hex 4 is not only useful in the diagnosis of Pompe but also in monitoring the response to ERT [10].

Patients with LOPD present later in life with proximal muscle weakness, gait abnormalities, respiratory insufficiency, poor weight gain, and swallowing difficulties [11]. Individuals with LOPD do not typically develop hypertrophic cardiomyopathy, but some experience arrhythmias. LOPD patients who are diagnosed clinically often, but not always, have elevated CK and Hex 4 levels. Baseline evaluation of Hex 4 levels in LOPD cases detected through NBS have been reported to be within normal range [10].

Diagnostic Odyssey: Before implementation of newborn screening, there was, on average, a 3 month-delay in diagnosing IOPD after the onset of symptoms [12]. In LOPD, symptoms may begin anytime from infancy to adulthood. In pediatric onset cases, symptom onset occurs at an average of 6 years of age, yet the diagnosis is made at an average of 18 years of age. Therefore, on average, there is a 12-year delay in diagnosis [12]. The average age of symptom onset in adult-onset LOPD is 35 years of age, with a 7-year delay in diagnosis after symptom onset [12]. Non-specific symptoms, seen in other more common disorders, coupled with lack of knowledge about this rare disorder usually result in significant diagnostic delays. These factors importantly shape an individual patient's odyssey and outcomes with all forms of Pompe disease.

Enzyme replacement therapy (ERT) has been available since 2006 for all forms of Pompe disease. It has dramatically changed patient outcomes. [13]. ERT improves cardiac and skeletal symptoms and slows down the progression of disease. Patients with severe disease, who cannot produce any natural GAA enzyme, are classified as Cross-Reactive Immunological Material (CRIM) negative. In such CRIM negative patients, the immune system identifies the administered enzyme as foreign and produces antibodies that make the enzyme therapy less effective [14]. Immune modulation therapy can be used to inhibit the development of antibody response in CRIM negative patients at the time of the start of their ERT [15–17].

This life-changing therapy is more effective when initiated before the onset of symptoms [18–22]. When we consider that (a) pathology begins long before patients present with symptoms and (b) many patients have a protracted diagnostic odyssey, shortening the diagnostic delay through newborn screening and beginning treatment as soon as possible is crucial for all forms of Pompe disease.

A pilot newborn screening (NBS) was launched in Taiwan in 2005. Chien et al. demonstrated the importance of NBS not only for IOPD but also for LOPD [19–21]. Between 2005 and 2009, 344,056 newborns were screened in Taiwan, and 13 cases of LOPD were detected [21]. A total of 4 of 13 patients were put on ERT because of hypotonia, muscle weakness, delayed developmental milestones/motor skills, or elevated CK levels starting at the ages of 1.5, 14, 34, and 36 months. Muscle biopsy specimens obtained from the treated patients revealed increased storage of glycogen and lipids [21]. Soon after Taiwan, several pilot programs in Italy, Australia, Japan, Korea, USA, and Hungary tested the feasibility of Pompe NBS and reported the incidence of and the impact of the disease [23].

In the USA, Pompe disease was added to the recommended universal newborn screening panel (RUSP) in February 2015 [24]. Some states such as Missouri, Illinois, and New York started screening for Pompe before the RUSP recommendation. Pennsylvania started Pompe screening in February 2016.

In this paper, we present Pennsylvania data and experience on Pompe NBS. Our aim is three-fold: to augment state-based knowledge of the disease and its diagnosis through NBS; to document the benefits and challenges of NBS for Pompe disease in Pennsylvania; and to encourage the speedy adoption of NBS for Pompe by other states and countries.

2. Materials and Methods

In Pennsylvania, NBS testing is done by PerkinElmer newborn screening laboratory in Pittsburgh, PA. GAA enzyme activity is measured by flow-injection tandem mass spectrometry (FIA/MS/MS) using the algorithm shown in Figure 1 [25]. Blood is obtained at around 36 h of life. A second sample is requested if the first GAA enzyme activity is below the cutoff value. If this second GAA enzyme activity is below the cutoff, the second-tier test, *GAA* full gene sequencing (Next Generation Sequencing), is performed. In Pennsylvania, newborn screening is free, and both GAA enzyme level and full gene sequencing are done as part of Pompe NBS without any charges. The cutoff was established at ~18% of the apparently normal newborn mean GAA activity and is based on the analysis of ~1000 apparently normal newborns as well as 9 confirmed positive Pompe patients. In PerkinElmer laboratory, it was determined that the daily patient means are stable, and thus, the use of a fixed cutoff has been utilized and has been shown to be effective. The use of fixed cutoffs also makes the daily evaluation of data much less complex. Results falling below this cutoff are considered abnormal.

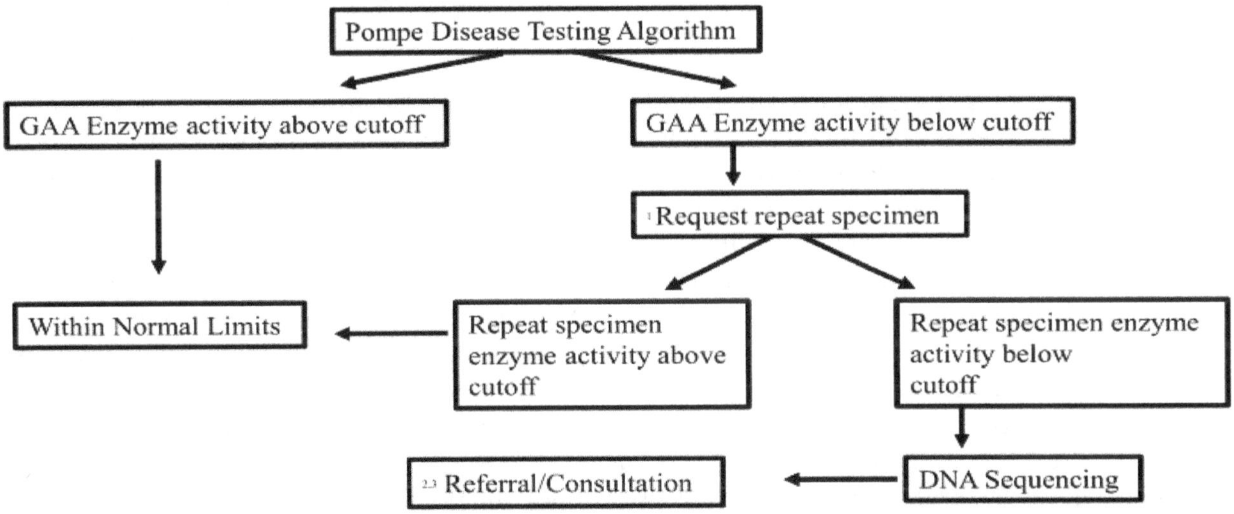

Figure 1. Flow chart of screening algorithm. [1] Pompe Repeat Request: Results show decreased enzyme activity for lysosomal alpha-glucosidase (GAA). We recommend a repeat dried filter paper blood specimen within 48 hours after the reporting of the first abnormal test. You should discuss the case with one of the metabolism referral centers if newborn has cardiomyopathy or symptoms of Pompe disease such as hypotonia and feeding issues. [2] Pompe Referral (Sequencing positive): Results continue to show decreased enzyme activity for Lysosomal alpha-Glucosidase (GAA). This result may be associated with Pompe disease. We recommend referral to a metabolic specialist. [3] Pompe Consult (Sequencing pseudodeficiency or no variant): Results continue to show decreased enzyme activity for Lysosomal alpha-Glucosidase (GAA). Consultation with a metabolic specialist may be considered to review and interpret these results in context with the patient's clinical presentation.

A single 1/8-inch (3mm) Dried Blood Spot (DBS) disc is extracted with 30 μL of cocktail solution containing β-Glucocerebrosidase (ABG), Acid Sphingomyelinase (ASM), Alpha-Glucosidase (GAA), Alpha-Galactosidase (GLA), Galactocerebrosidase (GALC) and Alpha-Iduronidase (IDUA) substrates and internal standards (in a buffer of pH 4.8) at 37 °C for 18 h +/− 2 h. The enzymatic reactions are quenched with 50% ethyl acetate: methanol followed by a liquid–liquid extraction using 50% ethyl acetate: water.

An aliquot of the organic top layer is transferred into a clean deep well plate, dried under a gentle stream of nitrogen gas, reconstituted in 80%/20%/0.2% acetonitrile/water/formic acid solution, and subjected to flow-injection tandem mass spectrometry (FIA/MS/MS). The electrospray source is operated in positive mode, and the analytes are interrogated in multiple reaction monitoring (MRM) mode. Blank filter paper spots are analyzed for background correction.

Enzyme activities (in units of μmol/L/h) are defined as the amount of substrate hydrolyzed by the enzyme in the reaction and are determined by calculating the ion abundance ratio of product to internal standard, multiplied by the volume and concentration of internal standard, divided by the response factor ratio of product to internal standard, sample incubation time, and sample blood volume (Enzyme activity = $(P/IS)*[IS]*V_{IS}/RF/3.1$ μL/time). A sample volume of 3.1 μL is assigned to a 1/8-inch DBS punch. A fixed GAA enzyme activity cutoff of 2.10 micromole/L/h is utilized. A repeat specimen is requested on an initial GAA enzyme result of <2.10 μmol/L/h. A repeat specimen with a second GAA enzyme level of <2.10 μmol/L/h is reflexed to full *GAA* gene sequencing. Turn-around-time for GAA enzyme testing is <72 h from specimen receipt. Full *GAA* sequencing turn-around time is 7–10 days from reflex.

Newborns with low enzyme activity (<2.10 μmol/L/h) and at least one variant [pathogenic, likely pathogenic, or variant of unknown significance (VUS)] are referred to one of the seven metabolic referral centers in Pennsylvania by pediatricians and department of health newborn screening program. Newborns with low enzyme activity and sequencing revealing only pseudodeficiency allele(s) are not referred to metabolic centers by the state. However, some pediatricians refer them to the metabolic centers for further clarification.

After the initial metabolic evaluation and confirmatory test results, patients are classified as IOPD, LOPD, "suspected" LOPD, or carrier. If patients carry one pathogenic variant and one VUS or two VUS, they are defined as "suspected" LOPD. After genetic counseling, carriers and those with pseudo-deficiency mutations are discharged with no further follow-up; all others are followed by a metabolic geneticist. Although there are slight differences among Pennsylvania centers in the initial work up, confirmatory GAA enzyme activity, aspartate aminotransferase (AST), alanine aminotransferase (ALT), creatine kinase (CK), urine glucose tetrasaccharide (Glc4 or Hex4) levels are tested in all cases. At the outset of NBS for Pompe, all centers performed electrocardiogram (ECG) and echocardiogram (ECHO) at the time of referral. As centers gained more experience, some decided not to perform ECG and ECHO at the first visit in cases with late onset mutations. Patients with LOPD and suspected LOPD are usually seen every 3 months in the first year and subsequently, every 6 months. In IOPD patients, treatment, including appropriate immunomodulation, is initiated immediately.

Statistical Analysis: The demographic and laboratory data were summarized by median and interquartile range (IQR) for continuous variables and frequency and percentage for categorical variables. Wilcoxon rank sum test was used to compare the GAA enzyme activity, as well as AST, ALT, CK, Hex4 levels between groups, either disease groups or genotype groups. Two-sided p values less than 0.05 were considered statistically significant. All data analyses were performed using SAS 9.4.

The Institutional Review Board reviewed and deemed this study exempt (IRB 20-017914).

3. Results

Between February 2016 and December 2019, 531,139 newborns were screened for Pompe disease. A total of 180 newborns (0.03%) had a low GAA enzyme activity on the first NBS. Repeat GAA enzyme activity from a second filter paper specimen was lower than the cutoff in 115 newborns (0.02%), and subsequently full *GAA* gene sequencing was performed. The screening algorithm is shown in Figure 1. Final diagnosis, screening and biochemical data from patients with a confirmed diagnosis are summarized in Tables 1–3. All positive cases were referred to one of the seven metabolic centers. The incidence of IOPD + LOPD was 1:16,095 and IOPD + LOPD + suspected LOPD was 1:8431 in PA.

Based on the PA DOH records, 5 newborns with positive screening were lost to follow up and never seen in metabolic centers. All 5 newborns were carriers based on the genetic test result.

Table 1. Final diagnosis of newborn screening for Pompe disease.

Pompe Disease	*n*	Incidence
IOPD	2	1:265,570
LOPD	31	1:17,134
Suspected LOPD	30	1:17,705
IOPD+LOPD	33	1:16,095
IOPD+ LOPD+ suspected LOPD	63	1:8431
Carriers	35	1:15,175
Pseudodeficiency	15	1:35,409
False positive (Normal confirmatory GAA activity, negative GAA full gene sequencing)	2	1:265,570

Total newborns screened: 531,139, Total positive *n* (%):115 (0.02).

IOPD: Two patients were diagnosed with IOPD. Their GAA enzyme levels were both 0.65 micromole/L/h at the first screening and 0.22 and 0.34 at the second screening, respectively. They both had lower GAA enzyme activities compared to carriers and pseudodeficiency; yet, there was overlap with other forms of Pompe disease. Both patients were compound heterozygous for mutations previously reported in patients with IOPD (Table 2).

The first patient was in the hospital and admitted for hypertrophic cardiomyopathy when the NBS was reported. He had elevated CK, AST, ALT, BNP, and Hex4 levels. ECG showed biventricular hypertrophy. ECHO findings included (1) moderately to severely decreased left ventricular systolic wall motion, (2) moderate hypertrophy of the left ventricle, and (3) severe right ventricular hypertrophy. The CRIM status was determined based on the genotype. ERT with immunomodulation (CRIM negative protocol) was started at 21 days of age [16]. At 31 months of age, he has normal cardiac functions but global developmental delay. He has obstructive sleep apnea and requires BiPAP at night. He continues to receive physical, occupational, and speech therapies.

The second patient had elevated CK, AST, ALT, BNP, and Hex4 levels. ECG showed short PR interval and biventricular hypertrophy. ECHO findings were (1) severe septal left ventricular hypertrophy and (2) mildly hypertrophied right ventricle. He was CRIM positive based on his genotype. ERT with immuno-modulation (methotrexate only) was started at 10 days of life [17]. His cardiac functions stabilized by 4 weeks on this regimen and normalized within 3 months. His CK never rose above 900, and down trended after the 3rd infusion and has been normal since then. He had mild motor delay on exam at 6 months old.

LOPD: Thirty-one newborns were identified to have LOPD (Table 2). Twelve of them (39%) were homozygous for the most common splice site mutation (c.-32-13T>G). A total of 16 patients were compound heterozygous, and 11 of them carried the splice site mutation (c.-32-13T>G). Three cases were homozygous for c.2238G>C mutation.

Table 2. Biochemical Parameters of Screened Patients confirmed IOPD and LOPD.

	Newborn Screening			Confirmatory Testing				
	GAA#1 (>2.10 micromole/L/h)	**GAA#2 (>2.10 micromole/L/h)**	**Genotype**	**GAA**	**AST and ALT (Normal Range for Lab, U/L)**	**CK (Normal Range for Lab, U/L)**	**BNP (Normal Range for Lab, pg/mL)**	**Hex4 (Normal Range for Lab, (mmol/mol Creatinine)**
IOPD Patients								
1	0.65	0.22	**c.759delC/c.1551+1G>C**	4.4 (>6.7)	AST: 103 (30–100)	923 (60–305)	1080 (0.0–100.0)	24.7
2	0.65	0.34	**c.525delT/c.1694_1697delTCTC**	0.4 (<3.88)	AST: 189 (22–71); ALT: 91 (7–50)	846 (60–305)	1232.5 (0.0–100.0)	30.2 (<20)
LOPD Patients								
1	1.86	0.78	**c.-32-13T>G/c.-32-13T>G**	3.1 (>6.7)	AST: 72 (24–72); ALT: 41 (17–63)	530 (28–300)	ND	4.9 (≤20)
2	1.86	1.44	**c.2238G>C/c.1552-3C>G**	5.3 (>6.7)	AST: 21 (24–72); ALT: 23 (17–63)	72 (28–300)	ND	4.2 (≤20)
3	1.73	1.08	**c.-32-13T>G/c.-32-13T>G**	3.6 (>6.7)	AST: 56 (24–72); ALT: 49 (17–63)	125 (28–300)	ND	4.5 (≤20)
4	1.24	0.67	**c.-32-13T>G/c.-32-13T>G**	2.4 (>6.7)	AST: 66 (24–72); ALT: 52 (17–63)	361 (28–300)	ND	3.9 (≤20)
5	1.82	0.94	**c.-32-13T>G/c.-32-13T>G**	6.9 (>6.7)	AST: 52 (24–72); ALT: 46 (17–63)	333 (28–300)	ND	4.4 (≤20)
6	1.32	0.88	**c.-32-13T>G/c.-32-13T>G**	0.7 (>6.7)	AST: 61 (24–72); ALT: 39 (17–63)	176 (28–300)	ND	5.9 (≤20)
7	1.05	0.19	**c.-32-13 T>C/c.546 G>A**	2.2 (>3.88)		283 (30–135)	ND	2.6 (<3.0)
8	0.83	0.85	**c.-32-13 T>G/c. 1655 T>C**	0.93 (>3.88)		365 (60–305)	ND	5.23 (<−8.9)
9	0.97	0.33	**c.2238G>C/c.2281delGinsAT/***c.2065G>A*	0.93 (>3.88)	AST: 72 (22–71); ALT: 43 (7–50)	145 (60–305)	13.0 (0.0–100.0)	5.3 (≤20)
10	0.84	0.49	**c.1438-1G>C/c.-32-13T>G**	2.1 (>3.88)	AST: 168 (20–64); ALT: 104 (12–42)	617 (60–305)	-	6.6 (≤20)
11	-	0.63	**c.-32-13T>G/c.2560C>T**	3.00 (>3.88)	AST: 125 (22–71); ALT: 50 (7–50)	421 (60–305)	-	-
12	-	-	**c.-32-13T>G /c.2238G>C**	2.60 (>3.88)	AST: 112 (22–71); ALT: 50 (7–50)	464 (60–305)	51.6 (0.0–100.0)	6.1 (≤20)
13	0.56	0.62	**c.-32-13T>G/c.-32-13T>G**	3.80 (>3.88)	AST: 78 (20–64); ALT: 42 (12–42)	122 (60–305)	71.8 (0.0–100.0)	4.8 (≤20)

Table 2. *Cont.*

	Newborn Screening			Confirmatory Testing				
	GAA#1 (>2.10 micromole/L/h)	**GAA#2 (>2.10 micromole/L/h)**	**Genotype**	**GAA**	**AST and ALT (Normal Range for Lab, U/L)**	**CK (Normal Range for Lab, U/L)**	**BNP (Normal Range for Lab, pg/mL)**	**Hex4 (Normal Range for Lab, (mmol/mol Creatinine)**
14	1.68	0.79	**c.156_157delTC/c.-32-13T>G**	2.40 (>3.88)	AST: 166 (20–64); ALT: 73 (12–42)	467 (60–305)	-	7.0 (≤20)
15	1.11	0.5	**c.2238G>C/c.-32-13T>G/***c.2065G>A*	1.60 (>3.88)	AST: 49 (20–64); ALT: 27 (12–42)	68 (60–305)	-	2.8 (≤20)
16	1.06	0.26	**c.-32-13T>G/c.-32-13T>G**	6.4 (>3.88)	AST: 73 (22–71); ALT: 39 (7–50)	140 (60–305)	99.8 (0.0–100.0)	8.5 (≤20)
17	1.04	0.77	**c.-32-13T>G/c.-32-13T>G**	1.80 (>3.88)	AST: 150 (22–71); ALT: 42 (7–50)	275 (60–305)	44.5 (0.0–100.0)	5.2 (≤20)
18	0.7	0.34	**c.-32-13T>G/c.2560C>T**	1.40 (>3.88)	AST: 152 (22–71); ALT: 55 (7–50)	542 (60–305)	16.5 (0.0–100.0)	7.6 (≤20)
19	1.07	0.38	**c.456_458insGA/c.-32-13T>G**	1.10 (>3.88)	AST: 158 (22–71); ALT: 39 (7–50)	510 (60–305)	<10.0 (0.0–100.0)	8.1 (≤20)
20	0.88	0.77	**c.-32-13T>G/c.-32-13T>G**	3.50 (>3.88)	AST: 63 (20–64); ALT: 34 (12–42)	204 (60–305)	65.4 (0.0–100.0)	-
21	1.77	0.84	**c.-32-13T>G/c.-32-13T>G**	-	AST: 71 (22–71); ALT: 60 (7–50)	155 (60–305)	-	12.6 (≤20)
22	1.07	0.92	**c.-32-13T>G/c.-32-13T>G**	1.60 (3.88)	AST: 92 (22–71); ALT: 46 (7–50)	265 (60–305)	81.5 (0.0–100.0)	5.9 (≤20)
23	1.12	0.62	**c.2238G>C;** *c.2065G>A*/**c.2238G>C;** *c.2065G>A*	2.5 (3.88)	AST: 73 (22–71); ALT: 28 (7–50)	48 (60–305)	102.3 (0.0–100.0)	-
24		0.43	**c.1856G>A/c.2238G>C**			197 (60–305)		
25		0.95	**c.2238G>C/c.2238G>C**					
26		1.01	**c.2238G>C/c.2238G>C**					
27	1.1	0.42	**c.1441T>C/c.2238G>C/***c.2065G>A*	2.40 (>3.88)	AST: 32 (22–71); ALT: 29 (7–50)	108 (60–305)	35.7 (0.0–100.0)	3.3 (≤20)
28		1.06	**c.-32-13T>G/c.2238G>C/***c.2065G>A*					
29		0.48	**c.-32-13T>G/c.1547G>A**					
30		1.07	**c.32-13T>G/c.32-13T>G**					
31		0.94	**c.32-13T>G/c.2238G>C** /*c.2065G>A*					

Pathogenic or likely pathogenic variants are bolded; Pseudodeficiency mutations are made red and italicized. Transcript number: NM_000152.3; Genome build: GRCh37.

Table 3. Biochemical Parameters of Screened Patients defined as Suspected LOPD.

	Newborn Screening			Confirmatory Testing				
Suspected LOPD Patients	**GAA#1 (>2.10 micromole/L/h)**	**GAA#2 (>2.10 micromole/L/h)**	**Genotype**	**GAA**	**AST and ALT (normal range for lab, U/L)**	**CK (normal range for lab, U/L)**	**BNP (normal range for lab, pg/mL)**	**Hex4 (normal range for lab, (mmol/mol creatinine)**
1	0.91	0.2	**c.-32-13T>G**/c.692+3G>C	2.1	AST: 30 (24–72); ALT: 30 (17–63)	150	ND	3.3
2	2.06	1.99	**c.-32-13T>G**/c.1594G>A	3.8	AST: 41 (24–72); ALT: 30 (17–63)	134	ND	3.0
3	1.48	0.67	**c.-32-13T>G**/c.546G>A	1.6	AST: 42 (24–72); ALT: 37 (17–63)	ND	ND	6.0
4	1.85	0.98	**c.-32-13T>G**/c.266G>A;c.1377C>G	1.4	AST: 39 (24–72); ALT: 32 (17–63)	293	ND	8.3
5	1.04	0.53	**c.-32-13T>G**/c.2003 A>G	0.6 (>3.88)		107 (26-192)		2.4 (<20)
6	0.61	0.41	**c.-32-13T>G**/c.1721T>C	0.8	AST: 96 (24–72); ALT: 84 (17–63)	377	ND	4.9
7	0.52	0.45	**c.-32-13T>G**/c.1291_1299del9	1.9	AST: 83 (20–70); ALT: 48 (17–63)	486	ND	9.4
8	0.56	0.63	**c.-32-13T>G**/1655T>C	2.5	AST: 156 (24–72); ALT: 103 (17–63)	668	ND	6.0
9	ND	1.34	**c.-32-13T>G**/c.533G>A	3.7	AST: 25 (24–72); ALT: 19 (17–63)	86	ND	2.5
10	1.3	2.01	**c.-32-13T>G**/ c.862G>A;*c.271G>A*	2.0	AST: 32 (24–72); ALT: 31 (17–63)	406	ND	3.4
11	1.58	0.64	**c.-32-13T>G**/ c.841C>T	1.4	AST: 23 (24–72); ALT: 42 (17–63)	136	ND	6.4
12	0.58 umol/L/h	1.84 umol/L/h	**c.1A>G**/c.1345C>T	1.90 (>3.88)	AST: 44 (15–41 U/L) ALT: 26 (12–42)	241 (15-200 U/L)	-	8.4 (≤20 mmol/mol creatinine)
13	1.02 umol/L/h	1.22 umol/L/h	**c.2560C>T**/c.1888+5G>T;*c.2065G>A*	3.80 (3.88)	AST: 112 (20–64); ALT: 29 (12–42)	69 (60–305)	407.3 (0.0–100.0)	4.6 (≤20 mmol/mol creatinine)
14	<0.19 umol/L/h	0.12 umol/L/h	**c.2236T>C**/c.700A>G/C	0.90 (>3.88)	AST: 52 (22–71); ALT: 36 (7–50)	142 (60–305)	44.2 (0.0–100.0)	15.7 (≤20)
15	1.94 umol/L/h	2.06 umol/L/h	**c.1478C>T**/1194+3G>C	6.05 (>3.88)	-	86 (60–305)	-	<4.4 (≤20)
16	1.97 umol/L/h	1.16 umol/L/h	**c.784G>A/c.859-19G>A**/c.1392G>C	4.00 (>3.88)	AST: 92 (20–64); ALT: 42 (12–42)	201 (60–305)	55.3 (0.0–100.0)	6.1 (≤20)

Table 3. *Cont.*

	Newborn Screening			Confirmatory Testing				
Suspected LOPD Patients	**GAA#1 (>2.10 micromole/L/h)**	**GAA#2 (>2.10 micromole/L/h)**	**Genotype**	**GAA**	**AST and ALT (normal range for lab, U/L)**	**CK (normal range for lab, U/L)**	**BNP (normal range for lab, pg/mL)**	**Hex4 (normal range for lab, (mmol/mol creatinine)**
17	0.98 umol/L/h	0.58 umol/L/h	**c.2105G>T**/c.1124G>A	1.20 {>3.88)	AST: 64 (22–71); ALT: 20 (7–50)	85 (60–305)	-	3.0 (≤20)
18	1.59 umol/L/h	0.95 umol/L/h	**c.-32-13T>G**/c.692+3G>C	2.70 (>3.88}	AST:73 (22–71); ALT:19 (7–50)	65 (60–305)	52.7 (0.0–100.0)	3.3 (≤20)
19	1.19	1.27	**c.1655T>C**/c.1888+5G>T/*c.2065G>A*	0.43 (1.29-25.7)	AST: 60 (22–71); ALT: 25 (7–50)	110 (60–305)	19.3 (0.0–100.0)	-
20	-	1.27	**c.-32-13T>G**/c.705G>A/*c.(1726G>A;c.2065G>A)*	1.80 (3.88)	AST 80 (22–71); ALT: 41 (7–50)	86 (60–305)	30.0 (0.0–100.0)	3.3 (≤20)
21	1.64	1.1	**c.-32-13T>G**/c.650C>T	4.10 (>3.88)	AST: 65 (22–71); ALT: 35 (7–50)	68 (60–305)	33.8 (0.0–100.0)	5.7 (≤20)
22	1.02	0.85	**c.1655T>C**/c.664G>A	2.01 (>3.88)	AST:69 (20–64); ALT: 41 (12-42)	94 (60–305)	57.4 (0.0–100.0)	6.2 (≤20)
23	-	0.42	**c.-32-13T>G**/c.1103G>A	-	AST: 126 (20–64); ALT:85 (12–42)	407 {60–305)	-	7.2 (≤20)
24	-	1.08	**c.258dupC**/c.1909C>A/*c.(1726G>A;c.2065G>A)*	-	AST: 64 (22–71); ALT: 38 (7–50)	102 (60–305)	13.0 (0.0–100.0)	3.4 (≤20)
25	1.98	1.17	**c.1552-3C>G**/c.1378G>A	-	AST: 91 (22–71); ALT: 46 (7–50)	123 (60–305)	29.1 (0.0–100.0)	3.7 (≤20)
26	-	1.49	**c.1655T>C**/c.266G>A	2.10 (>3.88)	AST: 56 (22–71); ALT: 36 (7–50)	88 3 60–305)	-	3.8 (≤20)
27		0.42	**c.-32-13T>G**/c.2467A>T					
28		1.63	**c.1504A>G**/c.2467A>T					
29		1.36	**c.2560C>T**/c.726G>A					
30		0.93	**c.2238G>C**/c.2467A>T					

Transcript number: NM_000152.3; Genome build: GRCh37. Pathogenic or likely pathogenic variants are bolded; VUSs are normal; Pseudodeficiency mutations are made red and italicized; benign or likely benign are bolded and in blue. Variants were checked in the Pompe Disease Mutation Database, available at http://www.pompevariantdatabase.nl or https://www.ncbi.nlm.nih.gov/clinvar.

All patients had low confirmatory GAA enzyme activity except two patients who had levels within normal range (patient 5, and patient 16 in Table 2). Both of these patients were homozygous for the c.-32-13T>G mutation. CK levels ranged from 48 to 617 U/L, with 11 individuals demonstrating mildly elevated CK levels. Urine Hex4 levels were within normal range in all cases. All but 2 cases had ECGs at the initial visit. ECHO was done at the time of initial visit in 24 patients. Two cases had their first ECHO at 3 months and 6 months, respectively. One case showed mild ventricular septal hypertrophy and mild hypertrophy of the left ventricle at the time of confirmatory test but follow up ECG and ECHO were normal at 3 months of age. Otherwise, ECG and ECHO at the time of diagnosis were normal or demonstrated nonspecific findings. Chest radiograms were done only by one referral site, and they were normal.

Suspected LOPD: Thirty patients were compound heterozygous for one pathogenic variant and one variant of unknown significance (VUS) or two VUS and were defined as suspected LOPD (Table 3). A total of 16 of 30 carried the most common splice site (c.-32-13T>G) mutation. The confirmatory GAA enzyme activity was lower than normal in most cases; three individuals had levels within the low-end of the normal range (Table 3). CK levels ranged from 65 to 668 U/L. Six cases had slightly elevated CK levels at the time of initial visit. Urine Hex4 levels were normal in all suspected LOPD patients. ECGs were normal or showed non-specific findings. A total of 20 cases had ECHO at the time of diagnosis, and they were normal demonstrated non-specific findings such as PFO or secundum ASD.

Pseudodeficiency: Fifteen infants had one or two pseudodeficiency alles, and they were reported as pseudodeficiency carriers. Although a referral to a metabolic center was not made, PCPs were given an option to consult with a metabolic physician about these cases. A total of 8 of 15 newborns with pseudodeficiency were referred to metabolic centers to enhance families' understanding of the meaning of pseudodeficiency alleles.

Carriers: Thirty-five newborns had low enzyme activity and one mutation. Further work up, including deletion and duplication testing, confirmed that they were carriers for Pompe disease. Parents of these infants received genetic counseling in each case.

False positive: There were two newborns who had GAA enzyme activities 1.78 and 1.61 (>2.0 micromole/L/h) on the second NBS, respectively, but they had negative *GAA* gene sequencing. They were seen at a metabolism referral center, and their confirmatory enzyme levels were 4,6 (>3.88) and 5.6 (>3.88), respectively. Both were reported as false positive.

Questions raised by Screening Results

Biomarker data collected through NBS for Pompe disease raised several important questions.

Do NBS GAA and confirmatory GAA levels make it possible to distinguish different types of Pompe disease, pseudodeficiencies, and carriers?

The median level of GAA in LOPD patients was lower than those of suspected LOPD, carriers, and pseudodeficiency cases. Patients with LOPD had significantly lower levels of GAA enzyme activity compared to cases who are carriers or have pseudodeficiency alleles in all NBS and confirmatory tests ($p < 0.003$, 0 and 0.007). There was no statistically significant difference in GAA levels between LOPD and suspected LOPD cases except the second NBS ($p < 0.015$). Patients with suspected LOPD also had statistically lower GAA levels in all NBS and confirmatory tests compared to those of carriers/pseudodeficiency ($p < 0.029$, 0.002, 0.001) (Figure 2).

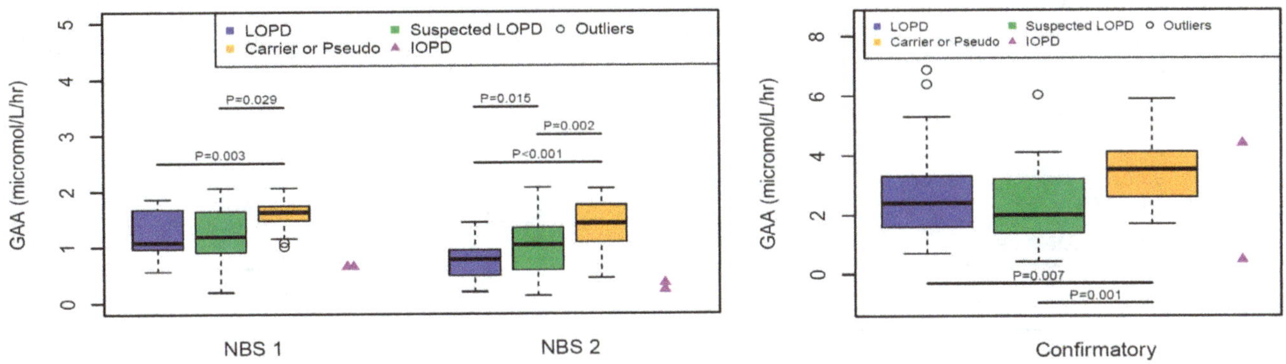

Figure 2. Comparing NBS and Confirmatory GAA enzyme activities of LOPD to Carriers/Pseudodeficiency or to Suspected LOPD patients, and suspected LOPD to carriers/pseudodeficiency) using Wilcoxon rank sum test. **NBS GAA#1** (Median: Min, Max): LOPD (*n*:22) (1.08:0.56,1.86); Suspected LOPD (*n*:21) (1.19: 0.19, 2.06); Carriers or Pseudo (*n*:30) (1.62: 1.01, 2.06), **NBS GAA#2** (Median: Min, Max): LOPD (*n*:30) (0.77:0.19, 1.44); Suspected LOPD (*n*:30) (1.03:0.12, 2.06); Carriers or Pseudo (*n*:43) (1.42:0.43, 2.04), **Confirmatory GAA** (Median, Min, Max): LOPD (*n*:23) (2.4:0.7, 6.9); Suspected LOPD (*n*:23) (2: 0.43, 6.05); Carriers or Pseudo (*n*:28) (3.5:1.7, 12.4).

Answer: In our cohort, the median value of GAA enzyme levels were statistically different, and it was possible to differentiate LOPD and suspected LOPD cases from pseudodeficiency and carriers. Two IOPD cases had much lower NBS GAA enzyme values compared to others. Although there were statistically significant differences, it is not always possible to utilize GAA levels to identify the Pompe disease status in individual newborns because of overlapping GAA values.

Do initial AST, ALT, CK, and Hex4 levels make it possible to distinguish different types of Pompe disease?

The median values of AST (72.5 U/L) and ALT (42.5 U/L) were higher in LOPD patients compared to those of suspected LOPD (AST: 64 U/L, ALT: 36 U/L) and carriers and pseudodeficiency (AST: 63.5 U/L, ALT: 32 U/L). The statistical difference was only noted in ALT values between LOPD and suspected LOPD ($p < 0.048$), and LOPD and carriers/pseudodeficiency ($p < 0.002$) (Figure 3).

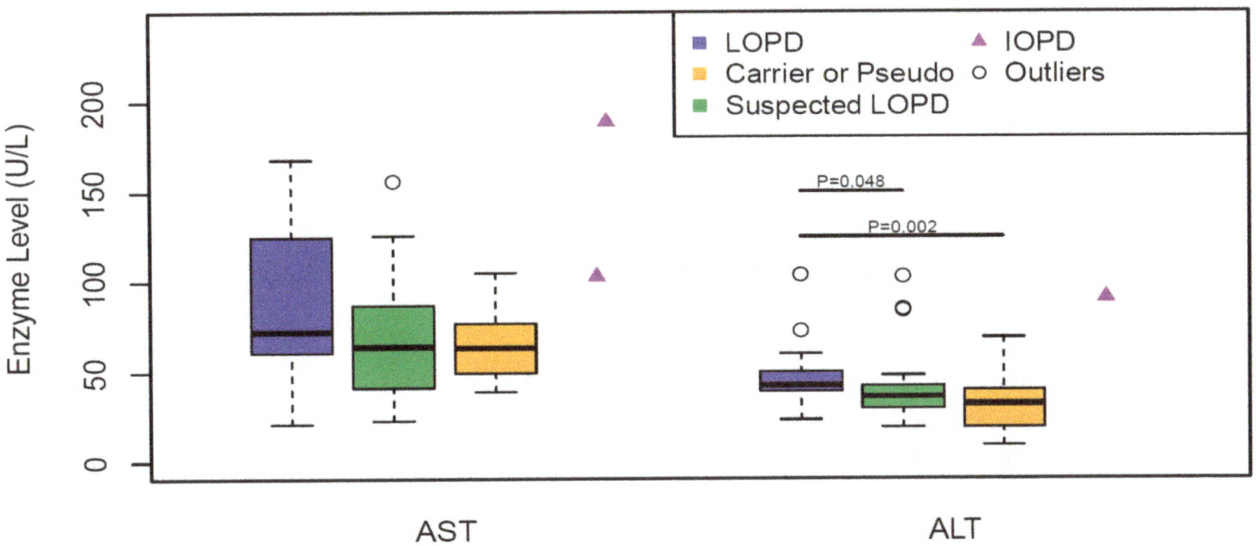

Figure 3. Comparing AST and ALT values of LOPD to Carriers/Pseudodeficiency or to Suspected LOPD patients, and suspected LOPD to carriers/Pseudodeficiency using Wilcoxon rank sum test. **AST** (U/L) (Median:Min, Max): LOPD (n:22) (72.5:21.1,168); Suspected LOPD (*n*:24) (64:23, 156); Carriers or Pseudo (*n*:20) (63.5:39, 105), **ALT**(U/L): LOPD (*n*:22) (42.5:23.1, 104); Suspected LOPD (*n*:24) (36:19, 103); Carriers or Pseudo (*n*:22) (32:9, 69).

The median value of CK (265 U/L) was significantly higher in LOPD patients compared to the median values of the suspected LOPD (123 U/L) or carriers/pseudodeficiency (107) ($p < 0.034$ and 0, respectively) (Figure 4).

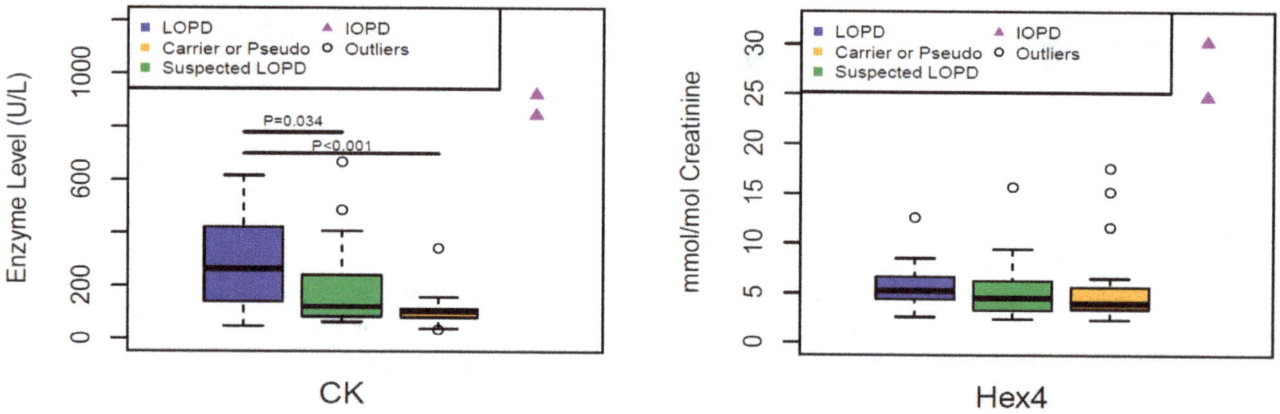

Figure 4. Comparing CK and Hex4 levels of LOPD to Carriers/Pseudodeficiency or to Suspected LOPD patients, and suspected LOPD to Carriers/Pseudodeficiency using Wilcoxon rank sum test. **CK** (U/L) (Median:Min, Max): LOPD (*n*:25) (265:48, 617); Suspected LOPD (*n*:25) (123:65, 668); Carriers or Pseudo (*n*:27) (107:35, 344), **Hex4** (mmol/mol creatinine): LOPD (*n*:21) (5.23:2.6, 12.6); Suspected LOPD (*n*:24) (4.5:2.4, 15.7); Carriers or Pseudo (*n*:26) (3.95:2.3, 17.6).

Although the median value of Hex 4 (5.23 mmol/mol creatinine) was higher in LOPD, it was not statistically different than those of suspected LOPD (4.5 mmol/mol creatinine) or carrier/pseudodeficiency (3.95 mmol/mol creatinine) (Figure 4).

None of these biomarkers were significantly different between suspected LOPD and carriers/pseudodeficiency (Figures 3 and 4).

Answer: In our cohort, the median values of CK and ALT (but not Hex4 or AST) levels were significantly higher in LOPD compared to other forms of Pompe disease detected by NBS. Two IOPD cases had much higher CK, AST, ALT and Hex4 levels compare to others. It is important to note that the analytes alone may not be used to make phenotyping or clinical decision in all cases.

Do cases homozygous for the common splice site mutation (c.-32-13T>G) have different GAA enzyme or CK levels compared to other LOPD patients?

The median values of GAA enzyme activity (NBS#2: 0.81 μmol/L/h, Confirmatory GAA: 3.3) were higher, and the median value of CK level (204 U/L) was lower in the patients homozygous for c.-32-13T>G mutation than those of other LOPD patients (NBS#2: 0.56 μmol/L/h, confirmatory GAA:2.2, CK:324 U/L), but we could not find any statistically significant difference (Figure 5).

Answer: No, GAA enzyme or CK levels do not help to differentiate cases homozygous for common splice site mutation from LOPD cases caused by other pathogenic mutations.

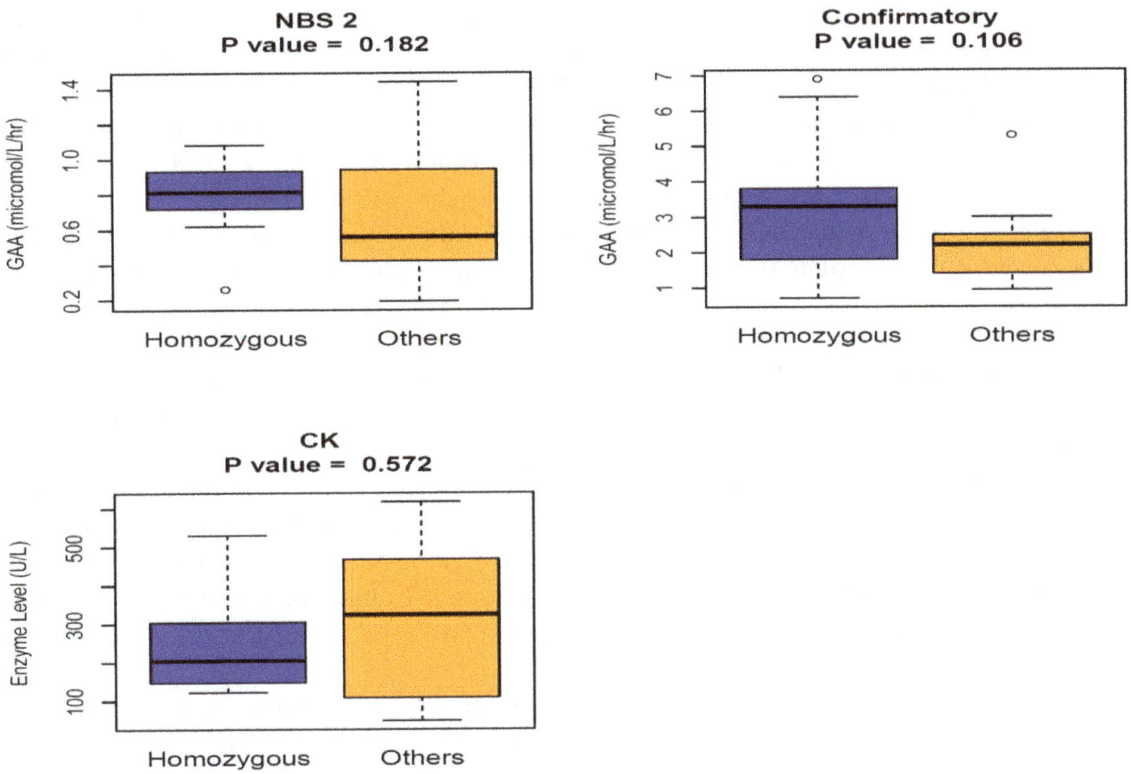

Figure 5. Comparison of NBS #2, Confirmatory GAA enzyme activities, and CK between c.-32-13T>G mutation homozygous patients and others in LOPD group, using Wilcoxon rank sum test. **NBS GAA#2** (Median:Min, Max): LOPD (homozygous for c.-32-13T>G) (*n*:12) (0.81:0.26, 1.08); LOPD-other pathogenic mutations (*n*:18) (0.56:0.19, 1.44); **Confirmatory GAA**: LOPD (homozygous for c.-32-13T>G) (*n*:10) (3.3:0.7, 6.9); LOPD-other pathogenic mutations (*n*:13) (2.2:0.93, 5.3); CK (U/L): LOPD (homozygous for c.-32-13T>G) (*n*:11) (204:122, 530); LOPD-other pathogenic mutations (*n*:14) (324:48, 617).

4. Discussion

Newborn screening detects all subtypes of Pompe disease. The reported incidence of the disease has increased since initiation of NBS, with values ranging from 1:8684 to 1:23,596 [23,26,27]. Increased incidence is largely due to improved detection of LOPD and suspected LOPD cases through NBS. In Pennsylvania, we found a similar increase with a combined incidence of IOPD and LOPD of 1:16,095 and a combined incidence of IOPD, LOPD, and suspected LOPD of 1:8,431. The incidence of IOPD by itself was 1:265,570 in Pennsylvania.

NBS for Pompe is done either by measuring only GAA enzyme activity or both GAA enzyme activity and full gene sequencing. In Pennsylvania, we chose to perform both GAA enzyme activity and gene sequencing in the NBS to increase certainty of diagnosis and provide a more detailed definition of positive screening at the initial patient visit [28]. Performing genetic testing as part of NBS has multiple advantages. The genetic test identifies those with pseudodeficiency alleles that are common in Pompe. Such patients do not need referral to a metabolic center for additional workup. Having a molecular diagnosis at the time of first visit informs the discussion of the different forms of the disease. It decreases anxiety by offering families a final diagnosis and a follow up plan based on the NBS test result. The availability of genotype at the time of reporting of abnormal NBS can also help in predicting CRIM status in IOPD patients and facilitates an informed and swift decision about the need for immunomodulation. In the absence of the results of genotype testing, families are subjected to uncertainty of diagnosis during the minimum two-week period required to order and receive the results of the genetic test. Including genetic testing with NBS for Pompe also circumvents the risk that insurance companies might deny coverage for it and guarantees that patients do not bear any additional financial burden.

NBS detects both IOPD and LOPD. Detecting IOPD cases in the first weeks of life is essential for initiation of therapy to yield optimal outcomes [21,29]. In our cohort, 2 patients with IOPD were detected (the incidence of IOPD by itself was 1:265,570 in Pennsylvania) and treated with ERT. The first patient was in the NICU of a local hospital and evaluated for feeding difficulty and cardiomyopathy. The physicians started a diagnostic work up to rule out potential etiologies and waited for the final result of Pompe NBS, which showed that he had IOPD at 19 days of age. This case showed us that there is a risk of delaying diagnosis of IOPD in the current Pompe algorithm in Pennsylvania. A second specimen is necessary to complete the sequencing test due to depletion of blood on the initial specimen on which all other newborn screening tests are performed. After detecting the first case of IOPD, we updated the NBS algorithm in Pennsylvania for Pompe to minimize delays in diagnosis of IOPD. The updated algorithm requires department of health (DOH) nurses to ask pediatricians if newborn has cardiomyopathy or symptoms of Pompe disease such as hypotonia and feeding issues when the first abnormal test is reported.

We identified 31 patients with LOPD. In addition to molecular testing results, biochemical findings such as GAA enzyme activity and CK level may help to differentiate LOPD cases from suspected LOPD or carriers/pseudodeficiency at the initial visit. In general, in LOPD cases as compared to suspected LOPD and carriers/pseudodeficiency carriers, GAA enzyme activities were lower, and CK levels were higher. Hex 4 levels were elevated and helpful biomarker for IOPD cases, but it was normal in LOPD cases at the time of diagnosis.

Since LOPD patients may present with symptoms at any age from infancy to adulthood, some may question the benefits and consequences of detection of LOPD patients via NBS. Early detection may increase family anxiety [30]. However, genetic counseling and clear explanations about LOPD along with a detailed follow-up plan reduce family anxiety accompanying initial diagnosis. We know that an extended delay in diagnosis occurs in most LOPD patients, which adversely impacts outcomes. Outcomes of early treatment of LOPD patients detected by NBS in Taiwan have been promising (21). Several metabolic centers in Pennsylvania closely follow patients with LOPD detected by NBS to make judgments about when to start treatment based on very early signs and symptoms of disease (biomarkers and developmental tests) in each individual patient.

The leaky *GAA* splice site variant, c.-32-13T>G in intron 1 is found on at least one allele in 68–90% of Caucasian patients [31]. In our NBS cohort, 74% had at least one c.-32-13T>G variant. There was no statistically meaningful difference in GAA enzyme or CK levels at the time of diagnosis between LOPD patients homozygous for c.-32-13T>G and other pathogenic mutations. Patients homozygous for c.-32-13T>G usually develop mild LOPD. However, recent reports described patients with more classical LOPD and highlighted the risk for arrhythmias in these patients [32–34]. These reports emphasize the importance of close follow up and detailed evaluations in all Pompe patients regardless of genotype.

We also identified 30 patients with suspected LOPD, i.e., they harbor two VUS or one pathogenic allele and one VUS. In this group, average GAA enzyme activity was significantly lower than those of carriers and cases with pseudodeficiency alleles on both NBS and confirmatory tests. The values of biomarkers such as CK, Hex4, AST, and ALT did not differ from those seen in carriers or pseudodeficiency carriers. This group poses a significant challenge. Some of these cases might never develop symptoms of Pompe disease; however, given our inability to fully assess disease risk in this cohort, they require ongoing monitoring. We follow up these patients every 6 months.

Pennsylvania data differ from those of Illinois and Missouri. In Illinois, a total of 684,290 infants were screened between 3 November 2014 and 30 September 2019 [27]. A total of 395 newborns with positive NBS were referred to metabolic centers. A total of 234 of 395 (59%) were false positive (normal confirmatory enzyme activity), and 62 (26%) carried pseudodeficiency alleles; this compares to only 1.7% and 13% in Pennsylvania, respectively. In Missouri, 467,000 newborns were screened for Pompe disease, and 274 had a positive test based on decreased GAA activity between January 2013 and December 2018 [35]. A total of 97 of 274 (35%) were false positive based on normal GAA activity, and 53 of 274 (19%) carried pseudodeficiency alleles; this compares to only 1.7% and 13% in Pennsylvania, respectively. These differences may arise from the fact that (1) Pennsylvania measures GAA activity twice on two different samples; Illinois and Missouri only test once; (2) each state makes its own decision about the chosen cutoff value for GAA; and (3) each state has different percentages of ethnic groups in the population.

5. Conclusions

The Pennsylvania experience shows that the overall incidence of Pompe cases increased after initiation of NBS compared to previously reported incidence [3–7] due to increased numbers of LOPD cases detected by screening. Furthermore, in our experience, NBS can detect suspected LOPD cases, some of whom may never go on to develop symptoms. Genotyping as a second-tier test was essential to inform the final diagnosis. This timely molecular diagnosis facilitated clear results disclosure at the first clinical visit and reduced parental anxiety. Finally, false positive and pseudodeficiency cases occurred at much lower rates than previously reported in other states.

Close monitoring and data collection on all patients detected through NBS is essential to assess the long-term outcomes and success of NBS for Pompe disease. NBS registries should be created and funded to enable data collection. Increased data collection will make it possible to identify and understand the pathogenic vs benign nature of VUS in cases defined as suspected LOPD.

Author Contributions: C.F., R.C.A.-N., J.B., S.R.C., B.S.D., P.L.G., N.H., C.M., N.L., and D.O. were involved in evaluation of patients with positive newborn screening tests, genetic counseling, and in treatment of those patients with a definitive diagnosis. J.C.D. performed and analyzed the newborn screening tests. R.X. analyzed the data and performed the statistical analysis. C.F., analyzed the data and wrote the first draft of manuscript. R.C.A.-N., J.B., S.R.C., B.S.D., J.C.D., P.L.G., N.H., C.M., N.L., D.O, and R.X. edited the manuscript. All authors have read and agreed to the published version of the manuscript.

Acknowledgments: The authors would like to acknowledge Jordan S Shover and Stacey Gustin from Pennsylvania Department of Health, Division of Newborn Screening, and Bethany Sgroi from Perkin Elmer, for their help in collection of newborn screening data.

References

1. Hirschhorn, R.; Reuser, A.J. Glycogen storage disease type II: Acid alpha-glucosidase (acid maltase) deficiency. In *The Metabolic and Molecular Bases of Inherited Disease*, 8th ed.; Scriver, C.R., Beaudet, A.L., Sly, W.S., Childs, B., Beaudet, A., Valle, D., Kinzler, K.W., Vogelstein, B., Eds.; McGraw-Hill: New York, NY, USA, 2001; pp. 3389–3420.
2. Hesselink, R.P.; Wagenmakers, A.J.; Drost, M.R.; Van der Vusse, G.J. Lysosomal dysfunction in muscle with special reference to glycogen storage disease type II. *Biochim. Biophys. Acta* **2003**, *1637*, 164–170. [CrossRef]
3. Ausems, M.G.; Verbiest, J.; Hermans, M.P.; Kroos, M.A.; Beemer, F.A.; Wokke, J.H.; Sandkuijl, L.A.; Reuser, A.J.; van der Ploeg, A.T. Frequency of glycogen storage disease type II in The Netherlands: Implications for diagnosis and genetic counselling. *Eur. J. Hum. Genet.* **1999**, *7*, 713–716. [CrossRef]
4. Martiniuk, F.; Chen, A.; Mack, A.; Arvanitopoulos, E.; Chen, Y.; Rom, W.N.; Codd, W.J.; Hanna, B.; Alcabes, P.; Raben, N.; et al. Carrier frequency for glycogen storage disease type II in New York and estimates of affected individuals born with the disease. *Am. J. Med. Genet.* **1998**, *79*, 69–72. [CrossRef]
5. Meikle, P.J.; Hopwood, J.J.; Clague, A.E.; Carey, W.F. Prevalence of lysosomal storage disorders. *JAMA* **1999**, *281*, 249–294. [CrossRef] [PubMed]
6. Pinto, R.; Caseiro, C.; Lemos, M.; Lopes, L.; Fontes, A.; Ribeiro, H.; Pinto, E.; Silva, E.; Rocha, S.; Marcão, A.; et al. Prevalence of lysosomal storage diseases in Portugal. *Eur. J. Hum. Genet.* **2004**, *12*, 87–92. [CrossRef] [PubMed]
7. Poorthuis, B.J.H.M.; Wevers, R.A.; Kleijer, W.J.; Groener, J.E.M.; de Jong, J.G.N.; van Weely, S.; Niezen-Koning, K.E.; van Diggelen, O.P. The frequency of lysosomal storage diseases in the Netherlands. *Hum. Genet.* **1999**, *105*, 151–156. [CrossRef] [PubMed]

8. Kishnani, P.S.; Howell, R.R. Pompe Disease in infants and children. *J. Pediatr.* **2004**, *144*, S35–S43. [CrossRef] [PubMed]
9. Young, S.P.; Zhang, H.; Corozo, D.; Thurberg, B.L.; Bali, D.; Kishnani, P.; Millington, D. Long-term monitoring of patients with infantile-onset Pompe disease on enzyme replacement therapy using a urinary glucose tetrasaccharide biomarker. *Genet. Med.* **2009**, *11*, 536–541. [CrossRef]
10. Chien, Y.H.; Goldstein, J.L.; Hwu, W.; Smith, P.B.; Lee, N.; Chiang, S.; Tolun, A.A.; Zhang, H.; Vaisnins, A.E.; Millington, D.S.; et al. Baseline Urinary Glucose Tetrasaccharide Concentrations in Patients with Infantile- and Late-Onset Pompe Disease Identified by Newborn Screening. *JIMD Rep.* **2015**, *19*, 67–73.
11. Van der Ploeg, A.T.; Reuser, A.J. Pompe disease. *Lancet* **2008**, *372*, 1342–1353. [CrossRef]
12. Kishnani, P.S.; Amartino, H.M.; Lindberg, C.; Miller, T.M.; Wilson, A.; Keutzer, J. Timing of diagnosis of patients with Pompe disease: Data from the Pompe registry. *Am. J. Med. Genet. A* **2013**, *161*, 2431–2443. [CrossRef] [PubMed]
13. Kishnani, P.S.; Corzo, D.; Nicolino, M.; Byrne, B.; Mandel, H.; Hwu, W.L. Recombinant human acid (alpha]-glucosidase: Major clinical benefits in infantile-onset Pompe disease. *Neurology* **2007**, *68*, 99–109. [CrossRef] [PubMed]
14. Kishnani, P.S.; Goldenberg, P.C.; DeArmey, S.L.; Heller, J.; Benjamin, D.; Young, S.; Bali, D.; Smith, S.A.; Li, J.S.; Mandel, H.; et al. Cross-reactive immunologic material status affects treatment outcomes in Pompe disease infants. *Mol. Genet. Metab.* **2010**, *99*, 26–33. [CrossRef] [PubMed]
15. Mendelsohn, N.J.; Messinger, Y.H.; Rosenberg, A.S.; Kishnani, P.S. Elimination of antibodies to recombinant enzyme in Pompe's disease. *N. Engl. J. Med.* **2009**, *360*, 194–195. [CrossRef] [PubMed]
16. Messinger, Y.H.; Mendelsohn, N.J.; Rhead, W.; Dimmock, D.; Hershkovitz, E.; Champion, M.; Jones, S.A.; Olson, R.; White, A.; Wells, C.; et al. Successful immune tolerance induction to enzyme replacement therapy in CRIM-negative infantile Pompe disease. *Genet. Med.* **2012**, *14*, 135–142. [CrossRef]
17. Kazi, Z.B.; Desai, A.K.; Troxler, R.B.; Kronn, D.; Packman, S.; Sabbadini, M.; Rizzo, W.B.; Scherer, K.; Abdul-Rahman, O.; Tanpaiboon, P.; et al. An immune tolerance approach using transient low-dose methotrexate in the ERT-naive setting of patients treated with a therapeutic protein: Experience in infantile-onset Pompe disease. *Genet. Med.* **2019**, *21*, 887–895. [CrossRef]
18. Chien, Y.H.; Hwu, W.; Lee, N.C. Pompe Disease: Early Diagnosis and Early Treatment Make a Difference. *Pediatr. Neonatol.* **2013**, *54*, 219–227. [CrossRef]
19. Chien, Y.H.; Lee, N.C.; Chen, C.A.; Tsai, F.S.; Tsai, W.H.; Shieh, J.Y.; Huang, H.J.; Hsu, W.C.; Tsai, T.H.; Hwu, W.L. Long-term prognosis of patients with infantile-onset Pompe disease diagnosed by newborn screening and treated since birth. *J. Pediatr.* **2015**, *166*, 985–991. [CrossRef]
20. Chien, Y.H.; Lee, N.C.; Thurberg, B.L.; Chiang, S.C.; Zhang, X.K.; Keutzer, J.; Huang, A.C.; Wu, M.H.; Huang, P.H.; Tsai, F.J.; et al. Pompe Disease in Infants: Improving the Prognosis by Newborn Screening and Early Treatment. *Pediatrics* **2009**, *124*, e1116. [CrossRef]
21. Chien, Y.H.; Lee, N.C.; Huang, H.S.; Thurberg, T.; Tsai, F.J.; Hwu, W.L. Later-Onset Pompe Disease: Early Detection and Early Treatment Initiation Enabled by Newborn Screening. *J. Pediatr.* **2011**, *158*, 1023–1027. [CrossRef]
22. Chien, Y.H.; Hwu, W.L.; Lee, N.C. Newborn screening: Taiwanese experience. *Ann. Transl. Med.* **2019**, *7*, 281. [CrossRef] [PubMed]
23. Bodamer, O.A.; Scott, C.R.; Giugliani, R. Newborn screening for Pompe disease. *Pediatrics* **2017**, *140*, S4–S13. [CrossRef] [PubMed]
24. Kemper, A.R.; Browning, M. Evidence Review: Pompe Disease. Available online: https://www.hrsa.gov/sites/default/files/hrsa/advisory-committees/heritable-disorders/rusp/previous-nominations/pompe-evidence-review-report-2008.pdf (accessed on 12 November 2020).
25. Tortorelli, S.; Turgeon, C.T.; Gavrilov, D.K.; Oglesbee, D.; Raymond, K.M.; Rinaldo, P.; Matern, D. Simultaneous Testing for 6 Lysosomal Storage Disorders and X-Adrenoleukodystrophy in Dried Blood Spots by Tandem Mass Spectrometry. *Clin. Chem.* **2016**, *62*, 1248–1254. [CrossRef] [PubMed]
26. Mechtler, T.P.; Stary, S.; Metz, T.F.; de Jesús, V.R.; Greber-Platzer, S.; Pollak, A.; Herkner, K.R.; Streubel, B.; Kasper, D.C. Neonatal screening for lysosomal storage disorders: Feasibility and incidence from a nationwide study in Austria. *Lancet* **2012**, *379*, 335–341. [CrossRef]
27. Burton, B.K.; Charrow, J.; Hoganson, G.E.; Fleischer, J.; Grange, D.K.; Braddock, S.R.; Hitchins, L.; Hickey, R.;

Christensen, K.M.; Groepper, D.; et al. Newborn Screening for Pompe Disease in Illinois: Experience with 684,290 Infants. *Int. J. Neonatal Screen.* **2020**, *6*, 4. [CrossRef]

28. Smith, L.D.; Bainbridge, M.N.; Parad, R.B.; Bhattacharjee, A. Second-Tier Molecular Testing in New-born Screening for Pompe Disease: Landscape and Challenges. *Int. J. Neonatal Screen.* **2020**, *6*, 32. [CrossRef]
29. Jang, C.F.; Jang, C.C.; Liao, H.C.; Huang, L.Y.; Chiang, C.C.; Ho, H.C.; Lai, C.H.; Chu, T.H.; Yang, T.F.; Hsu, T.R.; et al. Very Early Treatment for Infantile-Onset Pompe Disease Contributes to Better Outcomes. *J. Pediatr.* **2016**, *169*, 174–180.
30. Pruniski, B.; Lisi, E.; Ali, N. Newborn screening for Pompe disease: Impact on families. *J. Inherit. Metab. Dis.* **2018**, *41*, 1189–1203. [CrossRef]
31. Kroos, M.A.; Pomponio, R.J.; Hagemans, M.L.; Keulemans, J.L.M.; Phipps, M.; DeRiso, M.; Palmer, R.E.; Ausems, M.G.E.M.; van der Beek, N.A.M.E.; van Diggelen, O.P.; et al. Broad spectrum of Pompe disease in patients with the same c-32-13T->G haplotype. *Neurology* **2007**, *68*, 110–115. [CrossRef]
32. Rairkar, M.V.; Case, L.E.; Bailey, L.A.; Kazi, Z.B.; Desai, A.K.; Berrier, K.L.; Coats, J.; Gandy, R.; Quinones, R.; Kishnani, P. Insight into the phenotype of infants with Pompe disease identified by newborn screening with the common c.-32-13T>G "late-onset" GAA variant. *Mol. Genet. Metab.* **2017**, *122*, 99–107. [CrossRef]
33. Herbert, M.; Cope, H.; Li, J.S.; Kishnani, P. Severe Cardiac Involvement Is Rare in Patients with Late-Onset Pompe Disease and the Common c.-32-13T>G Variant: Implications for Newborn Screening. *J. Pediatr.* **2018**, *198*, 308–312. [CrossRef] [PubMed]
34. Musumeci, O.; Thieme, A.; Claeys, K.G.; Wenninger, S.; Kley, R.A.; Kuhn, M.; Lukacs, Z.; Deschauer, M.; Gaeta, M.; Toscano, A.; et al. Homozygosity for the common GAA gene splice site mutation c-32-13T>G in Pompe disease is associated with the classical adult phenotypical spectrum. *Neuromuscul. Disord.* **2015**, *25*, 719–724. [CrossRef] [PubMed]
35. Klug, T.; Swartz, L.B.; Washburn, J.; Brannen, C.; Kiesling, J. Lessons Learned from Pompe Disease Newborn Screening and Follow-up. *Int. J. Neonatal Screen.* **2020**, *6*, 11. [CrossRef] [PubMed]

13

A Multicentre Pilot Study of a Two-Tier Newborn Sickle Cell Disease Screening Procedure with a First Tier Based on a Fully Automated MALDI-TOF MS Platform

Pierre Naubourg [1], Marven El Osta [1], David Rageot [2], Olivier Grunewald [3], Gilles Renom [3], Patrick Ducoroy [1] and Jean-Marc Périni [3,*]

1 Biomaneo, 22B boulevard Winston Churchill, F-21000 Dijon, France; pierre.naubourg@biomaneo.com (P.N.); marven.elosta@biomaneo.com (M.E.O.); patrick.ducoroy@biomaneo.com (P.D.)

2 CLIPP, Clinical Innovation Proteomic Platform, Université de Bourgogne Franche Comté, F-21000 Dijon, France; david.rageot@clipproteomic.fr

3 Newborn Screening Laboratory, Biology and Pathology Center, Lille University Medical Centre, F-59000 Lille, France; olivier.grunewald@chru-lille.fr (O.G.); gilles.renom@chru-lille.fr (G.R.)

* Correspondence: jean-marc.perini@chru-lille.fr

Abstract: The reference methods used for sickle cell disease (SCD) screening usually include two analytical steps: a first tier for differentiating haemoglobin S (HbS) heterozygotes, HbS homozygotes and β-thalassemia from other samples, and a confirmatory second tier. Here, we evaluated a first-tier approach based on a fully automated matrix-assisted laser desorption/ionization time-of-flight mass spectrometry (MALDI-TOF MS) platform with automated sample processing, a laboratory information management system and NeoSickle® software for automatic data interpretation. A total of 6701 samples (with high proportions of phenotypes homozygous (FS) or heterozygous (FAS) for the inherited genes for sickle haemoglobin and samples from premature newborns) were screened. The NeoSickle® software correctly classified 98.8% of the samples. This specific blood sample collection was enriched in qualified difficult samples (premature newborns, FAS samples, late and very late samples, etc.). In this study, the sensitivity of FS sample detection was found to be 100% on the Lille MS facility and 99% on the Dijon MS facility, and the specificity of FS sample detection was found to be 100% on both MS facilities. The MALDI-MS platform appears to be a robust solution for first-tier use to detect the HbS variant: it is reproducible and sensitive, it has the power to analyze 600–1000 samples per day and it can reduce the unit cost of testing thanks to maximal automation, minimal intervention by the medical team and good overall practicability. The MALDI-MS approach meets today's criteria for the large-scale, cost-effective screening of newborns, children and adults.

Keywords: newborn screening; sickle cell disease; MALDI-TOF; mass spectrometry; thalassemia; prevention

---

1. Introduction

The use of mass spectrometry (MS) to screen newborns for haemoglobinopathies differs from the MS-based diagnosis of a broad range of clinically significant haemoglobin (Hb) variants. Newborn screening requires a robust, high-throughput and cost-effective MS method that solely detects the biomarkers of sickle cell disease (SCD) and β-thalassemia major. In contrast, the broader diagnostic procedure involves the detection of as many changes in globin proteins as possible in a single step. Newborn screening programs are typically organised as single-tier or two-tier procedures. In the two-tier procedure, the first tier is typically a routine MS method (electrospray ionization

(ESI)-MS [1–3] or matrix-assisted laser desorption/ionization (MALDI)-MS [4,5] capable of analysing intact globin chains. Pathological samples with a single mutation in the Hb β-chain can thus be unambiguously classified into three groups: heterozygotes without HbS variants, heterozygotes with HbS variants and HbS homozygotes [5]. Furthermore, β-globin production defects (β-thalassemia) can be detected [5]. The second tier is based on standard methods (such as HPLC, isoelectric focusing, and capillary electrophoresis (CE)) in order to distinguish between heterozygotes Hb F/AS (FAS) and compound heterozygotes (F/SC, F/SD, F/SE and F/S-OArab). In a single-tier procedure, only the most common variants (e.g., HbS, HbC, D^{Punjab}, OArab and HbE) are detected in a tryptic peptide analysis of haemoglobin using ESI-MS/MS [4,6–8] or the direct surface sampling of dried blood spots coupled to high-resolution MS [9–11].

In a multicentre pilot study, we evaluated a two-tier newborn SCD screening procedure in which the first tier is based on the fully automated MALDI-TOF MS classification of Hb profiles as FA, FS or FAS. To achieve this "plug-and-play" first tier, we maximised the performance levels of our previously described preanalytical and analytical procedures [5]. Likewise, we improved the software used for automatic data interpretation. Lastly, a laboratory information management system was set up to ensure data traceability. We investigated the usability of this MALDI-TOF MS newborn SCD screening platform by assessing its analytical throughput, user-friendliness, ease of implementation, potential interfering factors, MS spectral quality and percentage of correctly classified samples. We established quality criteria for standard and nonstandard MS profiles as a function of the newborn's phenotype, determined our algorithm's ability to correctly classify MS profiles and identified interfering factors and their causes. Lastly, we performed a preliminary analysis of the impact of β chain variants other than HbS on the MALDI-TOF profile. Newborns having received one or more blood transfusions were excluded from the present analysis, and are being assessed in a separate, dedicated study. Our results demonstrated the potential value of a MALDI-TOF MS approach for high-throughput newborn SCD screening.

2. Materials and Methods

2.1. Sample Collection

Residual blood spots from standard Guthrie cards (used in our laboratory's routine screening activity) were investigated with MALDI-TOF MS. All samples were collected with the parents' consent for use in the French national newborn screening programme. No additional consent was required because the specimens were not used for purposes other than for which the blood sample was initially collected. The source of the samples has been described previously [5]. The study was registered with the French National Consultative Committee on Information Processing in Medical Research (*Comité consultatif sur le traitement de l'Information en matière de recherche dans le domaine de la santé*; reference: 14.818 12/23/2014). After collection, the samples were anonymised and stored at +4 °C.

Sets of samples from our routine activity were selected each week, according to the following criteria: (i) samples presenting a β chain variant in CE and HPLC assays; (ii) samples from premature newborns (gestational age at delivery: 22–32 weeks); (iii) samples corresponding to late and very late screening; and (iv) and randomly selected samples of daily screening activity that had an interpretable CE profile.

We analyzed 6701 samples with full datasets (i.e., with clinical data as follows: N° of sample, sex, term, weight, name of maternity, transfusion, maternity location and date of screening, birth date plus validated results using CE in the first line and HPLC in the second line; Table 1). The percentage of FAS and FS phenotypes was higher for the premature newborns than for a standard population of newborns. The sample collection date was optimal (3–5 days after delivery) for the great majority of newborns.

Table 1. Characteristics of the newborns and samples.

Phenotype	Number	Characteristics of the Neonates and Samples						
		Term			Sample Collection Date			
		23–32 weeks	33–36 weeks	>37 weeks	3–5 day	6–10 day	11–30 day	>30 day
FS	71	0	5	66	67	3	1	0
F/A	2834	203	809	1822	2651	90	77	16
F/AC	576	13	50	513	547	20	2	7
F/AE	141	2	9	130	138	2	0	1
F/AO-Arab	21	0	2	19	19	2	0	0
F/AD	17	0	0	17	17	0	0	0
F/AKorle-Bu	10	0	0	10	10	0	0	0
F/AX	86	4	3	79	81	3	0	2
F/C	7	0	1	6	6	0	0	1
F/E	3	0	0	3	2	1	0	0
F/O-Arab	1	0	0	1	1	0	0	0
Corrected FA	3696	222	874	2600	3472	118	79	
F/AS	2894	57	247	2590	2763	89	23	19
F/SC	23	0	1	22	22	1	0	0
F/SE	1	0	0	1	1	0	0	0
F/SO-Arab	1	0	1	0	1	0	0	0
Corrected FAS	2919	57	249	2613	2787	90	23	19
S-β^+-thalassaemia	15	0	1	14	15	0	0	0

The number of corrected FA phenotype corresponding to the sum of all samples (FA, FAC, FAE, FAO-Arab, FAD, FAKorle-Bu, FAX, FC, FE, FO Arab where either β^A gene was duplicated [$\beta^A\beta^A$] or associated with other β chain variants ($\beta^A\beta^C$, $\beta^A\beta^E$, $\beta^A\beta^{O\text{-}Arab}$, $\beta^A\beta^D$, $\beta^A\beta^C$, $\beta^A\beta^X$) or where duplicate ß chain variants were found ($\beta^C\beta^C$, $\beta^E\beta^E$, $\beta^{O\ Arab}\beta^{O\text{-}Arab}$) that are detected FA by MALDI. The number of corrected FAS phenotype corresponding to the sum of all heterozygous (FAS) and composite heterozygous (FSC, FSE, FSO-Arab) samples where βS gene was associated respectively to βA gene or to other ß chain variants ($\beta^S\beta^C$, $\beta^S\beta^E$, $\beta^S\beta^{O\text{-}Arab}$) that are detected FAS by MALDI.

2.2. *Definition of Corrected Phenotypes*

Subjects who were heterozygous or homozygous for HbC, HbD-Punjab, HbE, HbO-Arab, HbKorle-Bu and some unidentified variants (HbX) according to conventional methods were detected as HbA by linear MALDI-TOF due to the technique's lack of mass resolution. Hence, these newborns were classified as having a corrected FA phenotype. Likewise, corrected FAS phenotypes included the composite heterozygous FSC, FSE and FS-OArab phenotypes.

2.3. *Sample Processing and Analysis*

In the present pilot study, all samples were measured with MALDI-MS at two analytical facilities (the University of Burgundy's CLIPP facility (Dijon, France) and Lille University Hospital's newborn screening laboratory (Lille, France)) after two chips (diameter: 3.5 mm) had been isolated from each blood spot.

2.4. *Sample Preparation for MS Measurements*

At both facilities, samples were prepared for MS measurements using a research version of the NeoSickle® kit (Biomaneo, Dijon, France) for an EVO 200 automated system in Dijon and an EVO 100 automated system in Lille (Tecan, Lyon, France). The NeoSickle® kit was used according to the manufacturer's instructions, which included a first step of solubilization of proteins by a specific solution, and a second step of mixing with the matrix that was specially adapted for the MALDI-TOF MS analysis of blood proteins. The sample–matrix mixture was then deposited in quadruplicate on a 384-spot polished steel MALDI target (Bruker Daltonik GmbH, Bremen, Germany).

2.5. *Mass Spectrometry Measurements*

At both facilities, MS was performed with a MALDI-TOF system (an AutoFlex™ Speed with a 2000 Hz Smartbeam™ II laser (Bruker Daltonik GmbH) in Dijon, and an AutoFlex™ III with a 200 Hz Smartbeam™ laser (Bruker Daltonik GmbH) in Lille.

2.6. Data Processing

Mass spectrometry acquisitions were analyzed by the algorithm if (i) the whole spectrum and the region of interest were sufficiently intense, (ii) the baseline was not too noisy and (iii) at least three of the four profiles per sample could be interpreted automatically. After evaluation of the quality of each spectrum, the spectra were normalized, smoothed and underwent baseline subtraction. The four spectra obtained of the same sample were then averaged to obtain a mean profile, which was submitted to the algorithm.

2.7. Analytical Data Flow

An algorithm for automatic discrimination between normal samples and samples containing an HbS variant had been developed using spectra from an initial cohort of phenotyped samples by CE and HPLC. It has since been improved as further data are acquired. All of the analytical results were centralized via a secure data collector and submitted to the algorithm. The median newborns' profiles were automatically classified as FA, FAS or FS.

2.8. Visual Assessment of MS Profiles

In order to evaluate the algorithm's ability to classify a newborn's profile as FA, FAS or FS, all of the following profiles were visually inspected: (i) samples classified as FS or FAS by CE/HPLC, (ii) samples for which MALDI-MS and CE/HPLC gave conflicting results, (iii) samples with abnormal CE and/or HPLC profiles, (iv) samples from premature newborns, (v) samples with β chain variants other than HbS, (vi) samples with low-intensity MS signals at 15,850 m/z and 15,880 m/z [5], (vii) samples with a "low HbA" warning and (viii) samples for which the Dijon and Lille facilities gave conflicting results. Lastly, half the remaining samples (classified as FA by both HPLC and CE) were checked at random.

2.9. The Data Collector

Sickle Cell Anemia Collect & Compare (SCACC) is a web application developed by Biomaneo to help biologists compare MS screening results with those of the reference screening methods (CE and HPLC). Within a single application, SCACC can store, group and present heterogeneous data in a user-friendly way, including clinical data on the sample donor, the experimental data from CE and HPLC analyses, the experimental data from the MS analysis and the validation files (i.e., the screening results sent to the paediatrician).

The SCACC application contains a table in which all of the information available for a given sample is shown on a single line. Along with a filter system for each variable, this layout makes it easy to create pools of interest (preterm samples, pathologic results, etc.) for the analysis of any misinterpreted results.

3. Results

3.1. Optimization of Preanalytical and Analytical Procedures

In France, newborn SCD screening is centralized at a few specialist analytical centres. This centralisation requires a very-high-throughput system capable of analyzing 600–1000 samples per day. The MALDI-TOF MS approach meets this requirement: for each run, it takes 1 h to deposit 288 samples in quadruplicate on three 384-spot MALDI targets.

Using an AutoFlex™ Speed system, it took 22 min to analyze a MALDI target containing 96 samples. Hence, the analytical throughput was estimated to be around 210 samples/hour; it took 5 h to analyze 1056 samples.

One of the essential criteria for automation was easy operation of the software that controlled the platform and displayed the results. A technician with little experience of MS could perform analyses on the MALDI-TOF MS system interfaced with the workstation. Another strong point is that all of the data from an analytical run were published and aggregated into a 96-well plate format. Abnormal profiles were differentiated from normal profiles by a colour code. Three different icons can be showed within a given coloured square: a cross indicating that the profile could not be interpreted, an exclamation mark indicating that the profile's initial automatic classification has been modified manually or a question mark indicating that the profile did not match the phenotype and must be checked by the operator. The spectrum's region of interest can be displayed in a mode in which β, βS and γ chains are seen or in a zoom mode in which only the β and βS chains are seen (Figure 1). The abnormal MS profiles were assessed visually by the operator. When applicable, two decision-support warnings could be displayed by the algorithm: "low HbA concentration" or "newborn having received a blood transfusion". The data for a given newborn (ID number, demographic data, zoom mode or not, classification changes and non-hidden alerts) can be displayed by clicking on a well.

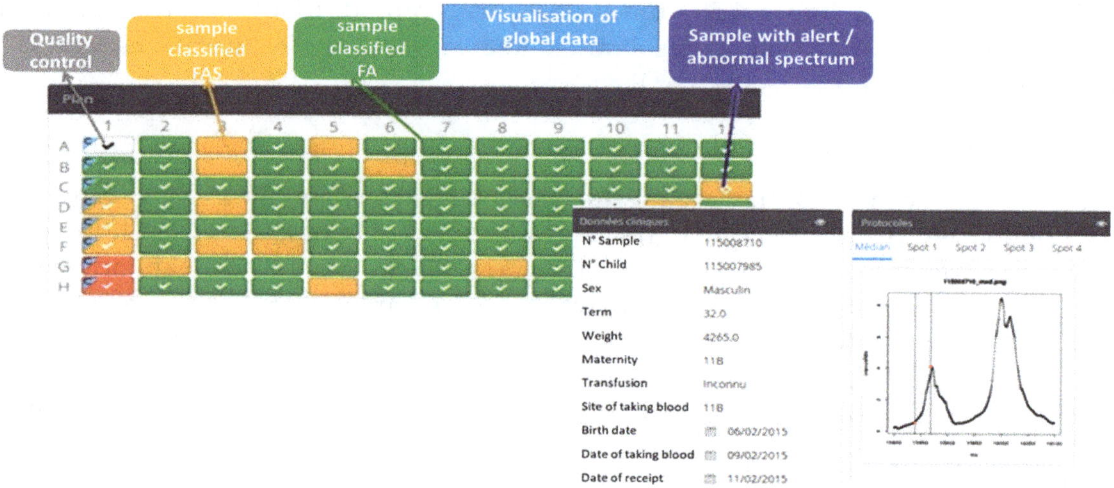

Figure 1. A screen display from the Sickle Cell Anemia Collect & Compare (SCACC) web application. Each box corresponds to a position of a sample on the 96-well plate. The green box corresponds to one sample classified FA, the orange box corresponds to one sample classified FAS and the red boxes are samples detected as FS. The software presents on the same page the clinical data (N° of sample, sex, term, weight, name of maternity, transfusion, location and date of taking blood, birth date) and the spectra of one sample.

3.2. *Spectral Quality of MALDI-TOF Data*

Taken as a whole, our results show NeoSickle®'s ability to correctly classify 97% of the samples tested in Lille and 98.8% of the samples tested in Dijon. The sensitivity of the NeoSickle® approaches to detect the FA samples is 99.2% and 97.2% with a specificity of 99% and 99.3% on the Lille and the Dijon MS facility, respectively. The detection of an HbS chain in samples is obtained on the Lille and the Dijon MS facility with a sensitivity of 98.4% and 97% and with a specificity of 99.8% and 99%, respectively.

The positive predictive value of FS profiles detection was 96.6% and 97.7% with the results obtained by the Lille and the Dijon MS facility, respectively. The negative predictive value of FS profiles detection obtained at Lille and the Dijon MS facility was 100% and 99.9%, respectively.

It is important to note that these results were obtained with biased blood samples that were enriched in FS and FAS samples and difficult samples (premature newborns, very late screening).

3.2.1. Criteria Used to Define a Standard MALDI-TOF Profile

In 85.8% of the analyses in Dijon and 92.9% of the analyses in Lille, the median FA, FAS, FS and S-β^{+} MS profiles (Figure 2a,c,e,g, respectively) were considered to be standard and were automatically interpreted by the NeoSickle® software. Limits not to be exceeded were defined: an FA profile with a low-noise ascending or convex baseline was considered to be normal (Figure 2b); an FAS profile was considered to be standard as long as a plateau separated the β^{S} and β^{A} chain peaks (Figure 2d);

and, lastly, an FS profile with a low-noise ascending or convex baseline to the right of the β^S chain peak was considered to be interpretable (Figure 2f). The profile of a newborn with S-β^+-thalassemia was characterized by a much more intense β^S peak, relative to the β^A peak (Figure 2g,h).

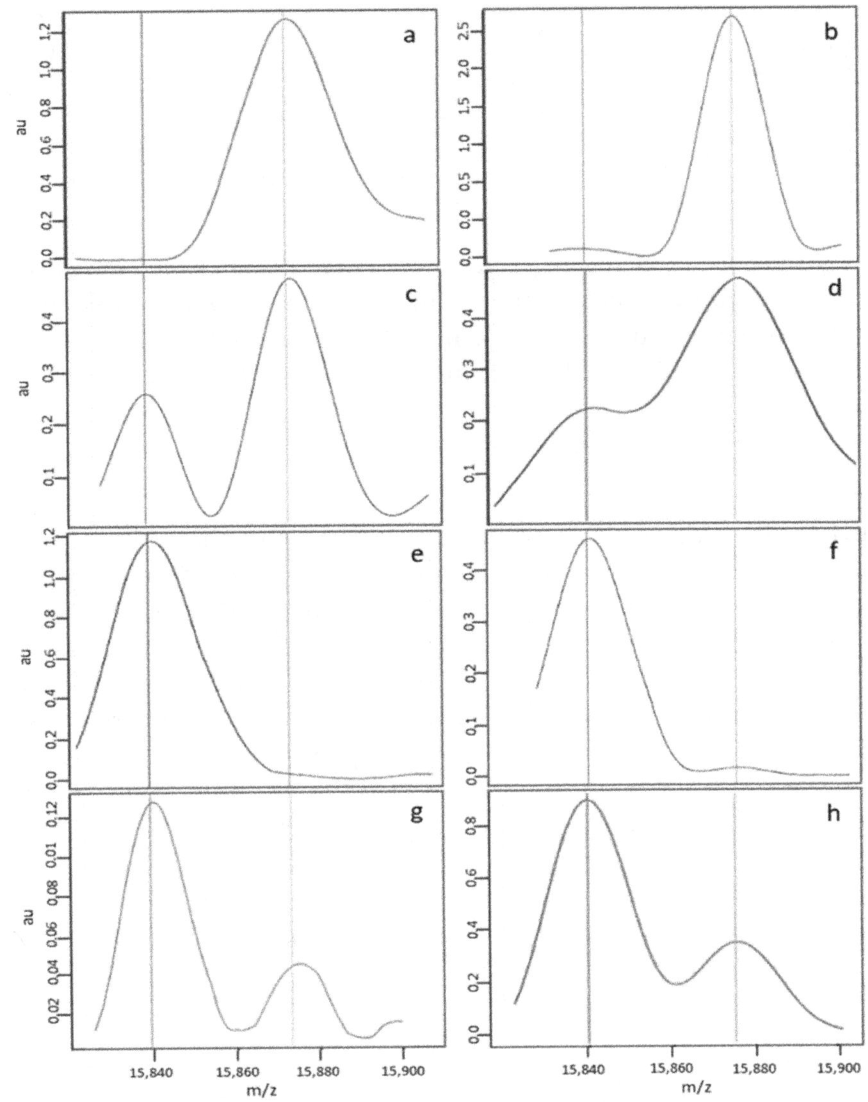

Figure 2. Examples of standard MS profiles correctly classified by the NeoSickle® software, from newborns with the following phenotypes: FA (**a**,**b**), FAS (**c**,**d**), FS (**e**,**f**) and S-β + (**g**,**h**).

3.2.2. Classification by the Algorithm of "Standard" Profiles, as a Function of the Newborn's Corrected Phenotype

There were no classification errors among the corrected FA and FS samples (Table 2). Concerning the corrected FAS samples, only 2 of the 2753 standard profiles from Lille were misclassified (as FS) by MS, and 17 of the 2507 standard profiles from Dijon were misclassified (16 cases classified as FA by MS, and 1 case classified as FS by MS). Although the spectra of the FAS samples misclassified as FA showed a shoulder with a plateau at 15,850 $m/z \pm 10$ m/z, the signal intensity was too low. This characteristic should be introduced in the criteria for a nonstandard MS profile.

The FAS samples misclassified as FS by MALDI-MS came from composite heterozygous newborns classified as FS-O Arab and FSE by CE and HPLC. Regular peaks at 18,850 and 1880 m/z were observed; however, the error was induced by the low intensity of the peak at 15,880 m/z. A profile with asymmetry for the β^A and β^S chains (a more intense β^S peak) prompted its classification as FS by the e-NeoSickle software.

Table 2. The number of standard MS profiles correctly classified (+) or misclassified (−), according to the newborn's corrected phenotype.

	Lille MS Facility						Dijon MS Facility					
Number of Standard Profiles	**6181**						**5698**					
Corrected Phenotype	**FA**		**FAS**		**FS**		**FA**		**FAS**		**FS**	
Number of samples	3386		2753		37		3161		2507		35	
classification by the algorithm	+	−	+	−	+	−	+	−	+	−	+	−
	3386	0	2751	2	37	0	3161	0	2490	17	35	0

The 16 samples misclassified in Dijon gave good results in Lille, indicating that the errors were probably due to a temporary lack of spectrum quality and not a sample or detection problem. The quality of the Dijon data was not as high as in Lille because the number of nonstandard spectra was higher; this finding agrees with the higher misclassification rate observed in Dijon.

3.2.3. Description of a Nonstandard MALDI-MS Profile

A nonstandard median MS profile was detected in 14.7% of the analyses in Dijon and 7.6% of the analyses in Lille. The MS profiles were considered to be nonstandard (Figure 3) for one of three reasons. Firstly (cause 1, see Table 3), some profiles had a nonregular baseline or a slightly distorted peak; this applied to (i) FA MS profiles with a variably broad/sharp/distorted peak but very low intensity at 15,837 $m/z \pm 5$ Da, relative to the β^A peak (Figure 3a,b); an FAS MS profile with minor deformation of the β^S peak (Figure 3c); and FS and S-β^+-thalassemia MS profiles with an irregular baseline (data not shown) and a deformation of the β^A peak (Figure 3d). Secondly (cause 2), some profiles had a low, broad peak at 15,837 m/z; this applied to (i) FA MS profiles with a variably shifted peak or (ii) FAS MS profiles characterized by a broad, well-centred peak at 15,837 $\pm$ 5 m/z but that was much less intense than the β^A chain peak at 15,867 m/z (data not shown). Thirdly (cause 3), some FA MS profiles had a broader β^A peak that variably overlapped with the region of interest at 15,837 m/z and led to misclassification as "FAS" (Figure 3e), whereas other FAS MS profiles showed a low resolution and thus poor separation of the β^A and β^S peaks, giving a single large peak as a shoulder and no plateau between the peaks (Figure 3f).

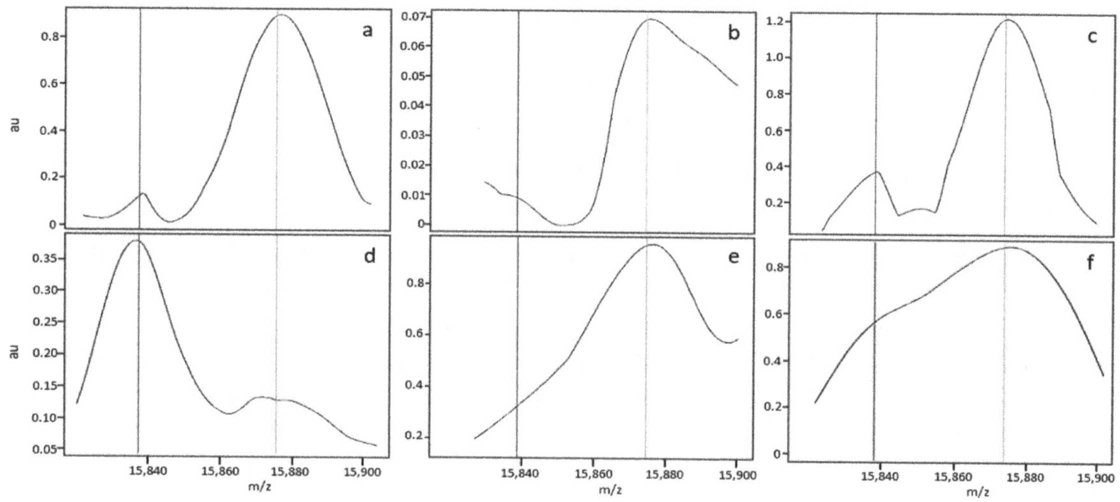

Figure 3. Zoom of MS profiles on the zone of interest for nonstandard FA (**a**,**b**,**e**), FAS (**c**,**f**) and FS (**d**) samples.

3.2.4. Classification by the Algorithm of Profiles Considered to be Nonstandard in a Visual Assessment, as a Function of the Newborn's Corrected Phenotype

The data in Table 3 show that the great majority of nonstandard profiles (84.5% in Lille and 81.2% in Dijon) were nevertheless correctly classified by the e-NeoSickle® algorithm. Furthermore, 7.5% of the nonstandard profiles in Lille and 4.6% of the nonstandard profiles Dijon were misclassified, and 8% of the nonstandard profiles in Lille and 14.2% of the nonstandard profiles in Dijon were uninterpretable.

It is important to note that the nonstandard profiles accounted for less than 14% of the analyses in Dijon and 7% of the analyses in Lille. Overall, only 2% of the profiles in Dijon and 0.6% of the profiles in Lille were uninterpretable, and 0.9% of the profiles in Dijon and 0.6% of the profiles in Lille were misclassified.

Table 3. Classification by the algorithm of profiles considered to be nonstandard in a visual assessment. Some spectra could not be interpreted by the algorithm (IN). The percentage is based on the number of profiles considered to be nonstandard (780 profiles at Lille and 985 at Dijon).

			Corrected Phenotypes		
			FA	**FAS**	**FS**
MALDI-TOF MS classification of non-standard profiles	Lille	FA	282 (54.7%)	30 (5.9%)	0 (0%)
MALDI-TOF MS classification of non-standard profiles	Lille	FAS	7 (1.4%)	118 (23.2%)	0 (0%)
MALDI-TOF MS classification of non-standard profiles	Lille	FS	0 (0%)	1 (0.2%)	34 (6.7%)
MALDI-TOF MS classification of non-standard profiles	Lille	IN	21 (4.5%)	17 (3.4%)	0 (0%)
MALDI-TOF MS classification of non-standard profiles	Dijon	FA	446 (45%)	22 (2.2%)	0 (0%)
MALDI-TOF MS classification of non-standard profiles	Dijon	FAS	21 (2.2%)	323 (32.7%)	1 (0.2%)
MALDI-TOF MS classification of non-standard profiles	Dijon	FS	0 (0%)	1 (0.2%)	36 (3.7%)
MALDI-TOF MS classification of non-standard profiles	Dijon	IN	68 (7.2%)	67 (6.8%)	0 (0%)

The frequencies of "nonregular baseline" (cause 1) and "low/broad peak" (cause 2) features were similar at the two MS facilities. Our analysis showed that most of the nonstandard spectra in Dijon (54%) were due to a lack of resolution (cause 3), whereas this was the case for only 13% in Lille. Proportionally, the corrected phenotype FS ($n = 71$) was more likely to be labelled as "low resolution", with respectively 31 and 36 abnormal spectra in Lille and Dijon. However, this low resolution had very little impact on the automatic classification, since less than 1% of all spectra labelled as "low resolution" were misclassified.

Sixteen percent of the spectra with a low, broad peak at 15,837 m/z were misclassified by the algorithm (Table 4). Of the 21 spectra of this type misclassified in Lille, 20 (95%) came from newborns with a corrected FAS phenotype. Likewise, of the 20 spectra of this type misclassified in Dijon (Table 4), 18 (90%) came from newborns with a corrected FAS phenotype. These spectra were very difficult to classify because the ratio between the β^S and β^A peaks was abnormal. A very low β^S peak (relative to the β^A peak) can be interpreted as a sample with high background noise or as a sample from an S homozygote or an AS heterozygote having received a blood transfusion (which induces a strong imbalance). Given that these spectra have low peak intensities, we recommend repeating the analysis or depositing a new sample.

Table 4. (A) Numbers and proportions of nonstandard spectra by corrected phenotype and by cause. (B) Numbers and proportions of correctly classified and misclassified spectra by cause. Cause 1 resulted in spectra with an irregular baseline, cause 2 resulted in spectra with a low, broad peak and cause 3 resulted in spectra with a low resolution. The percentage is based on the number of profiles considered to be nonstandard (780 profiles at Lille and 985 at Dijon).

A		Corrected Phenoztype		
		FA	FAS	FS
Lille	Cause 1	179 (37%)	90 (19%)	3 (0%)
	Cause 2	98 (21%)	28 (5%)	0 (0%)
	Cause 3	12 (3%)	31 (7%)	31 (7%)
Dijon	Cause 1	193 (23%)	69 (8%)	0 (0%)
	Cause 2	103 (12%)	24 (3%)	0 (0%)
	Cause 3	171 (20%)	253 (30%)	36 (4%)

B		Correctly Classified	Misclassified
Lille	Cause 1	252 (94%)	17 (6%)
	Cause 2	105 (84%)	21 (16%)
	Cause 3	77 (100%)	0 (0%)
Dijon	Cause 1	248 (95%)	14 (5%)
	Cause 2	107 (84%)	20 (16%)
	Cause 3	449 (98%)	11 (2%)

3.2.5. Causes of Abnormal Spectral Features in Nonstandard MS Profiles

A spectral analysis showed that nonstandard profiles mainly resulted from the compilation of differing spectra within a quadruplicate. Figure 4 shows the variability in the raw data and its impact on data processing. The spectra in Figure 4a,b,e,f correspond to the raw data generated for the first (Figure 4a,b) and third (Figure 4e,f) of the quadruplicate sample depositions. The two depositions varied markedly in terms of the raw spectral intensity (less than 40 ua for deposition 1, and 200 ua for deposition 3). The data processing steps (including peak alignment and baseline normalisation and subtraction) normalise the spectrum intensity but also remove differences (see Figure 4c,g, corresponding to the normalized spectra, and a blow-up view of the zone of interest Figure 4d,h). The compilation of normalized data introduces a bias, and might lead to misinterpretation of the results by the software. Figure 4i shows a median spectrum with an irregular baseline; this "pseudo β^S peak" can be confused with a true β^S peak. However, the relative intensity of the pseudo β^S peak differed from that of a true β^A peak.

The analysis of each individual spectrum enabled us to affirm that at least one good-quality, high-resolution spectrum was obtained for each biological sample. The sample deposition method for MALDI-MS is known not to be highly reproducible, and thus makes it difficult to obtain very homogeneous results. Even though our study highlighted this difficulty, our analysis also showed that a high-quality result can be obtained systematically.

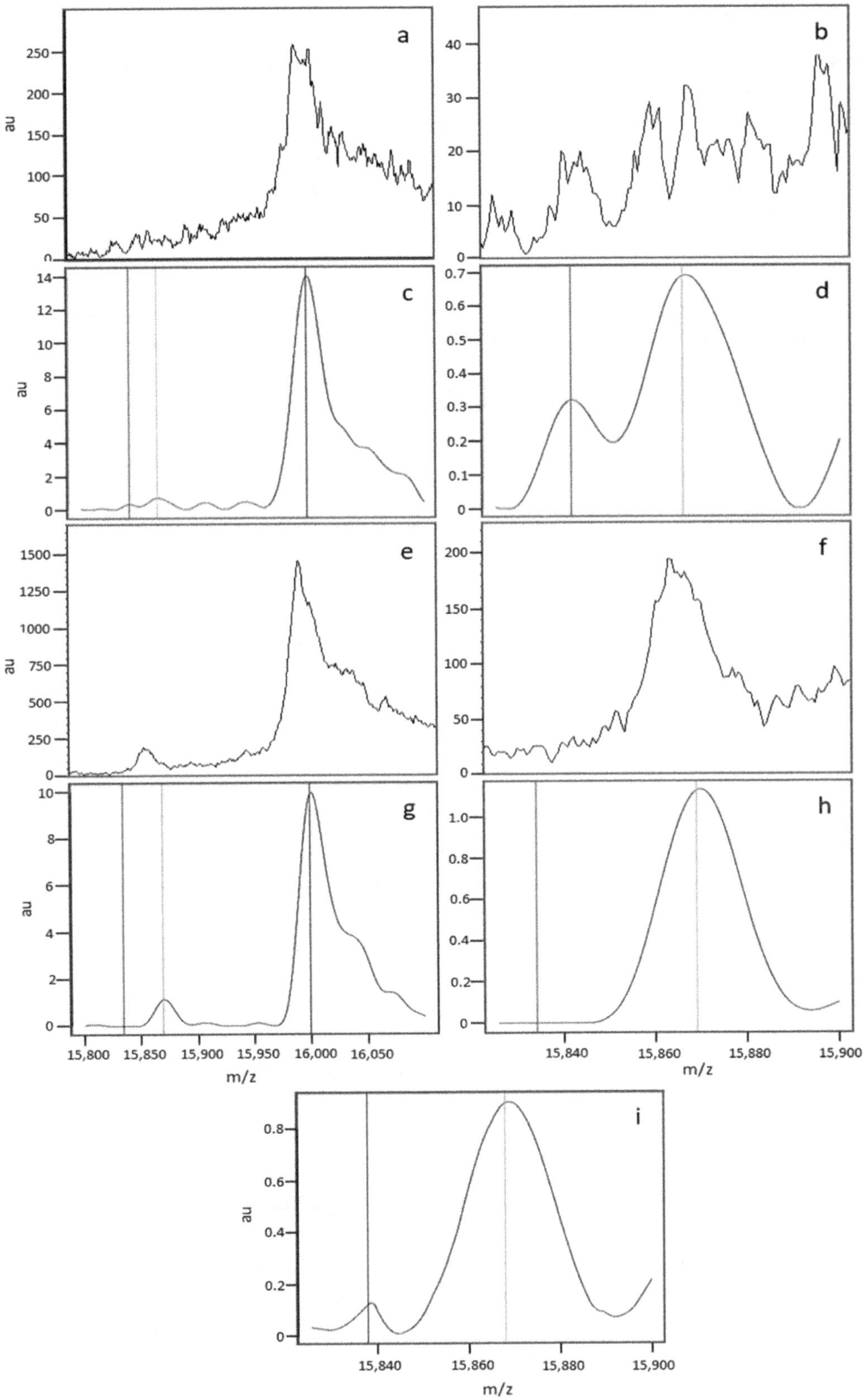

Figure 4. The spectra in (**a**,**b**,**e**,**f**) correspond to the raw data generated for the first (**a**,**b**) and third (**e**,**f**) of the quadruplicate depositions from the same sample. (**a**,**c**,**e**,**g**) show the whole spectrum (15,800–16,100 Da), and (**b**–**f**,**h**,**i**) show the region of interest (15,820–15,900 Da). The spectra in (**c**–**h** correspond to the processed spectra after alignment, baseline subtraction, and normalisation. The median spectrum (**i**) was obtained by compiling the individual normalized spectra.

4. Occasional Misclassifications

The analysis of samples that were classified differently by the two analytical facilities confirmed that MALDI-MS can provide an interpretable result for each sample. In fact, the data in Table 5 showed that the 68 samples with a corrected FA phenotype that could not be interpreted in Dijon were correctly classified in Lille (67 standard spectra and 1 low-resolution spectrum). Likewise, the 21 samples with a corrected FA phenotype and that could not be interpreted in Lille were correctly classified at Dijon. Identical results were obtained with the corrected FAS samples.

Table 5. Paired classification of the samples by the two analytical facilities. Relationship with the spectral quality. This table summarizes the number of profiles correctly classified, misclassified and uninterpretable for each category of profile quality and for the two analytical laboratories.

Profile Abnormalities at 15,850 ± 10 *m/z*											
Neonates with a Corrected FA Phenotype											
Automatic Classification of Matched Profiles		**Irregular Base Line**		**Low, Broad Peak**		**Low Resolution**		**Regular Base Line**		**Uninterpretable**	
Lille	**Dijon**	**Lille**	**Dijon**	**Lille**	**Dijon**	**Lille**	**Dijon**	**Lille**	**Dijon**	**Lille**	**Dijon**
correctly classified	uninterpretable	1	0	0	0	0	0	67	0	0	68
correctly classified	Misclassified	4	10	7	0	1	5	17	0	0	0
uninterpretable	correctly classified	0	0	0	0	0	0	0	21	0	0
Misclassified	correctly classified	4	0	3	0	0	0	0	7	0	0
Neonates with a Corrected FAS Phenotype											
Automatic Classification of Matched Profiles		**Irregular Base Line**		**Low, Broad Peak**		**Low Resolution**		**Regular Base Line**		**Uninterpretable**	
Lille	**Dijon**	**Lille**	**Dijon**	**Lille**	**Dijon**	**Lille**	**Dijon**	**Lille**	**Dijon**	**Lille**	**Dijon**
correctly classified	uninterpretable	0	0	0	0	0	0	68	0	0	68
correctly classified	Misclassified	0	4	0	14	1	5	23	0	0	0
uninterpretable	correctly classified	0	0	0	0	0	1	0	16	17	0
Misclassified	correctly classified	12	0	12	0	0	4	6	26	0	0

When a profile was misclassified or uninterpretable at one MS facility, the corresponding profile at the other MS facility was correctly classified and was less likely to be a nonstandard profile. Only one sample with a nonstandard profile was misclassified at both MS facilities (data not shown). A good classification with a standard spectrum was obtained for each sample on at least one of the MS facilities, which indicates that a low HbA concentration was not the main cause of misclassifications or uninterpretable results. Misclassifications or uninterpretable results were mainly due to the absence of a high-quality spectrum induced by technical incidents (tip blockage and non-deposition of the sample). Consequently, repeating the analysis of a sample with a nonstandard profile was the best way of obtaining a standard profile and a correct classification. Different data, such as peak intensities or the ratio between different peaks of β^A and β^S chains, allow for us to detect the nonstandard profile and to add an alert to the results.

5. Discussion

Newborn disease screening programmes are front-line public health measures, and as such must be based on robust analytical methods and data-processing software. Cost effectiveness is a further requirement, prompting the implementation of high-throughput screening units that reduce unit costs. Lastly, the maximal use of automation enables the analytical results to be validated with as little intervention as possible by the medical team. Our MALDI-MS platform and the associated data-processing and interpretation software were designed to address these challenges.

In newborn SCD screening with a MALDI MS system, the user-friendliness of the software interface and a high-throughput analysis coupled to automatic sample classification and traceability are directly related to practicability. As mentioned above, newborn SCD screening in France is centralised at a few specialist analytical centres. This centralisation requires a throughput of up to 600–1000 samples per day. The MALDI-TOF MS approach meets this requirement.

The next performance criterion of note concerns the method's robustness: in other words, its ability to generate good-quality standard MS profiles that enable correct classification in agreement with the sample's validated phenotype, whatever the newborn's clinical status. In order to test our MALDI-MS under extreme conditions, we increased the proportion of difficult samples in the presently analyzed cohort; this corresponds to pathological specimens and specimens collected and/or stored under non-optimal conditions (samples from premature newborns, samples collected long after delivery, samples collected from France's overseas regions and dependencies that may have been stored for a long time in a tropical atmosphere before delivery to the screening laboratory in continental France, etc.). In the present study, only samples from newborns having received one or more blood transfusions were discarded. The impact of blood transfusion will be described in a specific study of the effect of high HbA levels on the method's sensitivity, specificity and resolution as a function of the β^s chain concentration. Moreover, we evaluated the MALDI-TOF method's robustness by visually checking the spectral quality as well as by considering its ability to correctly classify the newborns as FA, FAS or FS. Benchmark MALDI-TOF MS spectra were thus established on the basis of the classification results and the visual quality of the spectra. The reference spectra correspond to all of the spectra defined as standard for which the information obtained is considered to be sufficient and of good quality. Indeed, visual spectral validation has proved to be most effective for revealing shot-to-shot variations.

Using this strategy, we determined the percentages of newborns with a standard profile and who were correctly classified (relative to their validated phenotype). The highest level of efficiency was obtained in the set of newborns with a corrected FA phenotype; around 85% of these analyses could be validated directly. A similar percentage was obtained for newborns with a corrected FAS phenotype. Moreover, nonstandard MS spectra were not systematically misclassified, and most were correctly classified. We consider these results to be very promising because it should be possible to further improve the procedures for sample deposition, raw data analysis and selection of the mass spectra to which the classification algorithm is applied.

None of the samples from FS newborns were misclassified, and a sample with an FAS-corrected phenotype was misclassified as an FA sample. This type of misclassification can lead to false negatives for newborns with an FSC phenotype. This major error required us to set up a strategy for correcting the automatic classification. The development and characteristics of tracking alerts for the nonstandard MS profiles will be described elsewhere. This approach should enable an occasional lack of reproducibility, sensitivity or resolution in Hb profiling to be detected.

There were two main reasons for the incorrect automatic classification of newborn phenotypes. Firstly, a low signal intensity at 15,850 and/or 15,880 m/z (i.e., similar to background noise) was intensified by the data processing (normalisation and alignment). Secondly, poor resolution of the ß and/or β^S chains generated signal overlap. The quadruplicate sample analysis improved the results, but was not always able to counterbalance shot-to-shot variability.

In a previous article [5], very poor spectral quality prevented the analysis of 20 of 844 samples (2.5%), even after several repeat analyses. The relatively high frequency of this incident was probably due to the inclusion of a high proportion of samples from premature newborns and/or HbS carriers. We have now resolved this problem. In most cases, a single repeat analysis was enough to obtain a standard profile. Some problems arose from time to time but were mainly related to robotic preparation of the blood spot samples. Further optimization of sample processing and the MS acquisition protocol should further improve the standardization of the MS profiles and reduce the frequency of repeat analysis.

Taken as a whole, our results for pooled standard and nonstandard spectra demonstrated NeoSickle®'s ability to classify correctly 97% of the samples tested in Lille and 98.8% of the samples tested in Dijon. Furthermore, only 2% of the nonstandard spectra in Dijon were uninterpretable, and less than 0.9% were misclassified. In Lille, 0.6% of the nonstandard spectra were uninterpretable and 0.6% were misclassified. It is important to note that these percentages were obtained with "difficult" blood samples (premature newborns, very late screening).

Our pilot study showed that the NeoSickle® approach can differentiate between heterozygous FSE, FSO-Arab and S-β + samples on one hand and heterozygous FAS and homozygous FS samples on the other. Indeed, the signal intensity of the β^E, $\beta^{O\text{-}Arab}$ variants was much weaker than that of the β chain.

In addition to classifying samples as FA, FAS or FS, studies of a larger cohort of patients might make it possible to clearly differentiate a fourth class (corresponding to heterozygous SX samples in which the β^X chain is E, O-Arab, a).

In conclusion, our new MALDI-TOF MS approach already meets today's requirements [12] for large-scale, cost-effective newborn SCD screening, and is well-positioned to address future requirements for even greater throughputs and total automation to detect the HbS variants.

Author Contributions: D.R. and M.E.O.: MALDI-TOF methodology; P.N.: software development; G.R. and O.G.: validation; P.D. and J.-M.P.: conceptualization, data curation, acquisition of funding and drafting of the manuscript.

References

1. Rai, D.K.; Griffiths, W.J.; Landin, B.; Wild, B.J.; Alvelius, G.; Green, B.N. Accurate mass measurement by electrospray ionization quadrupole mass spectrometry: Detection of variants differing by <6 Da from normal in human hemoglobin heterozygotes. *Anal. Chem.* **2003**, *75*, 1978–1982. [CrossRef] [PubMed]
2. Wild, B.J.; Green, B.N.; Cooper, E.K.; Lalloz, M.R.; Erten, S.; Stephens, A.D.; Layton, D.M. Rapid identification of hemoglobin variants by electrospray ionization mass spectrometry. *Blood Cells Mol. Dis.* **2001**, *27*, 691–704. [CrossRef] [PubMed]
3. Wild, B.J.; Green, B.N.; Stephens, A.D. The potential of electrospray ionization mass spectrometry for the diagnosis of hemoglobin variants found in newborn screening. *Blood Cells Mol. Dis.* **2004**, *33*, 308–317. [CrossRef] [PubMed]
4. Kiernan, U.A.; Black, J.A.; Williams, P.; Nelson, R.W. High-throughput analysis of hemoglobin from neonates using matrix-assisted laser desorption/ionization time-of-flight mass spectrometry. *Clin. Chem.* **2002**, *48*, 947–949. [PubMed]
5. Hachani, J.; Duban-Deweer, S.; Pottiez, G.; Renom, G.; Flahaut, C.; Périni, J.M. MALDI-TOF MS profiling as the first-tier screen for sickle cell disease in neonates: Matching throughput to objectives. *Proteomics Clin. Appl.* **2011**, *5*, 405–414. [CrossRef] [PubMed]
6. Daniel, Y.A.; Turner, C.; Haynes, R.M.; Hunt, B.J.; Dalton, R.N. Rapid and specific detection of clinically significant haemoglobinopathies using electrospray mass spectrometry-mass spectrometry. *Br. J. Haematol.* **2005**, *130*, 635–643. [CrossRef] [PubMed]
7. Boemer, F.; Ketelslegers, O.; Minon, J.M.; Bours, V.; Schoos, R. Newborn screening for sickle cell disease using tandem mass spectrometry. *Clin. Chem.* **2008**, *54*, 2036–2041. [CrossRef] [PubMed]
8. Moat, S.J.; Rees, D.; King, L.; Ifederu, A.; Harvey, K.; Hall, K.; Lloyd, G.; Morrell, C.; Hillier, S. Newborn blood spot screening for sickle cell disease by using tandem mass spectrometry: Implementation of a protocol to identify only the disease states of sickle cell disease. *Clin. Chem.* **2014**, *60*, 373–380. [CrossRef] [PubMed]
9. Edwards, R.L.; Griffiths, P.; Bunch, J.; Cooper, H.J. Compound heterozygotes and beta-thalassemia: Top-down mass spectrometry for detection of hemoglobinopathies. *Proteomics* **2014**, *14*, 1232–1238. [CrossRef] [PubMed]
10. Edwards, R.L.; Griffiths, P.; Bunch, J.; Cooper, H.J. Top-down proteomics and direct surface sampling of neonatal dried blood spots: Diagnosis of unknown hemoglobin variants. *J. Am. Soc. Mass Spectrom.* **2012**, *23*, 1921–1930. [CrossRef] [PubMed]
11. Edwards, R.L.; Creese, A.J.; Baumert, M.; Griffiths, P.; Bunch, J.; Cooper, H.J. Hemoglobin variant analysis via direct surface sampling of dried blood spots coupled with high-resolution mass spectrometry. *Anal. Chem.* **2011**, *15*, 2265–2270. [CrossRef] [PubMed]
12. Lobitz, S.; Telfer, P.; Cela, E.; Allaf, B.; Angastiniotis, M.; Backman Johansson, C.; Badens, C.; Bento, C.; Bouva, M.J.; Canatan, D.; et al. Newborn screening for sickle cell disease in Europe: Recommendations from a Pan-European consensus conference. *Br. J. Haematol.* **2018**. [CrossRef] [PubMed]

14

Processing Newborn Bloodspot Screening Results for CF

Jürg Barben [1,*] and Jane Chudleigh [2]

1 Division of Paediatric Pulmonology & CF Centre, Children's Hospital of Eastern Switzerland, 9006 St. Gallen, Switzerland
2 School of Health Sciences, City, University of London, London EC1V 0HB, UK; j.chudleigh@city.ac.uk
* Correspondence: juerg.barben@kispisg.ch;

Abstract: Every newborn bloodspot screening (NBS) result for cystic fibrosis (CF) consists of two parts: a screening part in the laboratory and a clinical part in a CF centre. When introducing an NBS programme, more attention is usually paid to the laboratory part, especially which algorithm is most suitable for the region or the country. However, the clinical part, how a positive screening result is processed, is often underestimated and can have great consequences for the affected child and their parents. A clear algorithm for the diagnostic part in CF centres is also important and influences the performance of a CF NBS programme. The processing of a positive screening result includes the initial information given to the parents, the invitation to the sweat test, what to do if a sweat test fails, information about the results of the sweat test, the inconclusive diagnosis and the carrier status, which is handled differently from country to country. The time until the definitive diagnosis and adequate information is given, is considered by the parents and the CF team as the most important factor. The communication of a positive NBS result is crucial. It is not a singular event but rather a process that includes ensuring the appropriate clinicians are aware of the result and that families are informed in the most efficient and effective manner to facilitate consistent and timely follow-up.

Keywords: cystic fibrosis; newborn screening; presumptive diagnosis; sweat test; parental information

---

1. Introduction

Many countries have now introduced newborn bloodspot screening (NBS) for cystic fibrosis (CF) using a large variety of protocols [1,2]. After proper collection of the dried blood spot specimen, each NBS programme consists of a screening part in the laboratory and a diagnostic part in a CF centre. Most NBS programmes use a 2- or 3-step procedure in the laboratory, with the measurement of immunoreactive trypsinogen (IRT) being the first step [2]. The choice of the second step depends on the presence of CF transmembrane conductance regulator (CFTR) mutations, the health care system and the legislation of a country. Most programs today have CFTR determination as the second step; some use pancreatitis-associated protein (PAP) determination or a second IRT measurement. Therefore, the definition of a positive NBS screening result is handled slightly differently depending on the algorithm used. Like any other screening programme, a positive NBS result requires a confirmatory diagnosis, which for CF is done by means of a sweat test [3]. In accordance with WHO screening guidelines [4], the aim of every NBS programme is to detect children with CF as early as possible and to initiate the appropriate treatment. This means that the sweat test and a clinical evaluation should be performed as soon as possible in an experienced CF centre so that children with a confirmed CF diagnosis can be treated as early as possible. According to the current ECFS guidelines, infants with a confirmed diagnosis after NBS should be seen by the CF specialist team within one month (and no later than 58 days after birth) [3,5]. At the same time, false-positive screening results leading to recalls and sweat tests should be minimised as far as possible. The procedure following a positive NBS result (initial information to parents, invitation to the sweat test, information on the results of the sweat test, inconclusive diagnosis and carrier status) is different from country to country. For parents, the waiting period until the final diagnosis and information adapted to their knowledge is the most important part of the screening process [6]. In a survey of CF specialists, timeliness was also deemed very important by all respondents to ensure that children and their families were seen as soon as possible after receiving the initial positive NBS result [7].

2. Sweat Test—The Gold Standard Confirmation Test of a Positive NBS Result

It has been acknowledged that diagnosing CF is complex and that despite consensus guidelines being published on the diagnosis of CF, there is evidence that these are not applied consistently [3,5]. To confirm a positive NBS result, the determination of chloride concentration in the sweat is still considered the gold standard, because it investigates the function of the chloride channel, which is crucial in CF [8,9]. Most screened infants have little or no clinical manifestation of the disease, making sweat testing the main diagnostic tool to discriminate between children with and without CF [3,5,8,10]. A positive NBS result always requires a confirmatory sweat test, as there may be laboratory errors (mix-up of samples) or the two CFTR mutations detected in the genetic test are on the same allele [3,11]. The diagnostic algorithm of sweat testing is shown in Figure 1 [12].

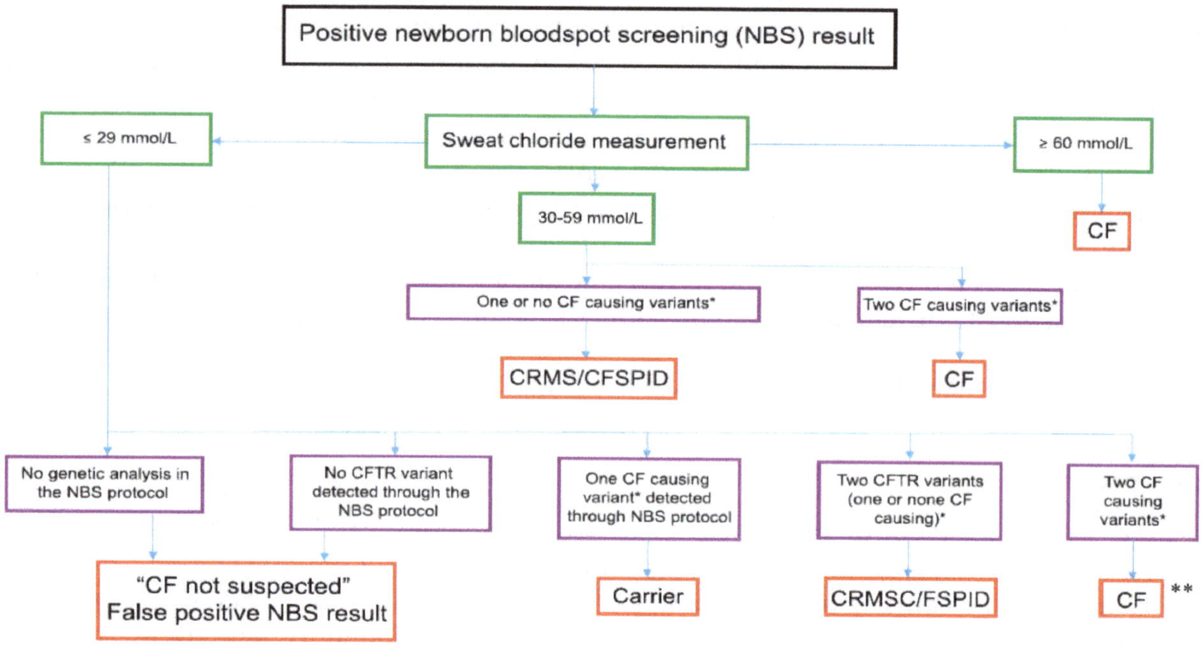

Figure 1. Adapted from reference [12] An algorithm for the designation of infants following a positive newborn bloodspot screening (NBS) result. (CF, cystic fibrosis; CFTR, CF transmembrane conductance regulator (gene); CRMS, CFTR-related metabolic syndrome; CFSPID, CF screen positive, inconclusive diagnosis; CRMS/CFSPID, harmonised definition). * Characterised by the CFTR2 website. ** If two CF causing mutations are present, a repetition of a sweat test is not necessary, but the parents should be genetically tested to exclude the presence of variants in the *cis* form.

However, sweat collection in infants is challenging and must be performed according to current guidelines [9,13,14]. A sufficient amount of sweat is needed to determine the chloride concentration; the smaller the children are or the lighter they are, the more difficult it is to obtain sufficient sweat. A sweat test should not be performed in children <2 kg, and the rates of sweat collections with insufficient volume (called Quantity Not Sufficient, QNS) are below 10% if the child weighs ≥4 kg [15,16]. Collecting sweat from two sites (left and right arm), as is recommended in the US, can reduce the QNS rate. The minimal standards and the diagnostic standards for laboratories performing sweat testing according to the recently revised ECFS best practice guidelines, are listed in Tables 1 and 2 [5].

Table 1. Minimal standards for laboratories performing sweat tests (according to the ECFS Guidelines, adapted from reference [5])

1	Sweat collection by experienced personnel (at least 150 sweat tests per annum) following national or international guidelines and subject to regular (at least annual) peer review.
2	Use of commercially available equipment approved for diagnostic use according to the national regulatory requirements or EU standards if no local ones are available.
3	Internal quality control (usually three samples) with acceptable limits of agreement for chloride before each sweat analysis.
4	Regular external quality assurance for the analyses according to national guidelines.
5	A high number of QNS (Quantity Not Sufficient) rates is a marker of technical issue. This necessitates renewing training for personnel experiencing sweat tests.

Table 2. Diagnostic standards of a sweat test (according to the ECFS Guidelines, adapted from reference [5])

1	The quantity of sweat should indicate an adequate rate of sweat production (15µL for Macroduct™ tube system).
2	The sweat sample should be processed immediately after sweat collection.
3	A sweat chloride value >59 mmol/L is consistent with a diagnosis of CF.
4	A sweat chloride value <30 mmol/L makes the diagnosis of CF unlikely. However, specific CF causing mutations can be associated with a sweat test below 30 mmol/L. These include c.3718-2477C N T (3849 + 10kbC N T) and mutations associated with varied clinical consequence, such as c.617T N G (L206W), c.1040G N A (R347H) and c.3454G N C (D1152H).
5	Individuals with sweat chloride values in the borderline range (30–59 mmol/L) should undergo a repeat sweat test and further evaluation in a specialist CF centre, including detailed clinical assessment and extensive CFTR gene mutation analysis.

The recommendations of the US Cystic Fibrosis Foundation (CFF) say that the proportion of unsuccessful sweat tests in infants should be less than 10% [9,17]. In reality, the failure rate can be as high as 40% during the first three months of life. The rates of QNS samples is higher the earlier you test these children [15,17–20]. More effective NBS protocols have earlier results but higher QNS rates as babies are lighter at the time of testing.

Nowadays, the sweat collection is more frequently undertaken with a capillary tube system (Macroduct™), which was introduced in 1986 and only needs 15 µL of sweat to perform a chloride analysis [21–24]. Measuring conductivity using the Sweat-Check™ analyser has been suggested to be as effective as chloride determination in discriminating healthy children from those with CF [21,25–27]. Nanoduct™ is a newer sweat conductivity analysis system that was specially developed for newborns as it requires only 3–5 µL of sweat and measures conductivity in situ [28]. A few studies have assessed and confirmed its ability to discriminate between those affected by CF and healthy children [16,29–33]. According to current guidelines, conductivity measurement is an accepted method to rule out CF, but for a definite diagnosis, the determination of sweat chloride is required as it is better validated [9,14,24]. As the Nanoduct™ system does not require further laboratory equipment and personnel, it could have a role in remote areas where resources are limited and for ambulatory sweat testing.

3. Presumptive Diagnosis or How to Proceed if a Sweat Test Fails

In some children, a determination of the sweat chlorides is not possible because of too little sweat production (QNS). So far, most algorithms do not explain what to do when sweat tests fail. Sometimes it is delayed until the child is older or heavier and this can take weeks before a sweat test is possible, and can lead to great uncertainty among parents [6]. In the Swiss NBS programme, if a sweat test was not possible, the sweat test was initially repeated after a few weeks or months until it was successful. However, this led to longer waiting times for definite diagnosis, and anxiety among families.

After one year, the algorithm was changed, and genetic testing was directly performed after a sweat test failure. This led to greater detection of unclear cases, now called CF Screen Positive Inconclusive Diagnosis (CFSPID), but no reduction in waiting time. After that, the algorithm was again changed, and measurement of faecal elastase (FE) was introduced that significantly reduced the number of CFSPID infants being identified and improved the timeliness to start pancreatic enzyme replacement therapy (PERT) [34]. This well-documented change in diagnostic procedure highlights the fact that the algorithm for the diagnostic part of the newborn screening used in the CF centres is also important and affects the performance of a CF–NBS programme with regard to the ratio CF:CFSPID and the time until definite diagnosis. In the case of a high clinical probability of a CF diagnosis, one should not wait until the chloride result of a sweat test is available. A positive NBS for CF and a high sweat conductivity make the diagnosis of CF very likely and further investigations (determination of faecal elastase, confirm CFTR variants if necessary) should be initiated at first clinical visit. If symptoms such as lack of weight gain or steatorrhoea are present, start of PERT and salt supplements should not be delayed. A possible pathway is shown in Figure 2. In case of two CFTR variants and a negative sweat test the parents should be genetically tested to exclude the presence of variants in *cis* form. The definite confirmation of the diagnosis with a sweat chloride measurement should be performed at a later stage, as soon as the child reaches a higher weight (>4000g) [34]. This is also important because in the future, sweat chloride values will be a surrogate marker to determine the effect of CFTR modulators in early childhood.

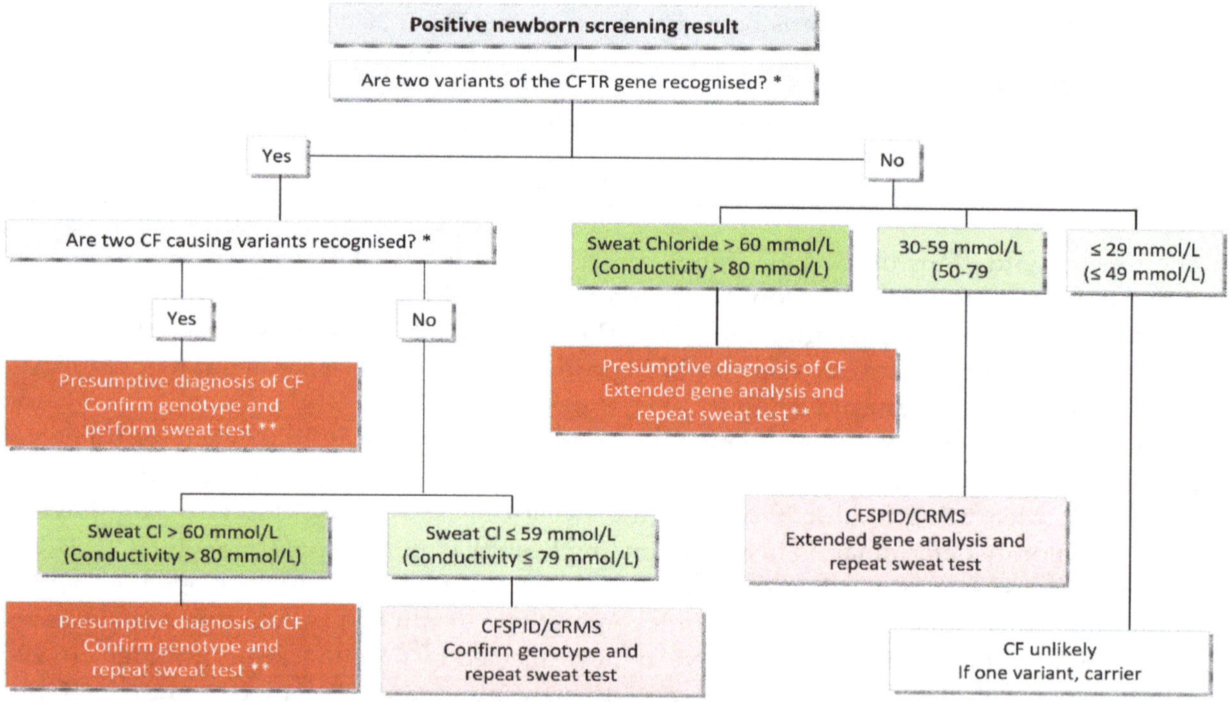

Figure 2. Diagnostic algorithm after a positive NBS result in the CF centre. * According to the CFTR2 website. ** Infants at this point have a presumptive diagnosis of CF and treatment should be established. Further testing is required to consolidate the diagnosis.

4. Unintended Effects of Newborn Screening for CF

Depending on the algorithm chosen, NBS for CF results in recognition of unclear cases, now called CFSPID. Evaluation and management of these infants can be quite challenging [35,36]. This is especially the case if the second step in the screening algorithm is to search for a large number of CFTR mutations whose clinical relevance is different or not yet known. Depending on the chosen algorithm in the diagnostic process in a CF centre, there are also more and more unclear cases [34]. These children have in most cases a favourable prognosis and there is no evidence for improvement through early treatment [37]. In these unclear cases, the disadvantages of early detection with unnecessary medicalisation and burden to the family may outweigh the benefits of early detection [38].

False-positive results are a challenge to every screening programme, since they cause parental anxiety and unnecessary medical examinations [39,40]. NBS programmes using DNA analysis in their algorithm have improved specificity but identify heterozygote carriers, which can cause some anxiety and depression in affected families [6].

False negative results are also a challenge for screening programmes, as parents may feel reassured that the screening did not show a positive result and may consider that CF has been ruled out and possibly be less likely to go to the doctor later if the symptoms are present. Even in the best performing NBS programmes, some CF-affected individuals will be missed. The extent depends on the chosen cut-off value of the initial IRT measurement (false negatives in up to 8%) and the selected algorithm in the screening phase, and needs to be balanced with achieving a reasonable positive predicted value (PPV). Children with meconium ileus may have a negative NBS result, but always require an assessment with sweat and genetic testing.

5. Consequences for Other Family Members

Once a CF diagnosis has been confirmed (or ruled out), the parents and other family members may be offered genetic screening and counselling. All siblings of a positively screened child need to be screened for CF with a sweat test. Asymptomatic adult family members may wish to be screened for carrier status to allow them to make informed choices about reproduction planning and prenatal screening. Adequate genetic counselling should also be arranged or made available to them.

6. Communicating Positive NBS Results for CF

Providing clear information to families is an important part of the NBS process to minimise unnecessary stress and anxiety. To date, there is no internationally accepted approach on how best to do this [7]. Communicating positive NBS results for any condition is not an event but a process that starts with the moment the result is identified as being above the agreed "cut off" and ends when the parents are given the definitive diagnosis for their child [41]. As a positive NBS result in itself is not diagnostic, and further tests are required to confirm or refute the NBS result before a definitive diagnosis is given to the family, this presents a period of uncertainty for families. This may be exacerbated in NBS for CF due to the range of possible outcomes, including a carrier result, confirmation of a diagnosis of CF or a designation of CFSPID, and the wide clinical spectrum that particularly the latter two presents.

Well-informed parents are less stressed by the screening process [6,39,40,42,43]. NBS programmes debate the antenatal information about the screened diseases in an NBS programme that should be given to new parents, who are already overloaded with information and brochures. In Switzerland, some parents felt that details about the screening test and the disease were missing when they were invited by phone for diagnostic evaluation. But information provided during this phone call is deliberately minimal without mentioning the respective disease, so as to reduce parental anxiety before they receive accurate information from a specialist [6].

When children with a positive NBS results are tested in a CF centre, their parents can feel anxious and depressed whilst awaiting definitive results [39,40]. CF specialists should be aware of the effect of the initial information given to parents and later in the CF centres, since this information can either reassure or cause anxiety to parents. The period between informing parents about a positive screening result and their appointment at the CF centre should be as short as possible. Parents should only be contacted when an appointment can be offered the following day.

According to the current ECFS best practice guidelines [5], a CF specialist should discuss a confirmed or inconclusive CF diagnosis in person with the parents (and not on the phone), and the family should receive written information to read after the consultation. Detailed information should also be sent to the family doctor or paediatrician. Families should be informed of further procedures and controls, the function and achievements of the CF research and made aware of opportunities for participation in clinical trials. In the case of a child identified to be a CF carrier, the family should receive a verbal report of the result, and written information should be sent to the family doctor or paediatrician. This information should be clear that (1) the infant does not have CF, (2) the baby is a healthy carrier of this mutation, (3) future pregnancies for the parents are not free of risk of CF and the parents may opt for genetic counselling, and (4) there are implications that could affect reproductive decision making for extended family members and the infant when they are of child-bearing age. A recently published US epidemiological study concluded that CF-related conditions, such as pancreatitis, infertility, diabetes, etc., were more prevalent among carriers than controls, whereas the individual-level risk remained low for most conditions [44]. This could have implications for future genetic counselling, but until these results are confirmed by other studies in other countries, CF carriers should not be medicalised unnecessarily.

A Swiss study exploring parents' perspective of NBS for CF found that parental dissatisfaction with the communication of the NBS result was associated with poor information provision about the NBS result and the actual disease, again demonstrating the importance of ensuring the information is delivered by someone who is well-informed [6]. An international study with CF clinicians found that in the EU, Australia and New Zealand, a range of professionals are responsible for communicating the positive NBS to families, including midwives, the CF centre, the CF nurse, the NBS laboratory as well as the primary care physician, which had the potential to influence the quality of the information provided to the family [7].

Regardless of who is responsible for communicating the positive NBS result for CF, provision of complete and accurate information reduced parental anxiety and facilitated better decision making regarding seeking diagnostic testing and support from the CF team thereafter. Therefore, whoever is responsible for the initial communication with families should have condition-specific knowledge and be familiar with the NBS algorithm being used [7].

7. Feedback and Tracking

Monitoring the performance of NBS is important as it ensures compliance with relevant guidelines and a high standard of care [5]. This requires good data collection to assess the success of the screening. Many countries have already implemented formal mechanisms to ensure that children are seen in time and that specific protocols are followed, and they report their quality and compliance data [2]. However, as the protocols and associated reported variables differ, it is difficult to draw comparisons between programmes.

In some countries, the process of following up a positive NBS result is less straightforward, which poses difficulties and concerns for CF clinicians. Data from an international study with CF clinicians highlighted concerns in certain countries (particularly Turkey and Germany) regarding ensuring all children who received a positive NBS result received the appropriate diagnostic testing and were followed up in a timely manner by the CF team [7]. This was attributed to the mechanisms in place for communicating the positive NBS result for CF to the child's family. In Germany, the NBS laboratory informs the birth clinic who then informs the parents about their child's positive NBS result. In Turkey, processes were governed by who was seen to "own" the information about the positive NBS result, which in turn determined who was responsible for communicating the positive NBS result to the family. This was considered to have the potential to influence parental perceptions of the urgency and/or necessity for their child to be followed up by the CF team. In addition, in Turkey and Germany, parents are expected to arrange the sweat test after they have been informed of their child's positive NBS result. In Germany, this was due to legal requirements that meant the CF centre could not be sent patient details. This raised concerns for CF clinicians in terms of ensuring that all babies who have a positive NBS result have a sweat test and are seen by the CF team in a timely manner.

8. Conclusions

Processing of a positive NBS screening result for CF has an important role in the success of a CF NBS programme, which is often underestimated when working out the optimal screening algorithm in the laboratory. It is a complex process not least because of the range of possible outcomes and the clinical uncertainty that this can present. Guidelines exist to assist clinicians but there is evidence these are used inconsistently for a range of reasons, including geographical, logistical, legal, financial and cultural constraints. Communication of positive NBS results is also challenging for many of the same reasons and presents a process rather than a singular event. However, whatever process is adopted must ensure this happens consistently and in a timely manner. Complete international harmonisation of NBS for CF is neither practical nor desirable but whatever processes are adopted must ensure outcomes for children, families and clinicians that are commensurate between programmes.

References

1. Castellani, C.; Massie, J.; Sontag, M.; Southern, K.W. Newborn screening for cystic fibrosis. *Lancet Respir. Med.* **2016**, *4*, 653–661. [CrossRef]
2. Barben, J.; Castellani, C.; Dankert-Roelse, J.; Gartner, S.; Kashirskaya, N.; Linnane, B.; Mayell, S.; Munck, A.; Sands, D.; Sommerburg, O.; et al. The expansion and performance of national newborn screening programmes for cystic fibrosis in Europe. *J. Cyst. Fibros.* **2017**, *16*, 207–213. [CrossRef] [PubMed]
3. Castellani, C.; Southern, K.W.; Brownlee, K.; Roelse, J.D.; Duff, A.; Farrell, M.; Mehta, A.; Munck, A.; Pollitt, R.; Sermet-Gaudelus, I.; et al. European best practice guidelines for cystic fibrosis neonatal screening. *J. Cyst. Fibros.* **2010**, *8*, 153–173. [CrossRef] [PubMed]
4. Wilson, J.M.G.; Jungner, G. *Principles and Practice of Screening for Disease*; Public Health papers, No.34; World Health Organization: Geneva, Switzerland, 1968.
5. Castellani, C.; Duff, A.J.; Bell, S.C.; Heijerman, H.G.; Munck, A.; Ratjen, F.; Sermet-Gaudelus, I.; Southern, K.W.; Barben, J.; Flume, P.A.; et al. ECFS best practice guidelines: The 2018 revision. *J. Cyst. Fibros.* **2018**, *17*, 153–178. [CrossRef] [PubMed]
6. Rueegg, C.S.; Barben, J.; Hafen, G.M.; Moeller, A.; Jurca, M.; Fingerhut, R.; Kuehni, C.E.; Group, T.S.C.F.S. Newborn screening for cystic fibrosis—The parent perspective. *J. Cyst. Fibros.* **2016**, *15*, 443–451. [CrossRef] [PubMed]
7. Chudleigh, J.; Ren, C.L.; Barben, J.; Southern, K.W. International approaches for delivery of positive newborn bloodspot screening results for CF. *J. Cyst. Fibros.* **2019**, *18*, 614–621. [CrossRef]
8. Farrell, P.M.; Rosenstein, B.J.; White, T.B.; Accurso, F.J.; Castellani, C.; Cutting, G.R.; Durie, P.R.; LeGrys, V.A.; Massie, J.; Parad, R.B.; et al. Guidelines for diagnosis of cystic fibrosis in newborns through older adults: Cystic Fibrosis Foundation consensus report. *J. Pediatr.* **2008**, *153*, S4–S14. [CrossRef]
9. LeGrys, V.A.; Yankaskas, J.R.; Quittell, L.M.; Marshall, B.C.; Mogayzel, P.J., Jr.; Cystic Fibrosis Foundation. Diagnostic sweat testing: The Cystic Fibrosis Foundation guidelines. *J. Pediatr.* **2007**, *151*, 85–89. [CrossRef]
10. Farrell, P.M.; White, T.B.; Ren, C.L.; Hempstead, S.E.; Accurso, F.; Derichs, N.; Howenstine, M.; McColley, S.A.; Rock, M.; Rosenfeld, M.; et al. Diagnosis of Cystic Fibrosis: Consensus Guidelines from the Cystic Fibrosis Foundation. *J. Pediatr.* **2017**, *181*, S4–S15. [CrossRef]
11. Bergougnoux, A.; Boureau-Wirth, A.; Rouzier, C.; Altieri, J.P.; Verneau, F.; Larrieu, L.; Koenig, M.; Claustres, M.; Raynal, C. A false positive newborn screening result due to a complex allele carrying two frequent CF-causing variants. *J. Cyst. Fibros.* **2016**, *15*, 309–312. [CrossRef]
12. Southern, K.W.; Barben, J.; Gartner, S.; Munck, A.; Castellani, C.; Mayell, S.J.; Davies, J.C.; Winters, V.; Murphy, J.; Salinas, D.; et al. Inconclusive diagnosis after a positive newborn bloodspot screening result for cystic fibrosis; clarification of the harmonised international definition. *J. Cyst. Fibros.* **2019**, *18*, 780. [CrossRef] [PubMed]
13. CLSI. *Sweat Testing: Sample Collection and Quantitative Chloride Analysis Approved Guideline*, 3rd ed.; Clinical and Laboratory Standards Institute: Wayne, PA, USA, 2009.
14. Royal College of Paediatrics and Child Health. Guidelines for the Performance of the Sweat Test for the Investigation of Cystic Fibrosis in the UK (Version 2). An Evidence Based Guideline 2014. Available online: http://www.acb.org.uk/docs/default-source/committees/scientific/guidelines/acb/sweat-guideline-v2-1.pdf (accessed on 25 March 2020).

15. Eng, W.; LeGrys, V.A.; Schechter, M.S.; Laughon, M.M.; Barker, P.M. Sweat-testing in preterm and full-term infants less than 6 weeks of age. *Pediatric Pulmonol.* **2005**, *40*, 64–67. [CrossRef] [PubMed]
16. Rueegg, C.S.; Kuehni, C.E.; Gallati, S.; Jurca, M.; Jung, A.; Casaulta, C.; Barben, J. Swiss Cystic Fibrosis Screening Group Comparison of two sweat test systems for the diagnosis of cystic fibrosis in newborns. *Pediatric Pulmonol.* **2019**, *54*, 264–272. [CrossRef]
17. LeGrys, V.A.; McColley, S.A.; Li, Z.; Farrell, P.M. The need for quality improvement in sweat testing infants after newborn screening for cystic fibrosis. *J. Pediatr.* **2010**, *157*, 1035–1037. [CrossRef]
18. Kleyn, M.; Korzeniewski, S.; Grigorescu, V.; Young, W.; Homnick, D.; Goldstein-Filbrun, A.; Schuen, J.; Nasr, S. Predictors of insufficient sweat production during confirmatory testing for cystic fibrosis. *Pediatric Pulmonol.* **2011**, *46*, 23–30. [CrossRef] [PubMed]
19. Laguna, T.A.; Lin, N.; Wang, Q.; Holme, B.; McNamara, J.; Regelmann, W.E. Comparison of quantitative sweat chloride methods after positive newborn screen for cystic fibrosis. *Pediatric Pulmonol.* **2012**, *47*, 736–742. [CrossRef] [PubMed]
20. Parad, R.B.; Comeau, A.M.; Dorkin, H.L.; Dovey, M.; Gerstle, R.; Martin, T.; O'Sullivan, B.P. Sweat testing infants detected by cystic fibrosis newborn screening. *J. Pediatr.* **2008**, *147*, S69–S72. [CrossRef] [PubMed]
21. Mastella, G.; Di Cesare, G.; Borruso, A.; Menin, L.; Zanolla, L. Reliability of sweat-testing by the Macroduct collection method combined with conductivity analysis in comparison with the classic Gibson and Cooke technique. *Acta Paediatr.* **2000**, *89*, 933–937. [CrossRef]
22. Baumer, J.H. Evidence based guidelines for the performance of the sweat test for the investigation of cystic fibrosis in the UK. *Arch. Dis. Child.* **2003**, *88*, 1126–1127. [CrossRef]
23. Cole, D.E.; Boucher, M.J. Use of a new sample-collection device (Macroduct) in anion analysis of human sweat. *Clin. Chem.* **1986**, *32*, 1375–1378. [CrossRef]
24. Coakley, J.; Scott, S.; Doery, J.; Greaves, R.; Talsma, P.; Whitham, E.; Winship, J. Australasian Guideline (2nd Edition): An Annex to the CLSI and UK Guidelines for the Performance of the Sweat Test for the Diagnosis of Cystic Fibrosis. *Clin. Biochem. Rev.* **2017**, *38*, 115–130.
25. Hammond, K.B.; Nelson, L.; Gibson, L.E. Clinical evaluation of the macroduct sweat collection system and conductivity analyzer in the diagnosis of cystic fibrosis. *J. Pediatr.* **1994**, *124*, 255–260. [CrossRef]
26. Heeley, M.E.; Woolf, D.A.; Heeley, A.F. Indirect measurements of sweat electrolyte concentration in the laboratory diagnosis of cystic fibrosis. *Arch. Dis. Child.* **2000**, *82*, 420–424. [CrossRef] [PubMed]
27. Lezana, J.L.; Vargas, M.H.; Karam-Bechara, J.; Aldana, R.S.; Furuya, M.E.Y. Sweat conductivity and chloride titration for cystic fibrosis diagnosis in 3834 subjects. *J Cyst. Fibros.* **2003**, *2*, 1–7. [CrossRef]
28. Webster, H.L.; Quirante, C.G. Micro-flowcell conductometric sweat analysis for cystic fibrosis diagnosis. *Ann. Clin. Biochem.* **2000**, *37*, 399–407. [CrossRef]
29. Barben, J.; Ammann, R.A.; Metlagel, A.; Schöni, M.H. Conductivity determined by a new sweat analyzer compared with chloride concentrations for the diagnosis of cystic fibrosis. *J. Pediatr.* **2005**, *146*, 183–188. [CrossRef]
30. Desax, M.C.; Ammann, R.A.; Hammer, J.; Schoeni, M.H.; Barben, J. Nanoduct sweat testing for rapid diagnosis in newborns, infants and children with cystic fibrosis. *Eur. J. Pediatr.* **2008**, *167*, 299–304. [CrossRef]
31. Sands, D.; Oltarzewski, M.; Nowakowska, A.; Zybert, K. Bilateral sweat tests with two different methods as a part of cystic fibrosis newborn screening (CF NBS) protocol and additional quality control. *Folia Histochem. Cytobiol.* **2010**, *48*, 358–365. [CrossRef]
32. Sezer, R.G.; Aydemir, G.; Akcan, A.B.; Paketci, C.; Karaoglu, A.; Aydinoz, S.; Bozaykut, A. Nanoduct sweat conductivity measurements in 2664 patients: Relationship to age, arterial blood gas, serum electrolyte profiles and clinical diagnosis. *J. Clin. Med. Res.* **2013**, *5*, 34–41. [CrossRef]
33. Vernooij-van Langen, A.; Dompeling, E.; Yntema, J.B.; Arets, B.; Tiddens, H.; Loeber, G.; Dankert-Roelse, J. Clinical evaluation of the Nanoduct sweat test system in the diagnosis of cystic fibrosis after newborn screening. *Eur. J. Pediatr.* **2015**, *174*, 1025–1034. [CrossRef]
34. Barben, J.; Rueegg, C.S.; Jurca, M.; Spalinger, J.; Kuehni, C.E.; Swiss Cystic Fibrosis Screening Group. Measurement of fecal elastase improves performance of newborn screening for cystic fibrosis. *J. Cyst. Fibros.* **2016**, *15*, 313–317. [CrossRef] [PubMed]
35. Munck, A.; Mayell, S.J.; Winters, V.; Shawcross, A.; Derichs, N.; Parad, R.; Barben, J.; Southern, K.W. Cystic Fibrosis Screen Positive, Inconclusive Diagnosis (CFSPID): A new designation and management

recommendations for infants with an inconclusive diagnosis following newborn screening. *J. Cyst. Fibros.* **2015**, *14*, 706–713. [CrossRef] [PubMed]

36. Ooi, C.Y.; Castellani, C.; Keenan, K.; Avolio, J.; Volpi, S.; Boland, M.; Kovesi, T.; Bjornson, C.; Chilvers, M.A.; Morgan, L.; et al. Inconclusive diagnosis of cystic fibrosis after newborn screening. *Pediatrics* **2015**, *135*, e1377–e1385. [CrossRef] [PubMed]
37. Barben, J.; Southern, K.W. Cystic Fibrosis Screen Positive, inconclusive Diagnosis (CFSPID). *Curr. Opin. Pulm. Med.* **2016**, *22*, 617–622. [CrossRef]
38. Massie, J.; Gillam, L. Uncertain diagnosis after newborn screening for cystic fibrosis: An ethics-based approach to a clinical dilemma. *Pediatric Pulmonol.* **2014**, *49*, 1–7. [CrossRef] [PubMed]
39. Tluczek, A.; Mischler, E.H.; Farrell, P.M.; Fost, N.; Peterson, N.M.; Carey, P.; Bruns, W.T.; McCarthy, C. Parents' knowledge of neonatal screening and response to false-positive cystic fibrosis testing. *J. Dev. Behav. Pediatr.* **1992**, *13*, 181–186. [CrossRef]
40. Tluczek, A.; Koscik, R.L.; Farrell, P.M.; Rock, M.J. Psychosocial risk associated with newborn screening for cystic fibrosis: Parents' experience while awaiting the sweat-test appointment. *Pediatrics* **2005**, *115*, 1692–1703. [CrossRef]
41. Chudleigh, J.; Chinnery, H.; Bonham, J.R.; Olander, E.K.; Moody, L.; Simpson, A.; Morris, S.; Ulph, F.; Bryon, M.; Southern, K.W. *A Qualitative Exploration of Health Professionals' Experiences of Communicating Positive Newborn Bloodspot Screening Results for Nine Conditions in England*; 2020. (In Press)
42. Dillard, J.P.; Shen, L.; Robinson, J.D.; Farrell, P.M. Parental information seeking following a positive newborn screening for cystic fibrosis. *J. Health Commun.* **2010**, *15*, 880–894. [CrossRef]
43. Ulph, F.; Cullinan, T.; Qureshi, N.; Kai, J. Informing children of their newborn screening carrier result for sickle cell or cystic fibrosis: Qualitative study of parents' intentions, views and support needs. *J. Genet. Couns.* **2014**, *23*, 409–420. [CrossRef]
44. Miller, A.C.; Comellas, A.P.; Hornick, D.B.; Stoltz, D.A.; Cavanaugh, J.E.; Gerke, A.K.; Welsh, M.J.; Zabner, J.; Polgreen, P.M. Cystic fibrosis carriers are at increased risk for a wide range of cystic fibrosis-related conditions. *Proc. Natl. Acad. Sci. USA* **2020**, *117*, 1621–1627. [CrossRef]

15

History of Newborn Screening for Cystic Fibrosis—The Early Years

Georges Travert [1,2,*], Mary Heeley [3] and Anthony Heeley [3]

1 University of Caen Normandy (UNICAEN), 14032 Caen, France
2 Caen University Hospital, 14040 Caen, France
3 East Anglian Biochemical Genetic Unit, Peterborough, UK
* Correspondence: georges.travert@wanadoo.fr

Abstract: This review summarises the trajectory of neonatal screening strategies for the detection of cystic fibrosis (CF) using the measurement of Immunoreactive Trypsin (IRT) in dried blood spots (DBS) from 1979 until the beginning of the 21st century when newborn screening (NBS) programmes started to spread throughout many countries, using IRT measurement combined with a CF genotype analysis of DBS.

Keywords: newborn screening; immunoreactive trypsin(ogen); dried blood spot; radioimmunoassay; DNA

---

1. The Background

In the 1950s, Dr. Harry Shwachman, paediatrician at Boston Children's Hospital, recognised that early diagnosis was an important factor underpinning the optimal outcome for cystic fibrosis (CF) patients, receiving both nutritional support and an aggressive treatment of lung infections [1]. However, at this time, no neonatal screening test had been described.

The first attempts at newborn screening (NBS) for CF were performed in the 1970s [2] and were based on a semi quantitative measurement of the albumin content in meconium (BM test). However, elevated meconium albumin levels are a consequence of exocrine pancreatic insufficiency, and pancreatic sufficient CF neonates could not be detected (false negatives). The test also had a very high false positive rate, especially among preterm newborns. Due to its lack of specificity and sensitivity, screening trials with this test were not widely implemented; the exception being where the meconium specimens could be delivered directly from the maternity ward to a laboratory, usually closely associated with a CF clinical centre, where more elaborate testing could take place [3].

The detection of faecal tryptic activity using artificial peptide substrates was next in line for promotion as a potential screening test [4]. Although this eliminated some of the problems associated with meconium testing, the inability to detect pancreatic sufficient neonates would remain a problem. However, two contemporary developments brought these lines of investigation to an abrupt end, as described in the next section.

These and other issues of the period have been reviewed in detail elsewhere [5].

2. New Neonatal Screening Strategies Emerge

Newborn population screening for inherited/congenital diseases such as phenylketonuria (PKU) and congenital hypothyroidism (CHT) had been widely implemented by the late 1970s. Biochemical screening on this scale had been enabled through the innovative work of Robert Guthrie [6], who demonstrated that phenylalanine could be measured accurately in minute amounts of blood that were obtained by heel-prick, collected, and dried on absorbent paper (DBS). Dried blood had the advantage of conferring good stability of the analyte during transport to the laboratory and for later storage. Moreover, these specimens were shown to be suitable for the measurements of analytes in the nanogramme range, such as hormones, using the relatively new techniques of radio-immunoassay (RIA) as Jean Dussault in Quebec, Canada, demonstrated in 1975 with a NBS test for CHT [7].

The 1970s also saw a surge of interest in the role of exocrine proteins in gastrointestinal physiology and pathology. RIA based methods were developed, which were sufficiently sensitive to detect the extremely low concentrations present in the circulation. The pancreatic zymogen trypsinogen was one of these proteins, and the immediate clinical interest in this assay stemmed from its potential for use in the differential diagnosis of pancreatic disease. With this objective in mind, a number of commercial diagnostic companies had, by the late 1970s, developed RIA reagents for serum trypsin(ogen) (IRT) measurement. Although older CF patients with overt pancreatic insufficiency had subnormal serum IRT levels, surprisingly, IRT levels in early infancy were elevated irrespective of the patient's pancreatic functional status.

The collection of liquid blood and the separation of serum was a cumbersome procedure for neonatal biochemical screening purposes. Would the use of DBS, of proven reliability in other established NBS protocols, also be suitable for the measurement of IRT? The answer to this question came in 1979 from the laboratory of the Department of Paediatrics at Auckland (NZ) Medical School.

The short report by Crossley and co-workers [8] was notable not only for their development of an assay of sufficient sensitivity to measure IRT in dried blood spots but also that IRT was sufficiently stable in DBS form for it to be measurable after storage for many months or even several years. In this study, DBS IRT levels were able to clearly distinguish each of 23 CF neonates from two controls randomly selected in the same batch of Guthrie cards, despite the cards having been stored at room temperature for up to seven years. Therefore the repositories of DBS cards which had been used for PKU/CHT screening would be a valuable resource for the retrospective testing of newborn DBS of infants whose later diagnosis of CF had been established solely on clinical grounds, and in whom the clinical history would be well documented.

The importance of this seminal paper and the almost instantaneous confirmation of its findings in several laboratories cannot be overestimated. The retrospective DBS testing of historical CF infants clearly demonstrated that pre-symptomatic detection of the condition was possible. Even so, it remained unclear how efficient the DBS IRT assay would be in the prospective NBS setting. Additionally, there were aspects of the assay described by Crossley which were unsuitable for routine newborn population screening purposes, i.e., the size of blood spot required. This problem was quickly overcome [9], and the scene was set for prospective screening trials to begin.

3. The Two-Stage IRT Prospective Screening Trials (IRT–IRT) 1979–1989

In 1980, apart from the ongoing work in Auckland, there were two European screening laboratories that had the necessary technical and clinical infrastructure in place to incorporate IRT screening alongside their established PKU/CHT programmes. These laboratories were at Caen (France) and at Peterborough (UK), responsible for screening the newborn population of Normandy and East Anglia respectively. At the time, there were two commercially available serum IRT assays, both of which had been independently adapted for DBS IRT screening in these French and UK laboratories (Hoechst Behring Germany in Caen and Sorin Biomedica Italy in Peterborough).

For various complex technical reasons, particularly the lack of an internationally accepted standard preparation of human trypsin(ogen) the results obtained by these different RIAs would not be directly comparable. Each laboratory had to determine, for its own newborn population, the DBS IRT concentration that would provide an optimal screening cut-off.

Moreover, it appeared that hypertrypsinaemia occurs frequently in non-CF neonates during the first days of life, declining rapidly thereafter, whereas the hypertrypsinaemia of CF persists to some degree for several months. Thus, a few infants would have to be re-tested, preferably within the following 1–2 weeks, and, again, an optimal screening cut-off would have to be established for these older infants; those infants with a DBS IRT level above this cut-off level would be referred for diagnostic sweat testing and clinical assessment. Carrying out a sweat test on 4–6 week-old infants by the standard Gibson–Cooke procedure is difficult, cumbersome, and time consuming. In the early 1980s, an innovative sweat collection system was developed commercially, which greatly facilitated the testing of small infants in screening trials [10].

It was gratifying to find, as early as 1980, that the results obtained from the trials in Normandy and East Anglia with different assays were producing similar results, in particular, acceptable sensitivity and specificity for the detection of CF infants with low retest rates [11,12]. These preliminary results had, quite independently, in 1980 been disseminated to audiences of paediatricians and clinical biochemists known to be interested in this field of investigation (at Caen in October and London in November). Together with the ongoing work in Auckland (NZ), this led to a burgeoning of two-stage IRT screening trials in other countries, and, as a result, data began to accumulate more rapidly, particularly from those laboratories whose screening hinterland was more populous. Among the latter were New South Wales, Australia, Colorado, USA, and Alto Adige/Veneto, Italy. Initiating these trials, respectively, were Bridget Wilken (Sydney), Keith Hammond (Denver), and Gianni Mastella (Verona).

Two other trials with different objectives, namely to determine whether NBS was clinically effective, began in the mid-1980s. One of these, carried out in Wales/the West Midlands region (UK), elected to screen a large neonatal population for CF using the two-stage IRT method but only on alternate weeks. The other, undertaken in Wisconsin (USA), was an ambitious randomised control trial (RCT) in which half the results of the initial IRT screening test were randomly and anonymously blinded for a period of four years. In the active group, infants with positive IRT singleton test results were immediately referred for sweat testing and, if appropriate, clinical follow-up. However, these trials contributed little useful information regarding the efficacy of the IRT–IRT protocol because, in the case of the former, IRT testing was delayed for 3 weeks after the blood had been drawn, and because of the latter's aforementioned design [13,14].

As work progressed, it became necessary to convene meetings that would allow investigators to compare results in a timely manner. The first international round table discussions occurred in Peterborough in 1987, but, unfortunately, the sponsorship was insufficient to bring colleagues from the Antipodes. A more generous sponsorship, probably combined with the certain prospect of better food in Normandy, resulted in a widely attended conference with exceptionally fruitful discussions in Caen 1988. The issues addressed at these meetings were as follows: (1) IRT assay methodology. (2) The early nutritional status and respiratory function of the screened cohorts. (3) Optimal shared care between regional CF clinical centres and local paediatricians.

At that time, 9 laboratories from 7 countries had each screened in excess of 100,000 newborns, and although a majority of these had consistently achieved satisfactory test specificity and sensitivity, others had not. (The data were collected personally by G. Travert and reported in the proceedings of the International Conference: Mucoviscidose, Dépistage néonatal et Prise en charge précoce. Travert G (ed) Université de Caen 1988). The predictive value of a positive (IRT–IRT) test result ranged from 25%–86%, and a retest rate of the initially screened population varying between 0.3%–4.7%.

The reasons for these discrepancies could not be attributed to the type of RIA employed; nevertheless, these assays were inherently prone to sporadic technical error. Other likely confounding variables were the age of the initial and recall testing, age-related screening cut-offs, and the quality of DBS provided for screening, including the very high risk of contamination.

These and other issues relating to DBS IRT screening have been reviewed in more detail elsewhere [15,16]. Whatever the reasons for the variable results, the need for a within- and between-laboratory performance indicator had been unanimously advocated at a meeting convened in 1985 by G. Mastella in Verona, the organization of which was entrusted to the laboratories of Caen and Peterborough.

The IRT International Quality Assurance Scheme (IRTIQAS) began in 1987 with 16 laboratories from 6 countries. Dried blood spots were prepared from the blood of pancreatitis patients for elevated levels, and often laboratory staff for the control levels, and were distributed monthly. Because different reagents, techniques, and variations of the trypsin antigen were being used by the 16 participants, absolute values could not be compared. However, the scheme gave an indication of within- and between-assay performance and an assurance that laboratories had chosen the appropriate cut-off to distinguish a CF neonate with a minimum proportion of false positives. By 1990 there were 40 laboratories from 8 countries, a clear indication that the scheme was beneficial to laboratories in determining whether their CV and bias were consistent, at which point the manufacturer's agreed to contribute to the running costs. IRTIQAS was not ideal because the utilized DBS could not be obtained from CF newborns because the volume of blood needed was prohibitive. The lack of an international reference standard was a major drawback. The preliminary results emanating from this scheme were presented at the 1988 Caen Conference and in more detail at the later (1990) International Conference organized by K. Hammond at Estes Park, Colorado [17].

In order to eliminate the multistep, error prone, manual process and radiochemical facilities required for RIA, alternative immunoassay technologies were being introduced in diagnostic clinical chemistry. One of these utilised solid phase monoclonal antibodies, a second chemically labelled antibody and an enzyme linked signal amplification system. Assays of this type could be carried out in multi well antibody-coated microtitre plates with much enhanced and simplified sample throughput. Biochemists at the Queensland (Australia) neonatal screening laboratory in Brisbane had developed such an assay for DBS IRT [18] and a commercial version was launched at the 1988 Caen meeting. The latter generated much interest and some CF screening laboratories changed to this methodology abruptly, causing further confusion in the quest to determine which screening modality was most efficacious in the long term.

In the concluding address of this conference in Caen, the eminent geneticist Jean Frezal predicted that in the future genetic analysis would underpin neonatal screening for CF; a prescient prediction, because, within twelve months, the *CFTR* gene and its main mutation F508del had been described [19]. New horizons for newborn CF screening had been opened up.

4. IRT-DNA from 1990

Polymorphic alleles closely associated with the *CFTR* gene had been studied as a potential adjunct to IRT screening in the Normandy neonatal population with some success [20]. However, it was the elucidation of the *CFTR* gene structure and the identification of the F508del mutation with high prevalence in the CF population that provided the stimulus for virtually every major screening centre to embrace molecular genetic analytical techniques. Would the introduction of DNA analysis into the IRT–IRT protocol improve the screening test performance? Would it enable the recall second IRT test to be abolished? Results from some preliminary work were presented at the 1990 International meeting in Colorado. Somewhat surprisingly, the Adelaide laboratory of the South Australian Regional Programme, reported that they had already implemented IRT-DNA screening [21]. They had used a low cut-off (99th centile) on 5-day old infants followed by DBS DNA analysis for the mutations F508del and I507del, i.e., on 1% of the neonatal population. Whilst this protocol eliminated the recall of infants for further IRT testing, it could be cogently argued that it posed a number of problems: (a) sensitivity was limited to 94% (gene prevalence related), (b) all heterozygous infants had to be sweat tested and the parents of those infants with normal results (86%) were offered genetic counselling, (c) those infants that screened IRT positive, in whom either of these mutations was absent (94%), were reported "CF not indicated"; rather tenuously in view of the imposed limit of sensitivity. Most centres running IRT–IRT protocols had, by this time, achieved better sensitivity, fewer infants were recalled for sweat testing, and none of the dilemmas associated with the detection of heterozygotes arose.

At the same meeting, the Caen laboratory group reported investigations, both retrospective and prospective, with IRT-DNA (F508del) and their results showed convincingly that the introduction of DNA analysis, with its present limitations, would not be beneficial as an adjunct to IRT screening if the primary purpose was to maximise the detection of CF infants as soon as possible after birth.

Nevertheless, the South Australian work was important in demonstrating the feasibility of IRT-DNA neonatal screening in a routine setting. Its effectiveness would undoubtedly be improved with the inclusion of more CF mutations in the IRT-DNA protocol or in the inclusion of a third stage IRT-DNA-IRT [22].

An equally important contemporary finding from the Caen laboratory resulted from their investigation of F508del in the DBS of infants who had screened IRT negative but whose DBS IRT levels approached that of the designated discriminatory cut-off, i.e., the 99.5th centile. In the general French population, the prevalence of F508del healthy carriers is 2.5%–3%. Amongst neonates with low IRT levels, it was 0.5% but progressively reached 10–11% in healthy newborns with IRT levels just below or just above the cut-off [23,24]. The practical consequence of these findings was that any trend to lower the IRT cut-off value, in order to improve the screening sensitivity, would inevitably result in an increased detection rate of healthy carriers. Therefore, as early as 1990, potential problems associated with IRT-DNA screening had emerged. It would take another decade of more adjustments to decide how many of the increasing number of known *CFTR* gene mutations should be included in the screening process.

Unsurprisingly, many of these problems remain unresolved, including the category of screened patients now called CFSPID (CF Screen Positive, Inconclusive Diagnosis) in Europe and CFTR-related Metabolic Syndrome (CRMS) in the USA.

5. The Tide Turns 1998

At the instigation of the directors of the Normandy and New South Wales screening laboratories, a further meeting was convened in 1998 at Caen to mark the approaching second decade of newborn screening for CF and to take stock of progress over this period.

From their inception these International conferences had included the work of clinical psychologists, nutritionists, paediatricians, and CF nurses who had been involved with the individual trials [25,26]. Much had been learned about managing the social and ethical issues of CF screening, of the early natural history of the disease and its clinical management, all of which is covered in Jim Littlewood's comprehensive on-line historic review of CF [27].

Throughout the 1990s, more robust screening strategies had emerged by increasing the number of CFTR mutations in the DNA analysis. The DBS IRT assay had been substantially improved by the Wallac Co. in Finland, using more selective monoclonal antibodies and an extremely sensitive labelling technology with an analytical system that was already widely used in neonatal screening laboratories for the detection of CHT.

On balance, it seemed that the work that began in the early 1980s had been successfully concluded. The way forward would, in part, depend on local population demographics, ethical considerations, and the ability of health services to deliver optimal treatment for the condition. All that remained to further the case for CF newborn screening was incontrovertible evidence that early diagnosis and clinical intervention conferred significant future health benefits for these infants. That evidence was provided in the long-awaited results of the meticulous RCT conducted by Philip M. Farrell and colleagues in Wisconsin. While presenting these results in Caen in 1998, he concluded that "the burden of proof is now on those who argue against neonatal screening for CF" [26] (p.250).

This gauntlet was unlikely to be taken up by any serious contenders; the results of the Wisconsin trial were confirmation of what a whole generation of paediatricians caring for these patients already knew instinctively. It was also unlikely that any government public health service agency would ignore the evidence. Several NBS laboratories, as early as 1988, had secured health service funding from their respective state/regional public health authorities for the inclusion of CF in their NBS programme, which was justified by the short term clinical and diagnostic cost benefits gained. Before commissioning new public health screening services, national government agencies would normally seek stakeholder consensus for the best practice guidelines; the inclusion of molecular genetic analysis in the current CF NBS protocol presented a novel and more complex issue than had hitherto arisen in NBS commissioning.

Unsurprisingly, the time taken to introduce CF NBS at a national level varied considerably, for example, in France by 2003 and four years later in the UK, but by the end of the decade all affluent countries had introduced CF NBS.

6. Conclusions

This historical review focuses on the crucial stages in the development of a reliable neonatal screening test for the early detection of cystic fibrosis in the pre-symptomatic stages of this debilitating disease. Initiating this endeavour was the conviction of many paediatricians with expertise in the treatment of these patients, as the earlier a diagnosis was made, the better the clinical outcome. It seemed particularly fitting that 20 years of work undertaken to justify CF NBS should come to fruition at the beginning of a new millennium and that it should coincide with recent advances in CFTR molecular genetics. The better understanding of CFTR structural/functional relationships would undoubtedly pave the way for new and more effective treatments for CF children born in the 21st century, in addition to the benefits that NBS would provide. The generation of paediatricians and clinical biochemists who had pioneered this work internationally had reason to be satisfied with the outcome of their efforts. CF NBS had at last come of age. The inclusion of DNA in the post 1990 CF NBS protocols, was primarily to overcome a problem inherent in IRT–IRT, i.e., the need to retest about 1 in 250 infants at 2–3 weeks of age. Unanswered was the question—could IRT-DNA in the longer term present its own problems? Perhaps a review of CF NBS in the following decades will reveal the answer.

References

1. Shwachman, H.; Kulczycki, L.L. Long-term study of 105 cystic fibrosis patients. *Am. J. Dis. Child.* **1958**, *96*, 6–15. [CrossRef] [PubMed]
2. Stephan, U.; Busch, E.W.; Kollberg, H.; Hellsing, K. Cystic fibrosis detection by means of a test-strip. *Pediatrics* **1975**, *55*, 35–38. [PubMed]
3. Evans, R.T.; Little, A.J.; Steel, A.E.; Littlewood, J.M. Satisfactory screening for cystic fibrosis with the BM meconium procedure. *J. Clin. Pathol.* **1981**, *34*, 911–913. [CrossRef] [PubMed]
4. Crossley, J.R.; Elliot, R.B.; Smith, P.A. Cystic Fibrosis screening in the newborn. *Lancet* **1979**, *i*, 1093–1095. [CrossRef]
5. Heeley, A.F.; Watson, D. Cystic Fibrosis—Its biochemical detection. *Clin. Chem.* **1983**, *29*, 2011–2018. [CrossRef]
6. Guthrie, R.; Susi, A. A simple phenylalanine method for detecting phenylketonuria in large populations of newborn infants. *Pediatrics* **1963**, *32*, 338–343.
7. Dussault, J.H.; Coulombe, P.; Laberge, J.; Guyda, H.; Khoury, K. Preliminary report on a mass screening program for neonatal hypothyroidism. *J. Pediatr.* **1975**, *86*, 670–674. [CrossRef]
8. Crossley, J.R.; Elliott, R.B.; Smith, P.A. Dried blood spot screening for cystic fibrosis in the newborn. *Lancet* **1979**, *i*, 472–474. [CrossRef]
9. King, D.N.; Heeley, A.F.; Walsh, M.P.; Kuzemko, J.A. Sensitive trypsin assay for dried blood specimens as a screening procedure for early detection of cystic fibrosis. *Lancet* **1979**, *ii*, 1217–1219. [CrossRef]
10. Carter, E.P.; Barrett, A.D.; Heeley, A.F.; Kuzemko, J.A. Improved sweat test method for the diagnosis of cystic fibrosis. *Arch. Dis. Child.* **1984**, *59*, 919–922. [CrossRef]
11. Heeley, A.F.; Heeley, M.E.; King, D.N.; Kuzemko, J.A.; Walsh, M.P. Screening for cystic fibrosis by dried blood spot trypsin assay. *Arch. Dis. Child.* **1982**, *57*, 18–21. [PubMed]
12. Travert, G.; Duhamel, J.F. Dépistage néonatal systématique de la mucoviscidose par dosage de la trypsine immunoréactive sanguine. Bilan de 80000 tests. *Arch. Fr. Pédiatr.* **1983**, *40*, 295–298. [PubMed]
13. Ryley, H.C.; Deam, S.M.; Williams, J.; Alfaham, M.; Weller, P.H.; Goodchild, M.C.; Carter, R.A.; Bradley, D.; Dodge, J.A. Neonatal screening for cystic fibrosis in Wales and the West Midlands: 1. Evaluation of immunoreactive trypsin. *J. Clin. Pathol.* **1988**, *41*, 726–729. [CrossRef] [PubMed]
14. Farrell, P.M.; Kosorok, M.R.; Rock, M.J.; Laxova, A.; Zeng, L.; Hoffman, G. Assessment of the benefits, risks and costs of cystic fibrosis screening in Wisconsin, USA. In Proceedings of the Neonatal Screening for Cystic Fibrosis, Caen, France, 10–11 September, 1998; Presses Universitaires de Caen, 1999; pp. 239–253.

15. Heeley, A.F.; Bangert, S.K. The neonatal detection of cystic fibrosis by measurement of immunoreactive trypsin in blood. *Ann. Clin. Biochem.* **1992**, *29*, 361–376. [CrossRef]
16. Wilcken, B. Newborn screening for cystic fibrosis; its evolution and a review of the current situation. *Screening* **1993**, *2*, 43–62. [CrossRef]
17. Heeley, M.E.; Travert, G.; Ferré, C.; Lemonnier, F. The International Quality Assurance Program for the assay of immunoreactive trypsin in dried blood spots. *Pediatr. Pulmonol.* **1991**, *11* (Suppl. 7), 72–75. [CrossRef]
18. Bowling, F.G.; Brown, A.R.D. Newborn screening for cystic fibrosis using an ELISA technique. *Clin. Chim. Acta* **1988**, *63*, 196–198.
19. Kerem, B.S.; Rommens, J.M.; Buchanan, J.A.; Markiewicz, D.; Cox, T.K.; Chakravarti, A.; Buchwald, M.; Tsui, L.C. Identification of the cystic fibrosis gene: Genetic analysis. *Science* **1989**, *245*, 1073–1080. [CrossRef]
20. Laroche, D.; Travert, G. The application of PCR amplification and the polymorphic marker KM19 to dried blood spots: Comparison with deletion F508 for the confirmation of the neonatal screening for cystic fibrosis. *Pediatr. Pulmonol.* **1991**, *11* (Suppl. 7), 19–22. [CrossRef]
21. Ranieri, E.; Ryall, R.G.; Robertson, E.E.; Pollard, A.C. A screening strategy for cystic fibrosis using immunoreactive trypsinogen and gene analysis. *Paediatric. Pulmonol.* **1991**, *Suppl 7*, 88. [CrossRef]
22. Pollitt, R.J.; Dalton, A.; Evans, S.; Boyne, J. *Three Stage Neonatal Screening (IRT-DNA-IRT) Neonatal Screening for Cystic Fibrosis*; Presses Universitaires de Caen: Caen, France, 1999; pp. 49–53.
23. Laroche, D.; Travert, G. Abnormal frequency of ΔF508 in neonatal transitory hypertrypsinaemia. *Lancet* **1991**, *337*, 55. [CrossRef]
24. Lecoq, I.; Brouard, J.; Laroche, D.; Férec, C.; Travert, G. Blood immunoreactive trypsinogen concentrations are genetically determined in healthy and cystic fibrosis newborns. *Acta Paediatr.* **1999**, *88*, 1–4. [CrossRef]
25. Kuzemko, J.A. Clinical Implications of screening for cystic fibrosis in the newborn. *Insights into Paediatr.* **1987**, *1*, 1–87, Gardiner-Caldwell, Macclesfield, UK.
26. *Neonatal Screening for Cystic Fibrosis*; Presses Universitaires de Caen: Caen, France, 1999; ISBN 2-84133-075-3.
27. Available online: http://cfmedicine.com/history (accessed on 30 January 2020).

16

The Role of Extended *CFTR* Gene Sequencing in Newborn Screening for Cystic Fibrosis

Anne Bergougnoux [1], Maureen Lopez [2] and Emmanuelle Girodon [2,*]

1 Molecular Genetics Laboratory, CHU Montpellier, EA7402 University of Montpellier, 34093 Montpellier CEDEX 5, France; anne.bergougnoux@inserm.fr
2 Molecular Genetics Laboratory, Cochin Hospital, APHP. Centre, University of Paris, 75014 Paris, France; maureen.lopez@aphp.fr
* Correspondence: emmanuelle.girodon@aphp.fr;

Abstract: There has been considerable progress in the implementation of newborn screening (NBS) programs for cystic fibrosis (CF), with DNA analysis being part of an increasing number of strategies. Thanks to advances in genomic sequencing technologies, *CFTR*-extended genetic analysis (EGA) by sequencing its coding regions has become affordable and has already been included as part of a limited number of core NBS programs, to the benefit of admixed populations. Based on results analysis of existing programs, the values and challenges of EGA are reviewed in the perspective of its implementation on a larger scale. Sensitivity would be increased at best by using EGA as a second tier, but this could be at the expense of positive predictive value, which improves, however, if EGA is applied after testing a variant panel. The increased detection of babies with an inconclusive diagnosis has proved to be a major drawback in programs using EGA. The lack of knowledge on pathogenicity and penetrance associated with numerous variants hinders the introduction of EGA as a second tier, but EGA with filtering for all known CF variants with full penetrance could be a solution. The issue of incomplete knowledge is a real challenge in terms of the implemention of NBS extended to many genetic diseases.

Keywords: cystic fibrosis; newborn screening; DNA analysis; next generation sequencing; extended genetic analysis

1. Introduction

For more than 40 years, newborn screening (NBS) programs for cystic fibrosis (CF) have been implemented across the world in Caucasian populations as pilot, regional, or national programs [1–6]. While early *CFTR* gene analysis is a key tool for the diagnosis of CF, for adapted follow-up, mutation-guided therapy, and genetic counseling, its place and extent in a core NBS program has long been a matter of debate. At present, there are a variety of established NBS programs [1], all starting with immunoreactive trypsinogen (IRT) measurement. DNA analysis is part of the majority of programs, most often performed in the second tier on the same dried blood spot as IRT measurement, and principally with search for a limited number of frequent variants. Some programs include extended *CFTR* gene analysis with next generation sequencing (NGS) focused on coding regions (referred to as extended genetic analysis (EGA)), mainly because of heterogeneous populations where the distribution and the frequency of CF-causing variants vary. These programs, however, lead to the detection of a high number of inconclusive cases, also referred to as Cystic Fibrosis Screen Positive, Inconclusive Diagnosis (CFSPID) in Europe or CFTR-related metabolic syndrome (CRMS) in the US, compared to the number of CF cases [1,7]. The definition of CRMS/CFSPID includes infants with a sweat chloride value between 30–59 mmol/L and zero or one CF-causing variant, or a sweat chloride value below 30 mmol/L and two *CFTR* variants, at least one of which has unclear phenotypic consequences [8,9].

Beyond technical and medical aspects, the choice of a NBS strategy is driven by the mutation spectrum in the screened population, the laboratory facilities, the health care system, the legal and economic aspects, and the acceptability by the population [10–13]. There is thus no universal model of NBS strategy. Nevertheless, there are minimal recommendations which have been issued by the European Society of Cystic Fibrosis (ECFS) [14], including, as performance criteria, a minimal positive predictive value (PPV) of 30% and a minimal diagnostic sensitivity of 95%. It is also an objective to minimize as much as possible the number of inconclusive cases and carrier detection. In the present article, we review the variety of NBS programs set up that include DNA analysis, along with their performance. The value, challenges, and drawbacks of *CFTR* EGA are then discussed, and then future prospects are eventually considered—in particular, in the view of a shift toward an extended NBS of a set of hereditary diseases by wide genomic analysis.

2. Overview of Newborn Screening Programs

A review of the literature was conducted to identify current NBS programs for CF and to update performance data, notably from the important review across Europe [1]. It is, however, possible that strategies have changed since the last available data. Where data were old and not detailed, they were not included in Table 1. In Europe, 22 countries have implemented NBS programs, 20 as national and two as regional programs. Fifteen programs use DNA analysis, mostly as a second tier after IRT measurement. Twelve countries use a variant panel only, and three have implemented EGA (Figure 1a). In North America, all Canada provinces follow an IRT/DNA panel strategy, as do the great majority of US states [5,6] (Figure 1b). Only six US states do not use DNA analysis in their core program. The states of California, Hawaii, and, recently, New York, which are composed of multi-ethnic and/or non-white populations, have introduced EGA as a third tier after analysis of a variant panel [5,7] (Personal Communication [15]). In Central and South America, some programs have been implemented, e.g., since 2001 in Brazil [16], but few have introduced DNA analysis in their strategy [17] (Figure 1c). In Australia and New Zealand, where NBS was implemented in 1989 and 1986, respectively, DNA analysis using mutation panels is now part of the strategy in the second tier [18,19] (Figure 1d).

(a)

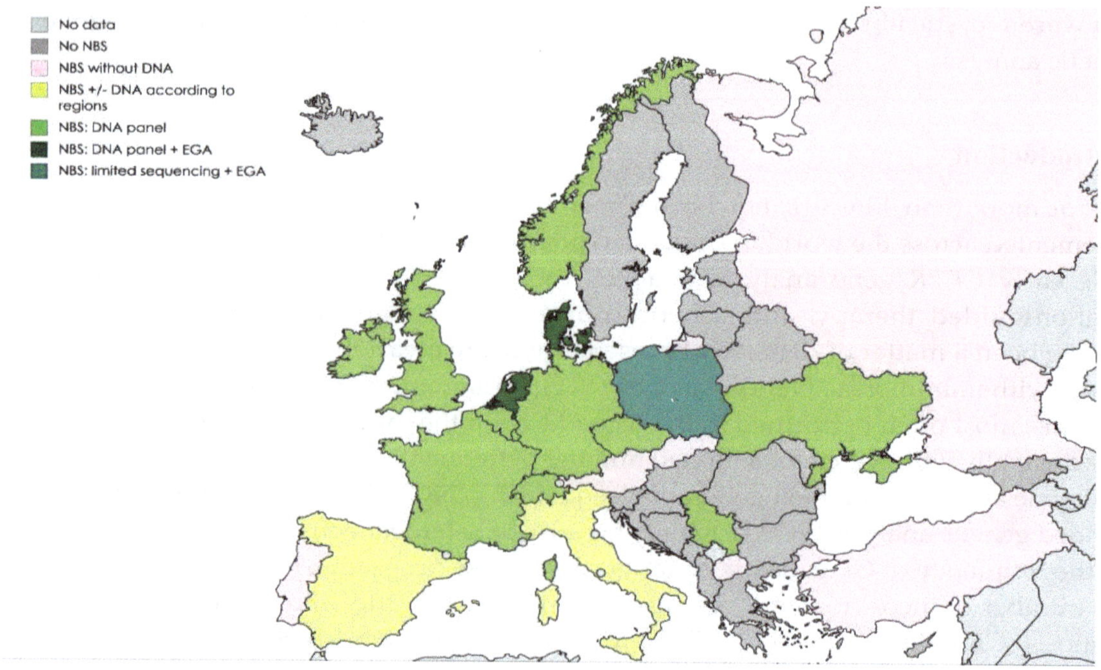

Figure 1. *Cont.*

(**b**)

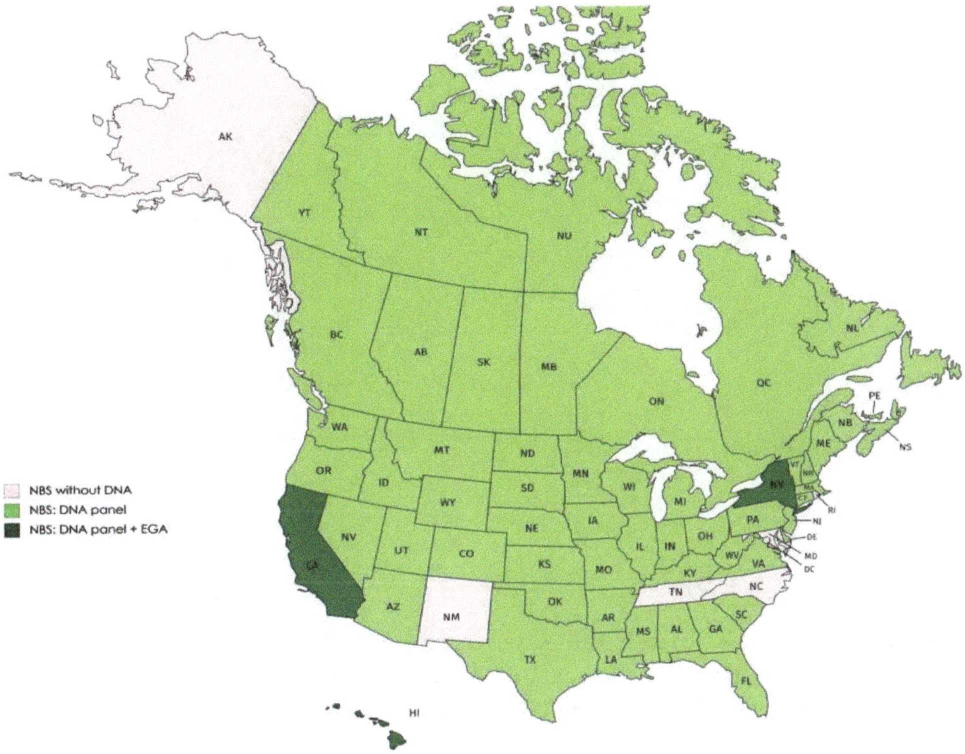

(**c**)

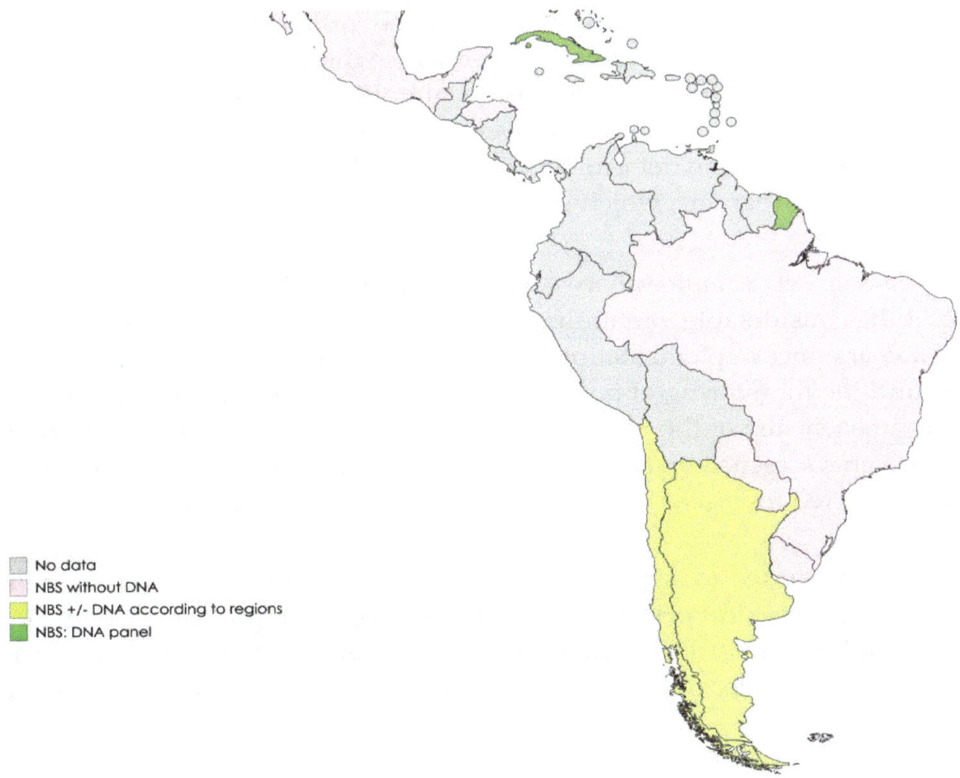

Figure 1. *Cont.*

(d)

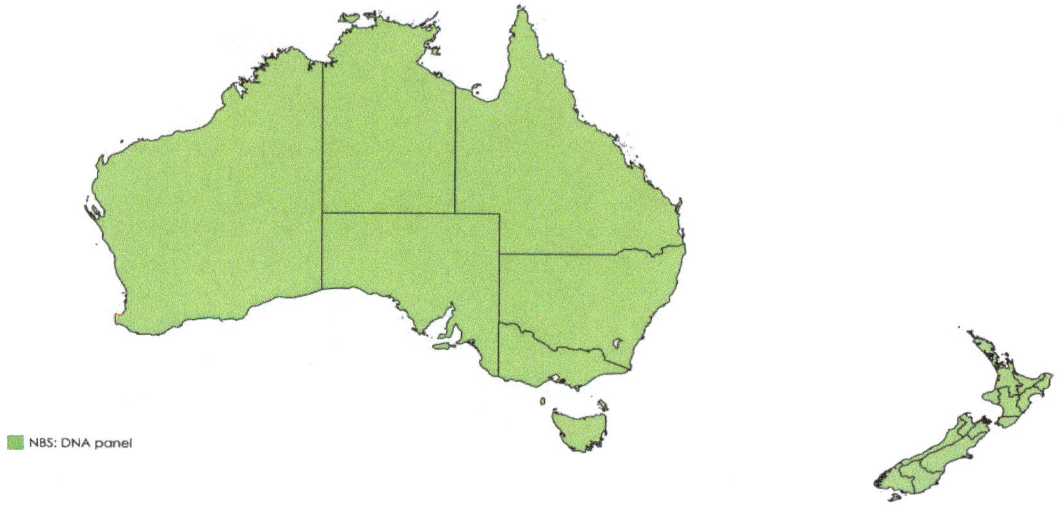

Figure 1. (**a**) In Europe, (**b**) in North America, (**c**) in South America, (**d**) in Australia and New Zealand. Newborn screening programs for cystic fibrosis (CF) according to the place of DNA analysis. NBS, newborn screening; EGA, extended *CFTR* genetic analysis.

Numerous programs have included a safety net protocol with the aim to identify CF infants who would be missed by testing variant panels because they carry two rare variants. Depending on the program, neonates with no variant but ultra-high IRT undergo either a second IRT measurement at 14–21 days or a direct sweat testing. In Denmark and the Netherlands, the safety net protocol leads to performing EGA. Safety net protocols lead to limiting false negatives cases, hence increasing the sensitivity of NBS programs, which is particularly effective in ethnic minority communities.

Comparing performances between different strategies using DNA analysis is a difficult task because of the considerable variability of protocols (Table 1), the changes over time in a country, the number of years since implementation, the duration of follow-up, the strategies and sensitivity of DNA analysis, and the monitoring of performance. Even when equivalent strategies are applied, there is variability in each step of the protocol, such as in the choice of the IRT cut-off value, the number of frequent variants screened by the panel, the use of a third or even fourth tier to minimize the number of children referred for sweat testing, or the safety net protocol (Table 1).

It is recommended to screen all pathogenic variants found at an incidence of 0.5% or higher according to geographical origins, or all variants accounting for more than 80% of CF alleles in the screened population [20]. The number of tested variants in NBS programs varies from 1 (F508del in Denmark and some states of the US [5,21]) to 388 (in New York State) (Personal Communication [15]).

Table 1. Strategies and performance of newborn screening programs for CF.

Countries/States	1st Tier	2nd Tier	3rd Tier	4th Tier	Safety Net	IRT1 > Cut Off	Sensitivity (wo MI)	PPV CF	Ratio CF:CFSPID	Carrier Frequency
Brazil (Sao Paulo) [16] Russia [22] Slovakia [1] Turkey [23] Spain (Andalusia) [24]	IRT	IRT				0.73–1.67%	86–100%	3–19%	ND 1.1:1 (Turkey)	NA
Austria [25]		PAP			IRT	0.97%		23%	25:1 *	NA
Portugal [26]						0.70%	94.4%	41%	ND	NA
Germany [27,28]		PAP	DNA (31)		ST	0.73%	96%	20%	5:1	1/44
US (Colorado, Texas, Wyoming) [29]		IRT	DNA (41–48)		ST	2.10%	96%	20%	10.8:1	1/13
US (Wisconsin) [30]		DNA (25)				ND	95%	9%	5.2:1	1/9.5
Australia (Victoria) [18]		DNA (12)				ND	96%	18.3%	7.8:1	ND
New Zealand [19]		DNA (3)				ND	100%	23%	ND	ND
Italy (Tuscany) [31]		DNA (66)				0.85%	89.5%	19.4%	2.85:1	1/16
France [32]		DNA (29)			IRT	0.50%	95%	34%	9:1	1/16
Switzerland [33]		DNA (7)			IRT	0.78%	97%	36%	17:1 *	1/11 *
Czech Republic [1,34]		DNA (50)			IRT	0.90%	94%	15%	7.5:1 *	1/21
Norway [35]		DNA (72)	DNA (20)		ST	0.8%	95%	43%	1:1	1/10
UK [1,36]		DNA (4)	DNA (29 or 31)	IRT	IRT	0.57% *	96%	76%	10.5:1 *	1/28 *
Denmark [21]		DNA (1)	EGA		EGA	3.70%	92%	85%	7:1	1/20
California [7]		DNA (40)	EGA			1.6%	92%	34%	0.65:1	1/25
Netherlands [37]		PAP	DNA (35)	EGA	EGA	0.98%	90%	63%	4:1	1/28
Poland [1,38]		DNA(limited seq)	EGA			0.6% *	100%	26%	1.2:1 *	1/15 *

CFSPID, CF screen positive, inconclusive diagnosis; DNA, refers to either variant panel analysis, with the number of variants screened indicated in brackets, or to limited *CFTR* gene sequencing (limited seq) in Poland; EGA, extended *CFTR* genetic analysis; IRT, immunoreactive trypsinogen; NA, not applicable; ND, not documented; ST, sweat test; PAP, pancreatitis-associated peptide; PPV, positive predictive value; wo MI, without meconium ileus. * Figures taken from [1]. Since the sensitivity of the panels used were not always available, they were not indicated in the table.

2.1. Programs Including Variant Panels Only

Most of the NBS protocols use a panel of frequent CF-causing variants after the first raised IRT value. Only Serbia, Ukraine, and some US states have included a second IRT measurement on a new blood sample before testing the panel, and Germany has included pancreatitis-associated peptide (PAP) measurement as a second tier before DNA analysis. The UK and Norway use a second DNA panel in neonates found to carry a variant of the first panel.

In most of these programs testing for a variant panel, infants carrying only one identified variant are referred for sweat testing in order to distinguish affected infants from healthy carriers. In the UK and Luxembourg, a second IRT measurement on a new sample is performed to select neonates found to carry one variant who will undergo sweat testing.

Inclusion into NBS programs of DNA analysis using variant panels appears to be at the benefice of both sensitivity and PPV compared to IRT/IRT protocols [1,11], with fewer false positive infants referred for sweat testing. However, despite the use of panels adapted to each population to achieve an optimal mutation detection rate, there remains disparity regarding sensitivity of the programs, with the majority above 95% (10/12 countries) according to ECFS recommendations [14]. Moreover, PPV varies from 3% to 76%. Of the 14 available PPV data sets, only four are above the ECFS target of 30%. Norway and the UK use DNA analysis in two successive panels, and the UK has also included a second IRT measurement after DNA analysis to select infants who will undergo sweat testing, which has raised the PPV up to 76%.

The CF:CFSPID ratio also varies between countries that use a DNA panel strategy, from 17:1 in Switzerland to 1:1 in Norway, along with the carrier frequency, from 1/9.5 in Wisconsin to 1/44 in Germany. This could be explained by different mutation detection rates of variant panels, implementation of a safety net protocol, IRT cut-off, and the frequency of carriers in each population. Indeed, the number of healthy carriers detected increases with the mutation detection rate [11].

2.2. Programs Including EGA

Six programs have implemented EGA in their strategy, applied after a first step of DNA analysis when one CF-causing variant is found. Denmark tests a single variant [21], the Netherlands a panel of 35 [37], California State tests a panel of 40 [7], Hawaii State a panel of 97 [5] and New York State a panel of 388 (Personal Communication [15]). Poland applies *CFTR* sequencing in two tiers: analysis of *CFTR* regions covering 77% of Polish variants, then all *CFTR* coding regions (Personal communication [39]). There is no available data on the performance of the programs in Hawaii State and in New York State where the strategy recently changed. While PPV in the Polish program is 26%, it is above 30% in the others, varying from 34% to 85% (Table 1). By contrast, the sensitivity displayed in the Polish program is 100%, compared with 90–92% for the other three.

Denmark have chosen a low IRT cut-off (50 ng/mL) and test for F508del which is carried by approximatively 96% of the CF patients on at least one allele [21]. F508del would be carried by only 79% of the CF patients in Poland on at least one allele, according to the 54.5% F508del allelic frequency among CF alleles [40]. The high frequency of F508del allele in Danish CF patients may also explain the better CF:CFSPID ratio in Denmark (7:1), compared with the ratio in California (0.65:1). The CF:CFSPID ratio of 4:1 in the Netherlands is probably due to the additional step of PAP measurement that minimizes the number of positive screened newborns.

The rate of CF carriers detected through NBS also varies, from 1/15 in Poland to 1/28 in the Netherlands.

3. Values and Challenges of *CFTR* Extended Genetic Analysis

Assessing the value of EGA in NBS strategies is not a simple matter, given the few experiences documented, the different protocols followed, and the variable number of years since implementation. The analysis and the discussion below take into account these experiences, as well as considerations beyond to assess the value and challenges of EGA, either as a third-tier step after testing for a variant panel or directly as a second-tier step. They are summarized in Table 2.

Table 2. Strengths and weaknesses of extended *CFTR* gene analysis in newborn screening programs for CF, as a second- or third-tier step (IRT/EGA or IRT/DNA panel/EGA), compared to strategies including tests for variant panels only (IRT/DNA panel).

Strengths	Weaknesses
High PPV	**but . . .**
• Reduction of false positive results of NBS strategy with EGA in the third tier, hence: • Reduction of unnecessary sweat tests with EGA in the third tier	• Low CF:CFSPID ratio, expected to be further lowered if using EGA in the second tier because of: • Numerous babies with two *CFTR* VUS or VVCC with EGA in the second tier, leading to unnecessary sweat tests, thus at the expense of PPV • The important need for follow-up of infants with CRMS/CFSPID
High Sensitivity	**but . . .**
• Highest expected sensitivity with EGA in the second tier • Best equity between populations, adapted for minorities carrying rare variants • Unmasking new couples at risk of having a CF child (carrier detection)	• Misdiagnosis of CF or CRMS/CFSPID if referring to CFTR2 only • Increased number of carriers detected, including carriers of VUS and VVCC, especially with EGA in the second tier
Technically feasible	**but . . . requires optimal healthcare system organization**
• NGS already in routine in laboratories for several years • Coverage of all known and unknown variants	• NBS sequencing platform development or reorganization, especially if EGA in the second tier • Questionable cost-effectiveness of the NBS program because of its impacts beyond • Technical limitations (homopolymers, large deletions, deep intronic variants) depending on the technique and the design
Increased knowledge on *CFTR* variants	**but . . . raises questions on variant interpretation**
• Database enrichment and genotype–phenotype studies • Genetic counseling for future cases/pregnancies	• Increased number of VUS • Need for additional in vitro/ex vivo experiments and clinical examinations for variant interpretation • Disease penetrance unknown for many variants
More precise medical care	**but . . . raises ethical questions**
• Detection of the two disease-causing variants in a single step • Earlier access to treatment	• Possible delay at the first medical visit according to ECFS recommendations [14] • Psychological impact of long-term follow up of infants with CRMS/CFSPID • Detection of patients who may not be symptomatic before adulthood and are at an unknown risk of developing a CFTR-related disorder

CFSPID, CF screen positive, inconclusive diagnosis; CRMS, CFTR-related metabolic syndrome; EGA, extended *CFTR* genetic analysis; IRT, immunoreactive trypsinogen; NBS, newborn screening; NGS, Next Generation Sequencing; VVCC, variant of varying clinical consequence; VUS, variant of uncertain or unknown significance.

3.1. Values of CFTR Extended Genetic Analysis in Newborn Screening Programs for CF

3.1.1. Reduction of NBS False-Positive Results and Improvement of the PPV

Inclusion of EGA as a third tier after testing a variant panel appears to reduce the number of NBS false-positive results, thus the consecutive number of unnecessary sweat tests, and to improve the PPV as compared to programs that include testing for variant panels only (Table 1) [41]. Sweat chloride measurement, a key component for confirmation of CF, indeed requires a specific local CF center organization with a dedicated laboratory, as well as strong experience and routine practice of physicians for optimal performance and high quality [42,43].

3.1.2. Best Equity of CF Screening between Populations

One of the main rationales and benefits of implementation of EGA in NBS programs for CF is better equity for multi-ethnic communities compared to variant panels [43]. Even if a unique panel has been initially designed to cover the most frequent CF variants of the local population, migration flows modifying the ethnic mix would require recurrent updates to maintain high sensitivity of the test. Any DNA panel, even of large size, will miss rare variants.

3.1.3. Increased Knowledge of the Phenotypical Spectrum of CFTR Variants

EGA also opens the opportunity to enrich our knowledge on the phenotypical spectrum and penetrance associated with *CFTR* variants, especially variants of varying clinical consequences (VVCC) and variants of unknown significance (VUS). Long term follow-up of patients who carry a VUS in *trans* of a CF-causing variant would help define variant pathogenicity and enrich locus-specific databases (CFMDB [44], CFTR2, [45], and *CFTR*-France, [46]).

3.1.4. Earlier Diagnosis and Access to Treatment

In the era of precision medicine, extended sequencing of the *CFTR* gene in IRT-positive neonates would detect all actionable variants for which efficient modulators of CFTR protein are now available. An early molecular diagnosis for CF would thus ensure early access to treatment. Comparison of the delay at the first medical visit may not seem better in programs that include EGA, but the delay until the two CF-causing variants are detected would be much shorter.

3.2. Challenges

3.2.1. Healthcare System Organization

Implementation of EGA in NBS programs for CF raises major challenges. Not only should the costs of the core strategy, which may vary considerably [7,13,47], be taken into consideration but so should those incurred by sweat testing if EGA is performed in the second tier, variant functional testing, genetic investigations in the parents, medical visits, and long-term follow-up of all screen-positive infants, either diagnosed with CF or with an inconclusive diagnosis.

3.2.2. Technical Issues

NBS Sequencing Platforms Development or Reorganization

Sequencing for NBS can be done on the same platform as for routine diagnosis already in place in laboratories. However, NBS requires a specific organization with optimized preanalytical protocols on dried-drop specimen and a specialized molecular genetics team for *CFTR* variant interpretation. Moreover, priority has to be given to the NBS process in order to respect ECFS recommendations about the timeliness of results.

Interestingly, the molecular strategy applied in the states of California and New York includes a single technical assay for DNA analysis, that is, NGS sequencing of all *CFTR* exons and recurrent deep intronic variants, with a two-step bioinformatic analysis: an initial, predefined variant panel is run simultaneously to a deep scan that is masked, and the mask is lifted if only one CF-causing variant is detected. This unique molecular strategy may further improve the timeliness of results as compared to other approaches.

Sequencing and Bioinformatics Limitations for Variant Detection

Technical limitations include sequencing errors in homopolymer-rich sequences or in pseudo-homologous genomic regions [48] and the risk of missing short insertions or deletions because of misalignment of sequence reads. It is thus recommended to use several variant callers in the NGS pipeline in order to maximize variant detection efficiency [49], and this should be considered in the evaluation of costs. Inappropriate or insufficient design coverage could lead to missing large deletions or insertions and variants located in deep intronic regions. The design should thus be adapted and continuously updated accordingly [50,51]. Low DNA quality and quantity extracted of dried-blot samples are other constraints for the detection of large deletions and insertions [52].

Positive results should be confirmed by an independent assay on a second DNA dilution for identity monitoring, as in other programs. Using EGA, a higher number of variants is expected to require confirmation because of an increased detection and the possible technical limitation of NGS. Familial segregation analysis is also essential to confirm compound heterozygosity and to avoid false-positive results due to numerous complex alleles reported in the *CFTR* gene [46,53,54]. Parents' blood sampling for DNA analysis should therefore be carried out optimally during the first visit so that medical care is not delayed. These essential experiments, whose numbers will inevitably increase with EGA being included in NBS, especially as a second-tier step, have to be considered for medico-economic studies.

3.2.3. Byproducts of NBS for CF and Ethical Issues

Increased Detection of Inconclusive Diagnosis

The identification of a substantial number of VUS or VVCC in neonates without any clinical symptoms and leading to an inconclusive diagnosis is a major drawback observed in the few experiences of EGA in NBS. In strategies that include EGA as a core component, neonates found to carry two variants (one of which being a VUS) and to have a negative sweat test fall into the category of inconclusive diagnosis, while in other strategies that include variant panels only, these neonates would be classified as healthy carriers. Indeed, since the sweat test is negative, DNA analysis stops at the step of variant panel and the VUS will not be identified. Implementation of EGA as a second-tier analysis after a raised IRT would lead to the further detection of infants with an inconclusive diagnosis who would have a negative sweat test and carry other kinds of genotypes, composed of two VVCC, a VVCC and a VUS, or two VUS.

Despite accumulation of considerable data on *CFTR* variants in locus-specific variant databases (CFMDB, CFTR2, *CFTR*-France), epidemiological data and genotype–phenotype correlations still miss most rare genetic *CFTR* variants, which are sometimes restricted to one family. Furthermore, the number of new variants is steadily increasing, as illustrated in the California program, where 78 out of 303 rare variants were novel [7]. On the other hand, databases may provide discordant information that one should be aware of, notably because of their different designs. Data in CFTR2 are provided from national registries of CF patients and thus represent the "tip of the iceberg" of all possible phenotypes associated with a given genotype. By contrast, *CFTR*-France collects genetic and clinical data from patients with CF and CFTR-RD and from asymptomatic individuals, and so some variants are differently classified in the two databases. In addition, variants that are not referred to in the list of 432 described in CFTR2 have been classified as VUS in several programs [7,55,56], despite their description in the literature and other databases, either as CF-causing or as non-CF-causing. As a consequence, the number of CRMS/CFSPID observed in programs that include EGA may be overestimated and the ratio of CF:CFSPID artificially biased.

The risk that neonates with an inconclusive diagnosis will develop symptoms consistent with CF, even in a less typical form, with a possible delayed positive conversion of the sweat test [57,58] is still unknown. Nevertheless, parents should be informed on the longer-term risks that their child may develop clinical symptoms of CF. Ex vivo electrophysiological explorations on nasal epithelium, organoids, or rectal biopsies and in vitro experiments on heterologous immortalized cell systems reproducing DNA changes may help interpret variant pathogenicity and better evaluate the risk of developing clinical CF. A follow-up longer than two years is then critical [56,58]. However, the full penetrance associated with some VVCC may not be apparent until adulthood [55]. One may wonder whether the detection of patients who will not be symptomatic before adulthood is desirable. The frequency of variants and genotypes in the general population should be considered to evaluate the risk of a particular genotype to cause clinical CF; in other words, the penetrance of clinical CF in individuals carrying a given genotype. This was previously shown to be very low for R117H [59], an observation which led to its withdrawal from NBS variant panels [27,32], and, more recently, for the T5 variants and other variants commonly identified in inconclusive cases [60]. Such epidemiological data emphasize the importance of documenting the penetrance of variants before widely implementing EGA in core NBS programs.

The increased detection of inconclusive cases when using EGA strategies should thus be anticipated with regard to the organization of CF centers, the costs of follow-up, and the additional investigations for variant interpretation. Moreover, additional studies on psychological consequences [61] of the long-term follow-up of these patients are needed before implementation of EGA as a global model.

Carrier Detection and Genetic Counseling

Detection of healthy carriers, heterozygous for one CF-causing variant, is another unwanted result of NBS, though it has been considered a benefit that enables reproductive planning [62]. It will inevitably be increased by a more extensive DNA analysis in NBS strategy [10] and will have a cost for increased referrals in the families. Indeed, once a CF-causing variant is detected, a "cascade" genetic screening is recommended in relatives [63,64].

Here, again, as for inconclusive cases uncertainty about VUS and VVCC is puzzling and complicates genetic counseling. It is thus not only the higher number of healthy carriers of known CF-causing variants that healthcare professionals have to deal with, but the even higher expected number of carriers of VVCC and VUS. Updated information should be provided to families as knowledge evolves on variant pathogenicity, but such recalls could also generate anxiety. Population genetics data should not be neglected, as it has been shown that a number of variants classified as VUS or VVCC in CFTR2 actually have a frequency in the general population that argues against a severe impact, as for c.2620-26A>G, R74W, R117H, I556V, or D1270N [65]. The risk is to consider neonates as carriers of a CF-causing variant and to offer inappropriate genetic counseling and testing in the family, and eventually inappropriate prenatal diagnosis. In view of the expanding strategies that include EGA, guidelines should be issued on these matters to minimize as much as possible these byproducts.

4. Conclusions and Perspectives

Considerable expansion has been observed in the implementation of NBS programs for CF, with DNA analysis being part of an increasing number of strategies. While testing for *CFTR* gene variant panels as a second tier has been proven to improve the performance and reduce the false-positive rates, the value and place of *CFTR* EGA before the diagnostic step of sweat testing is still not obvious. The performance is indeed the result of all steps, starting with IRT cut-off values. Implementation of EGA in the NBS process, which has been greatly facilitated by advances in genomic sequencing technologies, is expected to achieve an optimal sensitivity in ethnically diverse populations and a faster genetic diagnosis in CF infants without the need of another sample. EGA has been implemented in three European countries and three US states only, with different mutational backgrounds and different protocols, so that comparison remains difficult. The major drawback of approaches that include EGA is the unwanted detection of neonates with an inconclusive diagnosis, with a CF:CFSPID ratio varying from one program to another, but which is as low as 1.2:1 in Poland [1] and 0.65:1 in California [7]. This challenging situation, leading to uncertainty for healthcare professionals and families, also generates costs that should be considered in the health economic evaluation of a program before its implementation. Based on data indicative of a low penetrance for a set of variants identified in inconclusive cases [59,60], it is likely that the detection of neonates carrying a true CF-causing variant in *trans* of such a variant would considerably increase in a program based on IRT/EGA, thus finally requiring a high number of sweat tests to be performed, not to mention other tests, follow-up visits, and parents' resulting anxiety. Therefore, the significant risk reported for neonates with an inconclusive diagnosis to develop a CF disease [58] might be considerably lowered as many more cases are detected through EGA before sweat testing. By contrast, removal of R117H from the variant panel of the French NBS program led to dramatically improved performance, with the PPV increasing from 16% to 34% and the ratio CF:CFSPID from 6.3:1 to 9:1 [32].

Eventually, based on technological advances in genomic sequencing and the reduction of costs along with the steadily increasing implementation of NBS programs in multi-ethnic populations or populations where common variants are not included in current DNA panels, an optimal compromise to improve performance and minimize side effects would be to perform EGA with bioinformatics targeting a wide panel of fully penetrant CF-causing variants, including large deletions and deep-intronic variants, as recently implemented in New York State. EGA without applying any bioinformatic filter or without any additional step as IRT or PAP to limit the number of infants subjected to sweat testing might be detrimental, as long as the clinical impact and penetrance data associated with variants are not well documented. In view of this, the collection of data on the extended follow-up of neonates detected with an inconclusive diagnosis is of the utmost importance [58].

The question of the role of EGA in the context of NBS does not only focus on CF. Whole exome sequencing and whole genome sequencing are nowadays affordable due to a significant reduction of costs. The relevance of implementing extended NBS for numerous genetic diseases is currently debated [66–68], which again raises the unsolved question of the interpretation of rare variants all along the genome. In this respect, comprehensive information on genetic issues should be given to the parents prior to NBS. Expanded preconception carrier screening for recessive disorders is also under consideration in countries following an overall positive attitude of the general population [69], depending on ethnical and geographical origin, degree of consanguinity, and type of disorders. Preconception CF carrier screening has already been implemented in the US, Israël, and Northeast Italy [70]. Such a health public policy aims to detect most at-risk couples and this ineluctably impacts on the timing for a CF diagnosis and on the prevalence of CF births [71], which would then raise the question of the relevance of NBS. Reproductive attitudes would also inevitably change, as recently underlined [72]. Requests for prenatal diagnoses may increase, especially where non-invasive procedures have been recently available [73,74], but where a diagnosis of CF is made, with the growing availability of mutation-guided therapy the option of the continuation of pregnancy could be preferred over termination.

In conclusion, designation of an optimal NBS program remains necessarily country-dependent. The introduction of EGA as a second tier without filtering of CF variants has major drawbacks that are yet unsolved and may negatively impact the organization of care and the cost-effectiveness of NBS for CF. Consideration of any change in strategy should be carefully evaluated, planned, and monitored. This reinforces the need to adopt a standardized approach to collect data to the benefice of performance comparison. Taking all of these elements into account will ensure the sustainability of implemented NBS programs.

Author Contributions: Conception and design of the study, A.B. and E.G.; review of literature data, writing of the manuscript, A.B., M.L. and E.G. All authors have read and agreed to the published version of the manuscript.

Acknowledgments: The authors are grateful to Michele Caggana for recent data on the New York State program, Dorota Sands for data on the Poland program, and Carlo Castellani for valuable discussion.

References

1. Barben, J.; Castellani, C.; Dankert-Roelse, J.; Gartner, S.; Kashirskaya, N.; Linnane, B.; Mayell, S.; Munck, A.;

Sands, D.; Sommerburg, O.; et al. The expansion and performance of national newborn screening programmes for cystic fibrosis in Europe. *J. Cyst. Fibros.* **2017**, *16*, 207–213. [CrossRef] [PubMed]

2. NSWG Annual Report 2018. Available online: https://www.ecfs.eu/sites/default/files/general-content-files/working-groups/NSWG%20annual%20report%202018v2.pdf (accessed on 21 February 2020).
3. Massie, J.; Clements, B.; The Australian Paediatric Respiratory Group. Diagnosis of cystic fibrosis after newborn screening: The Australasian experience—twenty years and five million babies later: A consensus statement from the Australasian paediatric respiratory group. *Pediatr. Pulmonol.* **2005**, *39*, 440–446. [CrossRef] [PubMed]
4. Byrnes, C.A.; Vidmar, S.; Cheney, J.L.; Carlin, J.B.; Armstrong, D.S.; Cooper, P.J.; Grimwood, K.; Moodie, M.; Robertson, C.F.; Rosenfeld, M.; et al. Prospective evaluation of respiratory exacerbations in children with cystic fibrosis from newborn screening to 5 years of age. *Thorax* **2013**, *68*, 643–651. [CrossRef] [PubMed]
5. Pique, L.; Graham, S.; Pearl, M.; Kharrazi, M.; Schrijver, I. Cystic fibrosis newborn screening programs: Implications of the *CFTR* variant spectrum in nonwhite patients. *Genet. Med.* **2017**, *19*, 36–44. [CrossRef]
6. Mak, D.Y.F.; Sykes, J.; Stephenson, A.L.; Lands, L.C. The benefits of newborn screening for cystic fibrosis: The Canadian experience. *J. Cyst. Fibros.* **2016**, *15*, 302–308. [CrossRef]
7. Kharrazi, M.; Yang, J.; Bishop, T.; Lessing, S.; Young, S.; Graham, S.; Pearl, M.; Chow, H.; Ho, T.; Currier, R.; et al. Newborn Screening for Cystic Fibrosis in California. *Pediatrics* **2015**, *136*, 1062–1072. [CrossRef]
8. Farrell, P.M.; White, T.B.; Howenstine, M.S.; Munck, A.; Parad, R.B.; Rosenfeld, M.; Sommerburg, O.; Accurso, F.J.; Davies, J.C.; Rock, M.J.; et al. Diagnosis of Cystic Fibrosis in Screened Populations. *J. Pediatr.* **2017**, *181*, S33–S44. [CrossRef]
9. Southern, K.W.; Barben, J.; Gartner, S.; Munck, A.; Castellani, C.; Mayell, S.J.; Davies, J.C.; Winters, V.; Murphy, J.; Salinas, D.; et al. Inconclusive diagnosis after a positive newborn bloodspot screening result for cystic fibrosis; clarification of the harmonised international definition. *J. Cyst. Fibros.* **2019**, *18*, 778–780. [CrossRef]
10. Castellani, C.; Southern, K.W.; Brownlee, K.; Dankert Roelse, J.; Duff, A.; Farrell, M.; Mehta, A.; Munck, A.; Pollitt, R.; Sermet-Gaudelus, I.; et al. European best practice guidelines for cystic fibrosis neonatal screening. *J. Cyst. Fibros.* **2009**, *8*, 153–173. [CrossRef]
11. Castellani, C.; Massie, J.; Sontag, M.; Southern, K.W. Newborn screening for cystic fibrosis. *Lancet Respir. Med.* **2016**, *4*, 653–661. [CrossRef]
12. Castellani, C.; Linnane, B.; Pranke, I.; Cresta, F.; Sermet-Gaudelus, I.; Peckham, D. Cystic Fibrosis Diagnosis in Newborns, Children, and Adults. *Semin. Respir. Crit. Care Med.* **2019**, *40*, 701–714. [CrossRef] [PubMed]
13. Schmidt, M.; Werbrouck, A.; Verhaeghe, N.; de Wachter, E.; Simoens, S.; Annemans, L.; Putman, K. A model-based economic evaluation of four newborn screening strategies for cystic fibrosis in Flanders, Belgium. *Acta Clin. Belg.* **2019**, 1–9. [CrossRef] [PubMed]
14. Castellani, C.; Duff, A.J.A.; Bell, S.C.; Heijerman, H.G.M.; Munck, A.; Ratjen, F.; Sermet-Gaudelus, I.; Southern, K.W.; Barben, J.; Flume, P.A.; et al. ECFS best practice guidelines: The 2018 revision. *J. Cyst. Fibros.* **2018**, *17*, 153–178. [CrossRef] [PubMed]
15. Caggana, M. (New York State Department of Health, Albany, NY 12208, USA). Personal communication, 2020.
16. Rodrigues, R.; Magalhaes, P.K.R.; Fernandes, M.I.M.; Gabetta, C.S.; Ribeiro, A.F.; Pedro, K.P.; Valdetaro, F.; Santos, J.L.F.; de Souza, R.M.; Pazin Filho, A.; et al. Neonatal screening for cystic fibrosis in São Paulo State, Brazil: A pilot study. *Braz. J. Med. Biol. Res.* **2009**, *42*, 973–978. [CrossRef] [PubMed]
17. XI Congreso Latinoamericano de Errores Inatos del Metabolismo y Pesquisa Neonatal. 2019. Available online: http://www.sleimpn2019.org/index.php/trabajos/posters-pesquisa-neonatal (accessed on 21 February 2020).
18. Massie, R.J.H.; Curnow, L.; Glazner, J.; Armstrong, D.S.; Francis, I. Lessons learned from 20 years of newborn screening for cystic fibrosis. *Med. J. Aust.* **2012**, *196*, 67–70. [CrossRef]
19. Ministry of Health. *Newborn Metabolic Screening Programme: Annual Report 2017*; Ministry of Health: Wellington, New Zealand, 2018.
20. Ross, L.F. Newborn Screening for Cystic Fibrosis: A Lesson in Public Health Disparities. *J. Pediatr.* **2008**, *153*, 308–313. [CrossRef]
21. Skov, M.; Bækvad-Hansen, M.; Hougaard, D.M.; Skogstrand, K.; Lund, A.M.; Pressler, T.; Olesen, H.V.; Duno, M. Cystic fibrosis newborn screening in Denmark: Experience from the first 2 years. *Pediatr. Pulmonol.* **2020**, *55*, 549–555. [CrossRef]

22. Tolstova, V.D.; Kashirskaya, N.Y.; Kapranov, N.I.; Khodunova, A.A.; Denisenkova, E.V.; Smazhil, E.V. First results of newborn screening program for CF in Russia. *J. Cyst. Fibros.* **2008**, *7*, S13. [CrossRef]
23. Başaran, A.E.; Başaran, A.; Uygun, D.F.K.; Alper, Ö.; Acican, D.; BiNgöl, A. Initial regional evaluation of the Cystic Fibrosis Newborn Screening Program: Data from the Mediterranean coast of Turkey. *Turk. J. Med. Sci.* **2019**, *49*, 1655–1661.
24. Delgado Pecellín, I.; Pérez Ruiz, E.; Álvarez Ríos, A.I.; Delgado Pecellín, C.; Yahyaoui Macías, R.; Carrasco Hernández, L.; Marcos Luque, I.; Caro Aguilera, P.; Moreno Valera, M.J.; Quintana Gallego, M.E. Results of the Andalusian Cystic Fibrosis Neonatal Screening Program, 5 Years After Implementation. *Arch. Bronconeumol.* **2018**, *54*, 551–558. [CrossRef]
25. Renner, S.; Schanzer, A.; Metz, T.; Szépfalusi, Z.; Zeyda, M. CF newborn screening in Austria: After 20 years changing the algorithm from IRT/IRT to IRT/PAP/IRT. *J. Cyst. Fibros.* **2018**, *17*, S18. [CrossRef]
26. Marcão, A.; Barreto, C.; Pereira, L.; Vaz, L.; Cavaco, J.; Casimiro, A.; Félix, M.; Silva, T.; Barbosa, T.; Freitas, C.; et al. Cystic Fibrosis Newborn Screening in Portugal: PAP Value in Populations with Stringent Rules for Genetic Studies. *Int. J. Neonatal Screen.* **2018**, *4*, 22. [CrossRef]
27. Sommerburg, O.; Stahl, M.; Hammermann, J.; Okun, J.; Kulozik, A.; Hoffmann, G.; Mall, M. Neugeborenenscreening auf Mukoviszidose in Deutschland: Vergleich des neuen Screening-Protokolls mit einem Alternativprotokoll. *Klin. Padiatr.* **2017**, *229*, 59–66. [CrossRef] [PubMed]
28. Brockow, I.; Nennstiel, U. Parents' experience with positive newborn screening results for cystic fibrosis. *Eur. J. Pediatr.* **2019**, *178*, 803–809. [CrossRef]
29. Sontag, M.K.; Lee, R.; Wright, D.; Freedenberg, D.; Sagel, S.D. Improving the Sensitivity and Positive Predictive Value in a Cystic Fibrosis Newborn Screening Program Using a Repeat Immunoreactive Trypsinogen and Genetic Analysis. *J. Pediatr.* **2016**, *175*, 150–158. [CrossRef]
30. Rock, M.J.; Hoffman, G.; Laessig, R.H.; Kopish, G.J.; Litsheim, T.J.; Farrell, P.M. Newborn screening for cystic fibrosis in Wisconsin: Nine-year experience with routine trypsinogen/DNA testing. *J. Pediatr.* **2005**, *147*, S73–S77. [CrossRef]
31. Terlizzi, V.; Mergni, G.; Buzzetti, R.; Centrone, C.; Zavataro, L.; Braggion, C. Cystic fibrosis screen positive inconclusive diagnosis (CFSPID): Experience in Tuscany, Italy. *J. Cyst. Fibros.* **2019**, *18*, 484–490. [CrossRef]
32. Munck, A.; Delmas, D.; Audrézet, M.-P.; Lemonnier, L.; Cheillan, D.; Roussey, M. Optimization of the French cystic fibrosis newborn screening programme by a centralized tracking process. *J. Med. Screen.* **2018**, *25*, 6–12. [CrossRef]
33. Rueegg, C.S.; Kuehni, C.E.; Gallati, S.; Baumgartner, M.; Torresani, T.; Barben, J. One-Year Evaluation of a Neonatal Screening Program for Cystic Fibrosis in Switzerland. *Dtsch. Arztebl. Int.* **2013**, *110*, 356–363. [CrossRef]
34. Krulišová, V.; Balaščaková, M.; Skalická, V.; Piskáčková, T.; Holubová, A.; Paděrová, J.; Křenková, P.; Dvořáková, L.; Zemková, D.; Kračmar, P.; et al. Prospective and parallel assessments of cystic fibrosis newborn screening protocols in the Czech Republic: IRT/DNA/IRT versus IRT/PAP and IRT/PAP/DNA. *Eur. J. Pediatr.* **2012**, *171*, 1223–1229. [CrossRef]
35. Lundman, E.; Gaup, H.J.; Bakkeheim, E.; Olafsdottir, E.J.; Rootwelt, T.; Storrøsten, O.T.; Pettersen, R.D. Implementation of newborn screening for cystic fibrosis in Norway. Results from the first three years. *J. Cyst. Fibros.* **2016**, *15*, 318–324. [CrossRef] [PubMed]
36. Schlüter, D.K.; Southern, K.W.; Dryden, C.; Diggle, P.; Taylor-Robinson, D. Impact of newborn screening on outcomes and social inequalities in cystic fibrosis: A UK CF registry-based study. *Thorax* **2020**, *75*, 123–131. [CrossRef] [PubMed]
37. Dankert-Roelse, J.E.; Bouva, M.J.; Jakobs, B.S.; Janssens, H.M.; de Winter-de Groot, K.M.; Schönbeck, Y.; Gille, J.J.P.; Gulmans, V.A.M.; Verschoof-Puite, R.K.; Schielen, P.C.J.I.; et al. Newborn blood spot screening for cystic fibrosis with a four-step screening strategy in the Netherlands. *J. Cyst. Fibros.* **2019**, *18*, 54–63. [CrossRef] [PubMed]
38. Sands, D.; Zybert, K.; Mierzejewska, E.; Oltarzewski, M. Diagnosing cystic fibrosis in newborn screening in Poland—15 years of experience. *Dev. Period Med.* **2015**, *19*, 16–24.
39. Sands, D. (Zaklad Mukowiscydozy, Instytut Matki i Dziecka, Kasprzaka 17a, 01-211 Warsow, Poland). Personal communication, 2020.

40. Ziętkiewicz, E.; Rutkiewicz, E.; Pogorzelski, A.; Klimek, B.; Voelkel, K.; Witt, M. *CFTR* mutations spectrum and the efficiency of molecular diagnostics in Polish cystic fibrosis patients. *PLoS ONE* **2014**, *9*, e89094. [CrossRef]
41. Currier, R.J.; Sciortino, S.; Liu, R.; Bishop, T.; Alikhani Koupaei, R.; Feuchtbaum, L. Genomic sequencing in cystic fibrosis newborn screening: What works best, two-tier predefined *CFTR* mutation panels or second-tier *CFTR* panel followed by third-tier sequencing? *Genet. Med.* **2017**, *19*, 1159–1163. [CrossRef]
42. Cirilli, N.; Southern, K.W.; Buzzetti, R.; Barben, J.; Nährlich, L.; Munck, A.; Wilschanski, M.; De Boeck, K.; Derichs, N. Real life practice of sweat testing in Europe. *J. Cyst. Fibros.* **2018**, *17*, 325–332. [CrossRef]
43. Schrijver, I.; Pique, L.; Graham, S.; Pearl, M.; Cherry, A.; Kharrazi, M. The Spectrum of *CFTR* Variants in Nonwhite Cystic Fibrosis Patients: Implications for Molecular Diagnostic Testing. *J. Mol. Diagn.* **2016**, *18*, 39–50. [CrossRef]
44. Cystic Fibrosis Mutation Data Base (CFMDB). Available online: http://www.genet.sickkids.on.ca/ (accessed on 21 February 2020).
45. Sosnay, P.R.; Siklosi, K.R.; Van Goor, F.; Kaniecki, K.; Yu, H.; Sharma, N.; Ramalho, A.S.; Amaral, M.D.; Dorfman, R.; Zielenski, J.; et al. Defining the disease liability of variants in the cystic fibrosis transmembrane conductance regulator gene. *Nat. Genet.* **2013**, *45*, 1160–1167. [CrossRef]
46. Claustres, M.; Thèze, C.; des Georges, M.; Baux, D.; Girodon, E.; Bienvenu, T.; Audrezet, M.-P.; Dugueperoux, I.; Férec, C.; Lalau, G.; et al. *CFTR*-France, a national relational patient database for sharing genetic and phenotypic data associated with rare *CFTR* variants. *Hum. Mutat.* **2017**, *38*, 1297–1315. [CrossRef]
47. Wells, J.; Rosenberg, M.; Hoffman, G.; Anstead, M.; Farrell, P.M. A Decision-Tree Approach to Cost Comparison of Newborn Screening Strategies for Cystic Fibrosis. *Pediatrics* **2012**, *129*, e339–e347. [CrossRef] [PubMed]
48. Deeb, K.K.; Metcalf, J.D.; Sesock, K.M.; Shen, J.; Wensel, C.A.; Rippel, L.I.; Smith, M.; Chapman, M.S.; Zhang, S. The c.1364C>A (p.A455E) Mutation in the *CFTR* Pseudogene Results in an Incorrectly Assigned Carrier Status by a Commonly Used Screening Platform. *J. Mol. Diagn.* **2015**, *17*, 360–365. [CrossRef] [PubMed]
49. Hwang, S.; Kim, E.; Lee, I.; Marcotte, E.M. Systematic comparison of variant calling pipelines using gold standard personal exome variants. *Sci. Rep.* **2015**, *5*, 17875. [CrossRef] [PubMed]
50. Lefterova, M.I.; Shen, P.; Odegaard, J.I.; Fung, E.; Chiang, T.; Peng, G.; Davis, R.W.; Wang, W.; Kharrazi, M.; Schrijver, I.; et al. Next-Generation Molecular Testing of Newborn Dried Blood Spots for Cystic Fibrosis. *J. Mol. Diagn.* **2016**, *18*, 267–282. [CrossRef] [PubMed]
51. Bergougnoux, A.; Délétang, K.; Pommier, A.; Varilh, J.; Houriez, F.; Altieri, J.P.; Koenig, M.; Férec, C.; Claustres, M.; Lalau, G.; et al. Functional characterization and phenotypic spectrum of three recurrent disease-causing deep intronic variants of the *CFTR* gene. *J. Cyst. Fibros.* **2019**, *18*, 468–475. [CrossRef] [PubMed]
52. Boemer, F.; Fasquelle, C.; d'Otreppe, S.; Josse, C.; Dideberg, V.; Segers, K.; Guissard, V.; Capraro, V.; Debray, F.G.; Bours, V. A next-generation newborn screening pilot study: NGS on dried blood spots detects causal mutations in patients with inherited metabolic diseases. *Sci. Rep.* **2017**, *7*, 17641. [CrossRef] [PubMed]
53. Bergougnoux, A.; Boureau-Wirth, A.; Rouzier, C.; Altieri, J.-P.; Verneau, F.; Larrieu, L.; Koenig, M.; Claustres, M.; Raynal, C. A false positive newborn screening result due to a complex allele carrying two frequent CF-causing variants. *J. Cyst. Fibros.* **2016**, *15*, 309–312. [CrossRef]
54. Terlizzi, V.; Castaldo, G.; Salvatore, D.; Lucarelli, M.; Raia, V.; Angioni, A.; Carnovale, V.; Cirilli, N.; Casciaro, R.; Colombo, C.; et al. Genotype-phenotype correlation and functional studies in patients with cystic fibrosis bearing *CFTR* complex alleles. *J. Med. Genet.* **2017**, *54*, 224–235. [CrossRef]
55. Salinas, D.B.; Sosnay, P.R.; Azen, C.; Young, S.; Raraigh, K.S.; Keens, T.G.; Kharrazi, M. Benign and Deleterious Cystic Fibrosis Transmembrane Conductance Regulator Mutations Identified by Sequencing in Positive Cystic Fibrosis Newborn Screen Children from California. *PLoS ONE* **2016**, *11*, e0155624. [CrossRef]
56. Ren, C.L.; Borowitz, D.S.; Gonska, T.; Howenstine, M.S.; Levy, H.; Massie, J.; Milla, C.; Munck, A.; Southern, K.W. Cystic Fibrosis Transmembrane Conductance Regulator-Related Metabolic Syndrome and Cystic Fibrosis Screen Positive, Inconclusive Diagnosis. *J. Pediatr.* **2017**, *181*, S45–S51. [CrossRef]
57. Ooi, C.Y.; Castellani, C.; Keenan, K.; Avolio, J.; Volpi, S.; Boland, M.; Kovesi, T.; Bjornson, C.; Chilvers, M.A.; Morgan, L.; et al. Inconclusive Diagnosis of Cystic Fibrosis After Newborn Screening. *Pediatrics* **2015**, *135*, e1377–e1385. [CrossRef] [PubMed]

58. Munck, A.; Bourmaud, A.; Bellon, G.; Picq, P.; Farrell, P.M.; DPAM Study Group. Phenotype of children with inconclusive cystic fibrosis diagnosis after newborn screening. *Pediatr. Pulmonol.* **2020**, *55*, 918–928. [CrossRef] [PubMed]
59. Thauvin-Robinet, C.; Munck, A.; Huet, F.; Génin, E.; Bellis, G.; Gautier, E.; Audrézet, M.-P.; Férec, C.; Lalau, G.; Georges, M.D.; et al. The very low penetrance of cystic fibrosis for the R117H mutation: A reappraisal for genetic counselling and newborn screening. *J. Med. Genet.* **2009**, *46*, 752–758. [CrossRef] [PubMed]
60. Boussaroque, A.; Audrézet, M.-P.; Raynal, C.; Sermet-Gaudelus, I.; Bienvenu, T.; Férec, C.; Bergougnoux, A.; Lopez, M.; Scotet, V.; Munck, A.; et al. Penetrance is a critical parameter for assessing the disease liability of *CFTR* variants. *J. Cyst. Fibros.* **2020**, in press. [CrossRef]
61. Hayeems, R.Z.; Miller, F.A.; Barg, C.J.; Bombard, Y.; Carroll, J.C.; Tam, K.; Kerr, E.; Chakraborty, P.; Potter, B.K.; Patton, S.; et al. Psychosocial Response to Uncertain Newborn Screening Results for Cystic Fibrosis. *J. Pediatr.* **2017**, *184*, 165–171. [CrossRef]
62. McClaren, B.J.; Metcalfe, S.A.; Aitken, M.; Massie, R.J.; Ukoumunne, O.C.; Amor, D.J. Uptake of carrier testing in families after cystic fibrosis diagnosis through newborn screening. *Eur. J. Hum. Genet.* **2010**, *18*, 1084–1089. [CrossRef]
63. Dequeker, E.; Stuhrmann, M.; Morris, M.A.; Casals, T.; Castellani, C.; Claustres, M.; Cuppens, H.; des Georges, M.; Ferec, C.; Macek, M.; et al. Best practice guidelines for molecular genetic diagnosis of cystic fibrosis and CFTR-related disorders—updated European recommendations. *Eur. J. Hum. Genet.* **2009**, *17*, 51–65. [CrossRef]
64. Castellani, C.; Cuppens, H.; Macek, M.; Cassiman, J.J.; Kerem, E.; Durie, P.; Tullis, E.; Assael, B.M.; Bombieri, C.; Brown, A.; et al. Consensus on the use and interpretation of cystic fibrosis mutation analysis in clinical practice. *J. Cyst. Fibros.* **2008**, *7*, 179–196. [CrossRef]
65. Boussaroque, A.; Bergougnoux, A.; Raynal, C.; Audrézet, M.-P.; Sasorith, S.; Férec, C.; Bienvenu, T.; Girodon, E. Pitfalls in the interpretation of *CFTR* variants in the context of incidental findings. *Hum. Mutat.* **2019**, *40*, 2239–2246. [CrossRef]
66. Ceyhan-Birsoy, O.; Murry, J.B.; Machini, K.; Lebo, M.S.; Yu, T.W.; Fayer, S.; Genetti, C.A.; Schwartz, T.S.; Agrawal, P.B.; Parad, R.B.; et al. Interpretation of Genomic Sequencing Results in Healthy and Ill Newborns: Results from the BabySeq Project. *Am. J. Hum. Genet.* **2019**, *104*, 76–93. [CrossRef]
67. Kingsmore, S.F. Newborn testing and screening by whole-genome sequencing. *Genet. Med.* **2016**, *18*, 214–216. [CrossRef] [PubMed]
68. Wilcken, B.; Wiley, V. Fifty years of newborn screening. *J. Paediatr. Child Health* **2015**, *51*, 103–107. [CrossRef] [PubMed]
69. Nijmeijer, S.C.M.; Conijn, T.; Lakeman, P.; Henneman, L.; Wijburg, F.A.; Haverman, L. Attitudes of the general population towards preconception expanded carrier screening for autosomal recessive disorders including inborn errors of metabolism. *Mol. Genet. Metab.* **2019**, *126*, 14–22. [CrossRef] [PubMed]
70. Delatycki, M.B.; Alkuraya, F.; Archibald, A.; Castellani, C.; Cornel, M.; Grody, W.W.; Henneman, L.; Ioannides, A.S.; Kirk, E.; Laing, N.; et al. International perspectives on the implementation of reproductive carrier screening. *Prenat. Diagn.* **2020**, *40*, 301–310. [CrossRef] [PubMed]
71. Castellani, C.; Picci, L.; Tridello, G.; Casati, E.; Tamanini, A.; Bartoloni, L.; Scarpa, M.; Assael, B.M. Cystic fibrosis carrier screening effects on birth prevalence and newborn screening. *Genet. Med.* **2016**, *18*, 145–151. [CrossRef] [PubMed]
72. Bell, S.C.; Mall, M.A.; Gutierrez, H.; Macek, M.; Madge, S.; Davies, J.C.; Burgel, P.-R.; Tullis, E.; Castaños, C.; Castellani, C.; et al. The future of cystic fibrosis care: A global perspective. *Lancet Respir. Med.* **2020**, *8*, 65–124. [CrossRef]
73. Gruber, A.; Pacault, M.; El Khattabi, L.A.; Vaucouleur, N.; Orhant, L.; Bienvenu, T.; Girodon, E.; Vidaud, D.; Leturcq, F.; Costa, C.; et al. Non-invasive prenatal diagnosis of paternally inherited disorders from maternal plasma: Detection of NF1 and *CFTR* mutations using droplet digital PCR. *Clin. Chem. Lab. Med.* **2018**, *56*, 728–738. [CrossRef]
74. Guissart, C.; Tran Mau Them, F.; Debant, V.; Viart, V.; Dubucs, C.; Pritchard, V.; Rouzier, C.; Boureau-Wirth, A.; Haquet, E.; Puechberty, J.; et al. A Broad Test Based on Fluorescent-Multiplex PCR for Noninvasive Prenatal Diagnosis of Cystic Fibrosis. *Fetal. Diagn. Ther.* **2019**, *45*, 403–412. [CrossRef]

17

Sickle Cell Disease—Genetics, Pathophysiology, Clinical Presentation and Treatment

Baba P. D. Inusa [1,*], Lewis L. Hsu [2], Neeraj Kohli [3], Anissa Patel [4], Kilali Ominu-Evbota [5], Kofi A. Anie [6] and Wale Atoyebi [7]

1 Paediatric Haematology, Evelina London Children's Hospital, Guy's and St Thomas NHS Trust, London SE1 7EH, UK
2 Pediatric Hematology-Oncology, University of Illinois at Chicago, Chicago, IL 60612, USA; LewHsu@uic.edu
3 Haematology, Guy's and St Thomas NHS Trust, London SE1 7EH, UK; Neeraj.Kohli@gstt.nhs.uk
4 Holborn Medical Centre, GP, London WC1N 3NA, UK; Anissa.patel@nhs.net
5 Paediatrics Department, Basildon and Thurrock University Hospitals, NHS Foundation Trust, Basildon SS16 5NL, UK; Kilali.ominu-evbota@btuh.nhs.uk
6 Haematology and Sickle Cell Centre, London North West University Healthcare NHS Trust, London NW10 7NS, UK; kofi.anie@nhs.net
7 Department of Clinical Haematology, Cancer and Haematology Centre, Oxford University Hospitals NHS Foundation Trust, Churchill Hospital, Oxford OX3 9DU, UK; Wale.atoyebi@ouh.nhs.uk
* Correspondence: Baba.inusa@gstt.nhs.uk

Abstract: Sickle cell disease (SCD) is a monogenetic disorder due to a single base-pair point mutation in the β-globin gene resulting in the substitution of the amino acid valine for glutamic acid in the β-globin chain. Phenotypic variation in the clinical presentation and disease outcome is a characteristic feature of the disorder. Understanding the pathogenesis and pathophysiology of the disorder is central to the choice of therapeutic development and intervention. In this special edition for newborn screening for haemoglobin disorders, it is pertinent to describe the genetic, pathologic and clinical presentation of sickle cell disease as a prelude to the justification for screening. Through a systematic review of the literature using search terms relating to SCD up till 2019, we identified relevant descriptive publications for inclusion. The scope of this review is mainly an overview of the clinical features of pain, the cardinal symptom in SCD, which present following the drop in foetal haemoglobin as young as five to six months after birth. The relative impact of haemolysis and small-vessel occlusive pathology remains controversial, a combination of features probably contribute to the different pathologies. We also provide an overview of emerging therapies in SCD.

Keywords: sickle cell disease (SCD); pathophysiology; hydroxyurea/hydroxycarbamide; haemolysis; vaso-occlusive crisis; acute chest syndrome; end-organ damage; bone marrow transplant; anaemia; foetal haemoglobin; gene therapy for haemoglobinopathies

---

1. Introduction

Sickle cell disease (SCD) was first reported by Herrick in 1910 even though reports suggest prior description of the disorder [1]; it is the result of homozygous and compound heterozygote inheritance of a mutation in the *β-globin* gene. A single base-pair point mutation (GAG to GTG) results in the substitution of the amino acid glutamic acid (hydrophilic) to Valine (hydrophobic) in the 6th position of the β-chain of haemoglobin referred to as haemoglobin S (HbS) [2]. Phenotypic variation in clinical presentation is a unique feature of SCD despite a well-defined Mendelian inheritance, the first to be molecularly characterised as described by Pauling [3] and confirmed to be due to a single amino acid substitution by Ingram [3] almost 70 years ago. SCD is a multi-organ, multi-system disorder with both acute and chronic complications presenting when foetal haemoglobin (HbF) drops towards the adult level by five to six months of age [4].

2. Classification

The inheritance of homozygous HbS otherwise referred to as sickle cell anaemia (SCA) is the most predominant form of SCD, the proportion varies according the country of origin [5–7]. The next most common form of SCD is the co-inheritance of HbS and HbC—referred to as HbSC, this is most prevalent in Western Africa, particularly Burkina Fasso and Mali and the coastal countries including Ghana, Benin and Western Nigeria [5,7,8]. The co-inheritance with β thalassaemia results in a sickle β thalassaemia genotype (*HbS/βo or HbS/β+*), depending on the genetic lesion on the thalassaemia component, the clinical presentation may be mild or equally as severe as homozygous SCD (HbS/HbS) [9]. Those with *HbS/βo*-thalassaemia have a more severe course of disease similar to homozygous SS patients, while offspring with *HbS/β+*-thalassaemia depending on the β-globin mutation is associated with variable phenotype from mild to severe phenotypes SCD [3,10].

3. Epidemiology

SCD is one of the most common inherited life-threatening disorders in human, it predominantly affect people of African, Indiana and Arab ancestry [5,11,12]. It is estimated that over 80% of over 300,000 annual births occur in sub-Saharan Africa (SSA), the largest burden from Nigeria and Democratic Republic of Congo [13]. The gene frequency is highest in West African countries with 1 in 4 to 3 (25–30%) being carriers of HbS compared to 1/400 African Americans and is variable in European populations [14–16]. The prevalence of SCD in developed countries is increasing partly due to migration from high prevalent countries [17–20]. It is estimated that over 14,000 people live with SCD in the UK, similar to France, while countries like Italy, Germany have seen increasing numbers from Africa [21–24]. With increasing survival, the age distribution of SCD is changing from a childhood disorder pattern that patients now survive into adulthood and old age. It is now reported that over 94% of those born with SCD now survive into adulthood in the US, France and UK in contrast to the high mortality in SSA where 50–90% may die in the first five years of life [12,25,26]. In low resource settings and countries where newborn screening is not yet standard care, patients may die young even before diagnosis is confirmed [27]. Among the common causes of death in the absence of early diagnosis followed by education and preventive therapies such as penicillin prophylaxis and regular surveillance include infections, severe anaemia (acute splenic sequestration, aplastic anaemia) and multi-organ failure [28]. It is essential therefore that Newborn and Early Infant diagnosis is given the priority it deserves by those countries where SCD is a public health problem [28,29].The implementation of early infant diagnosis remains out of reach for the majority of countries in SSA despite multiple declarations by international organisations and public statements by politicians to honour such commitments. The benefits for screening can only become meaningful when such practice is embraced by policy-makers across the continent and India where the majority of SCD are born and live. Comprehensive care includes penicillin V prophylaxis, Hydroxycarbamide therapy and preventive therapies such as antimalarials and health promotion where relevant will improve outcomes and health related quality of life [30].

4. Pathophysiology

The schematic representation in Figure 1 highlights the pathophysiology of SCD [31]. Red blood cells (RBCs) that contain HbS or HbS in combination with other abnormal β alleles, when exposed to deoxygenated environment undergo polymerisation and become rigid. The rigid RBC's are liable to haemolysis, and due to increased density may affect blood flow and endothelial vessel wall integrity. The dense rigid RBC's lead to vaso-occlusion, tissue ischaemia, infarction as well as haemolysis [32]. The consequence of haemolysis is a complex cascade of events including nitric oxide consumption; haemolysis linked nitric oxide dysregulation and endothelial dysfunction which underlie complications such as leg ulceration, stroke, pulmonary hypertension and priapism [33]. Unlike normal RBC's with half-life of approximately 120 days, sickle RBC's (sRBC) may survive just 10–20 days due to increased haemolysis [34]. During deoxygenation; healthy haemoglobin rearranges itself into a different conformation, enabling binding with carbon dioxide molecules which reverts to normal when released [32]. In contrast, HbS tends to polymerise into rigid insoluble strands and tactoids, which are gel-like substances containing Hb crystals. During acute sickling, intravascular haemolysis results in free haemoglobin in the serum, while RBC's gaining Na^{+}, Ca^{2+} with corresponding loss of K^{+} [31]. The increase in the concentration of Ca^{2+} leads to dysfunction in the calcium pump. The calcium depends on ATPase but it is unclear what role calcium plays in membrane rigidity attributed to cytoskeletal membrane interactions. [35]. Furthermore, hypoxia also inhibits the production of nitric oxide, thereby causing the adhesion of sickle cells to the vascular endothelium [33]. The lysis of erythrocytes leads to increase in extracellular haemoglobin, thus increasing affinity and binding to available nitric oxide or precursors of nitric oxide; thereby reducing its levels and further contributing to vasoconstriction [32].

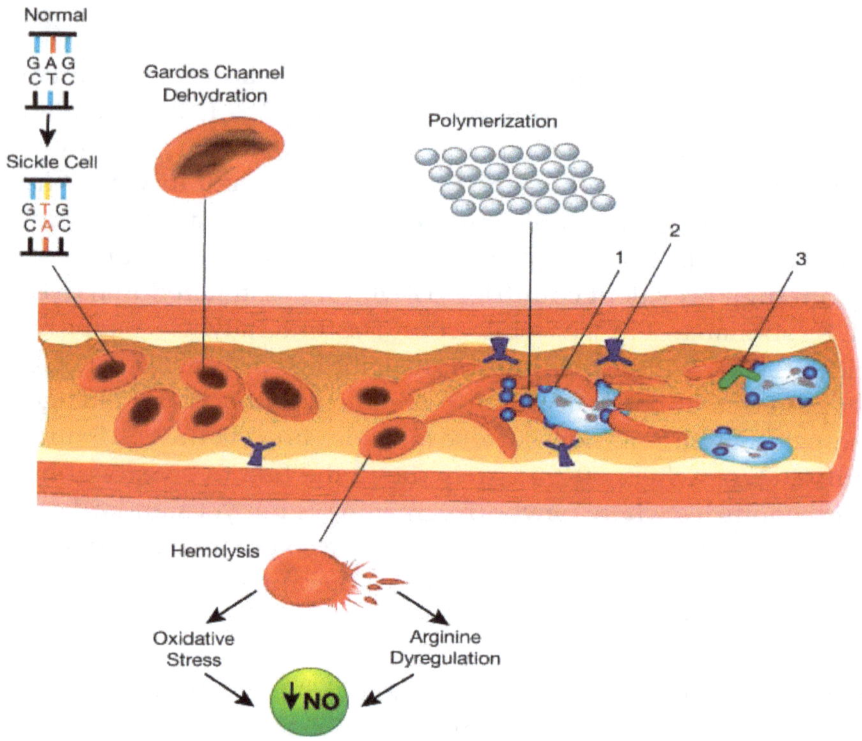

Figure 1. Schematic representation of the pathophysiology (in part) of sickle cell anemia. A single gene mutation (GAG→GTG and CTC→CAC) results in a defective haemoglobin that when exposed to de-oxygenation (depicted in the right half of the diagram) polymerizes (upper right of the diagram), resulting in the formation of sickle cells. Vaso-occlusion can then occur. The disorder is also characterized by abnormal adhesive properties of sickle cells; peripheral blood mononuclear cells (depicted in light blue; shown as the large cells under the sickle cells) and platelets (depicted in dark blue; shown as the dark circular shapes on the mononuclear cells) adhere to the sickled erythrocytes. This aggregate is labelled 1. The mononuclear cells have receptors (e.g., CD44 (labeled 3 and depicted in dark green on the cell surface)) that bind to ligands, such as P-selectin (labeled 2 and shown on the endothelial surface), that are unregulated. The sickle erythrocytes can also adhere directly to the endothelium. Abnormal movement or rolling and slowing of cells in the blood also can occur. These changes result in endothelial damage. The sickled red cells also become dehydrated as a result of abnormalities in the Gardos channel. Hemolysis contributes to oxidative stress and dysregulation of arginine metabolism, both of which lead to a decrease in nitric oxide (NO) that, in turn, contributes to the vasculopathy that characterizes SCD.

5. Disease Modifiers

The sickle β-globin mutation renders the sickle gene pleiotropic in nature, with variable phenotypic expression associated with complex genetic and environmental interactions, as well as disease modifiers that are increasingly being recognised. Sickle RBC (sRBC) polymerisation in deoxygenated environments is influenced by a number of factors including the co-inheritance of alpha thalassaemia, foetal haemoglobin (HbF) level which is determined by a number of genetic factors including genetic variations of BLC11A, HBS1L-MYB and HBB loci and hydroxycarbamide therapy amongst others [35]. The BCL11A and ZBTB7A genes (LRF protein) are responsible for the suppression of γ chains, and HbF production. HbF reduces sickle cell polymerisation due to reduction in HbS concentration and the fact that it is excluded from the sickle cell polymers. HbF also has high oxygen retention thereby ameliorating both the vaso-occlusive and haemolytic pathology in SCD. Among the four main sickle haplotypes, the level of HbF is highest in the Indian/Arab haplotype [8] predominantly found in the Arab Peninsula and India followed by the Senegal, and Benin haplotypes most predominant in Sub-Saharan Africa. The Bantu haplotype with the lowest HbF is predominantly found in Central African countries [8,36]. Alpha thalassaemia also modulates the expression of SCD. People with one or two α genes deleted have less haemolysis and fewer vasculopathy complications [8].

6. Clinical Manifestations

SCD is characterised by protean manifestations ranging from acute generalised pain to early onset stroke, leg ulcers and the risk of premature deaths from multi-organ failure [8]. As a result of the effect of HbF, clinical features do not begin until the middle to second part of the first year of post-natal life when this has predominantly switched to adult haemoglobin [36–40].

6.1. Vaso-Occlusive Crisis (Pain)

Patients with SCD may experience intense pain early in infancy, childhood and adulthood. Pain usually accounts for the majority of hospitalisations and overall negative impact in patients' health related quality of life. Pain is the cardinal feature of SCD and it is characteristically unpredictable, episodic in nature, described as one of the most excruciating forms of pain that affects human beings. Pain occurs due to stimulation of nociceptive nerve fibres caused by microvascular occlusion. The microcirculation is obstructed by sRBCs, thereby restricting the flow of blood to the organ and this results in (i) ischaemia, (ii) oedema, (iii) pain, (iv) necrosis, and (v) organ damage [10]. In the first year of life one of the cardinal features is the 'hand-foot syndrome' due to vaso-occlusion of post-capillary vasculature resulting in tissue oedema and pain of the extremities [41]. Infants display their pain nonverbally with irritability and apparent 'regression' tendencies such as inability to weight bear, walk or crawl. In older children and adults, vaso-occlusive pain can affect any part of the body. The onset of pain is spontaneous, usually no precipitating factors; well-known triggers include infections, fever, dehydration, acidosis, sudden change in weather including wind speed, cold, rain and air pollution. Resolution of pain is unpredictable. Acute pain might lead to chronic pain [42].

6.2. Anaemia

Symptomatic anaemia is the commonest symptom in SCD generally more common in SCA (Homozygous S), which usually runs the lowest haemoglobin level common to double heterozygous states. The steady state haemoglobin for asymptomatic patients varies according to the phenotype, ranging from levels as low as 60–80 g/L for homozygous S and /*Sβo* to 100–110 g/L in double heterozygous *SC* and *Sβ+* forms. However, the rate of fall from individual steady state haemoglobin level may trigger symptoms of hypoxia (aplastic crises) or a shock-like state (e.g., acute splenic sequestration) [4,43].

6.3. Acute Aplastic Crisis

The most common cause of acquired bone marrow failure in SCD and other haemolytic disorders is caused by Parvovirus B19 [44]. This virus causes the fifth disease and normally in healthy children is quite mild, associated with malaise, fever and sometimes a mild rash; the virus affects erythropoiesis by invading progenitors of RBCs in the bone marrow and destroying them, thus preventing new RBCs from being made. There's a slight drop in haematocrit in children with HbAA who are generally unaffected, however in SCD as the lifespan of RBC's is reduced to about 10–20 days, there is a significant drop in haemoglobin concentration. Parvovirus B19 infection usually takes about four days to one week to resolve and patients with SCD usually require a blood transfusion [39,44].

6.4. Infection

SCD increases susceptibility to infections, notably bacterial sepsis and malaria in children under five years [45]. Respiratory infections can trigger the sickle-cell acute chest syndrome, with a high risk of death. Risk factors for infections include: (i) functional asplenia/hyposplenia which present with reduced splenic immune response at a very young age, (ii) impaired fixation of complement, (iii) reduced oxidative burst capacity of chronically activated neutrophils, dysfunctional IgM and IgG antibody responses and defective opsonisation. The main pathogen of concern is *Streptococcus pneumoniae,* though severe and systemic infections arise with *Haemophilus influenzae*, *Neisseria meningitides*, and *Salmonellae* leads to osteomyelitis especially *Salmonella* due to bowel ischaemia and gut flora dissemination [46,47].

6.5. Splenic Sequestration Crisis

The main function of the spleen is the removal of defective red blood cells including sickled RBCs (sRBC) resulting in further haemolysis [48]. Blood flow through the spleen is slow reducing oxygen tension and increased polymerisation in HbS. As a result of the narrow capillaries in the splenic vascular bed, further hypoxia occurs with RBC polymerisation and entrapment of affected blood cells. This leads to a cycle of hypoxia, RBC polymerisation, and reduced blood flow causing the spleen to enlarge, for unexplained reasons, this may occur suddenly with pooling of blood within the vascular bed resulting in shock and circulatory failure. The rapidly increasing spleen size may lead to abdominal distension, sudden weakness, increased thirst, tachycardia and tachypnoea. Splenic sequestration crisis is an emergency because if left untreated, it can lead to death in 1–2 h due to circulatory failure [49].

6.6. Other Complications

The complications listed above are highlighted as those affecting babies and young children, because these are immediately relevant after newborn screening. Older children, adolescents, and young adults develop many chronic complications: stroke, cognitive dysfunction, priapism, leg ulcers, avascular necrosis (of the femoral head or humeral head), chronic pain, retinopathy, pulmonary hypertension, acute kidney injury, chronic kidney disease, thromboembolic events, and hepatic sequestration [50,51], cholelithiasis (gallstones) and cholecystitis as a result of excessive production and precipitation of bilirubin due to haemolysis. SCD also increases susceptibility to complications in pregnancy [52].

6.7. Psychosocial Impact

SCD has a significant psychosocial impact on patients and families [53]. This mainly results from the effect of pain and symptoms on their daily lives, and society's attitudes towards them. Cultural factors are particularly important to these problems because of beliefs and practices [54]. Furthermore, the ability of people with SCD to cope with their condition varies greatly because severity, general health, and quality of life varies greatly among individuals [55,56].

7. Treatment and Management

SCD causes a range of acute and long-term complications, requiring a multi-disciplinary approach, involving various medical specialists. In the United Kingdom, comprehensive SCD care is coordinated by specialist haemoglobinopathy teams [57]. Such teams play a key role in education about SCD for patients and their families, as well as guiding treatment with disease-modifying therapies, access to psychology, social and welfare support. Additionally, they coordinate screening services such as Transcranial Doppler (TCD) ultrasound monitoring in children, detection of iron overload or allo-antibody formation in individuals on transfusion programmes, and referral to specialists for major organ complications with an interest in SCD.

8. Management of Acute Vaso-Occlusive Crises (Pain)

Pain is the commonest acute complication of SCD, and significantly impact health-related quality of life [58]. Pain management may vary from patient to patient depending on family dynamics and individual patient thresholds or access to health care, however mild to moderate painful episodes may be treated in the home without the need of attending a health facility. Self-help psychological strategies including distraction techniques such as guided imagery can be a useful evidence-based adjunct to managing pain, and patients who utilise complementary coping strategies tend to require fewer hospitalisations [53,59]. The management strategy for pain includes 4 stages: which are assessment, treatment, reassessment, and adjustment [60]. It is also important to take into consideration (1) the severity of pain and (2) the patient's past response to different analgesics and to follow their regular protocols to alleviate the patient's pain.

Supportive Care

Given the fact that pain is often triggered by infection, exposure to cold or dehydration, supportive care during these episodes involves providing hydration, warmth and treating any treating the underlying infection. Simple devices such as incentive spirometry can be critical in preventing complications such as acute chest syndrome. Longer-term infection prevention varies regionally but can involve vaccination programs and penicillin prophylaxis [61].

9. Disease Modifying and Curative Treatments

Currently the only available disease-modifying medications for SCD are hydroxycarbamide and L-glutamine. Both are given daily to reduce the rate of acute complications, but results vary from person to person. Another effective disease modifying therapy is blood transfusion to raise the haemoglobin for improved oxygenation in severe anaemia and also to reduce the proportion of sickle haemoglobin (HbS%) may be give as a simple top-up blood transfusion or as exchange transfusion (manual or automated). The main curative therapy is stem cell transplantation while gene therapy is in the horizon in clinical Trials.

9.1. Hydroxycarbamide

Hydroxycarbamide has gained widely accepted use globally [62]. Although it was originally used as a cytoreductive agent by inhibiting ribonucleotide reductase, the main mechanism through which hydroxycarbamide works in SCD is through increasing total haemoglobin concentration and HbF production [63]. Hydroxycarbamide also reduces the number of leucocytes in blood, and reduces expression of surface adhesion molecules on neutrophils, red cells and vascular endothelium resulting in improved blood flow and reducing vaso-occlusion [62]. A number of trials in adults and children have shown beneficial effects of long-term hydroxycarbamide use, including reducing the severity and frequency of crisis in children with SCD [64]. The Multi-Centre Study of Hydroxycarbamide (MSH) showed that over a two-year follow-up period, adults on hydroxycarbamide had a significantly lower frequency of painful crises compared with placebo (median 2.5 versus 4.5 respectively, $p = 0.001$), as well as lower incidence of acute chest syndrome (25 versus 51, $p = 0.001$) and lower need for blood transfusion (48 patients versus 73, $p = 0.001$). A subsequent observational study following up on participants of the MSH study over a nine-year period showed a 40% reduction in mortality amongst patients on hydroxycarbamide. Patients with SCD who have increased HbF levels suffer less pain and live longer [62]. A meta-analysis in 2007 looked at effectiveness, efficacy and toxicity of hydroxycarbamide in children with SCD and they found that HbF levels increased by about 10% and also found a significant increase in haemoglobin concentration by approximately 1%; and on average there was a decrease in hospitalisation rates by 71% as well as a decrease in the frequency of pain crisis [62,65]. Indications for Hydroxycarbamide vary according to the phenotype, age and individual practice [65]. The US National Institute of Health (NIH) evidence-based guidelines and British Society of Haematology recommend offering Hydroxycarbamide to all HbSS and HbS/β0 thalassaemia genotype children from age of 1 year even though actual practice varies widely between continents.

In adults, indications for hydroxycarbamide may include [66–68]:

1. Frequent painful episodes (>3 per annum) or chronic debilitating pain not controlled by usual protocols.
2. History of stroke or a high risk for stroke or other severe vaso-occlusive events.
3. Severe symptomatic anaemia.
4. History of acute chest syndrome.

Patients on hydroxycarbamide undergo regular monitoring for the development of leucopenia and/or thrombocytopenia. Hydroxycarbamide can cause birth defects in animal models, hence the caution about its use during pregnancy, but hydroxycarbamide has not yet been linked to birth defects in humans. Short term research has shown only minor side effects and the benefits of using hydroxycarbamide outweigh any short-term adverse effects [62,65].

9.2. L-Glutamine

Glutamine is a conditionally essential amino acid, meaning that although the body normally makes sufficient amounts, at times of stress the body's need for glutamine increases, and in such instances, it also relies on dietary glutamine to meet this demand. The U.S. Food and Drug Administration (FDA) approved use of pharmaceutical-grade L-glutamine for sickle patients aged five years or older in July 2017 [69]. Formal clinical trials showed that this purified version of glutamine significantly reduced the frequency of acute complications of SCD. Side effects appear to be minor and do not require lab monitoring [31,69].

FDA approval was based on the results of two double-blind randomized placebo-controlled trials studying the effect of L-glutamine on clinical end-points in adults and children over five years old with HbSS or *HbS/βo* thalassaemia. A phase III double-blind placebo-controlled trial randomising two hundred and thirty patients aged 5 to 58 years in a 2:1 ratio to either 0.3 g/kg oral L-glutamine twice daily, rounded to 5 g doses to a maximum of 30 g, or placebo. Concerns around the study results are due to the high dropout rate, with 97 (63.8%) participants in the intervention group and 59 (75.6%) in the placebo group completing the eleven-month study. The researchers showed a 17.9% reduction in the mean frequency of sickle crises in the L-glutamine group (3.2 versus 3.9 in the L-glutamine and placebo groups respectively ($p = 0.0152$)) and significantly fewer pain crises in the L-glutamine group (median 3.0 in the L-glutamine group and 4.0 in the placebo group, $p = 0.005$). There was significantly fewer hospitalisations in the L-glutamine group (median 2.0 in the L-glutamine group and 3.0 in the placebo group, $p = 0.005$) [69]. There were also significant reductions in the frequency of acute chest crises (8.6% on the L-glutamine group versus 23.1% in the placebo group, $p = 0.003$), and duration of hospital admissions (median 6.5 in the L-glutamine group versus 11 in the placebo group, $p = 0.02$) [69]. Potential concerns around use include the lack of long-term follow up data, financial cost compared with hydroxycarbamide, and theoretical concern around reducing treatment concordance with hydroxycarbamide therapy amongst patients seeking more naturalistic medication [70].

9.3. Blood Transfusion

Individuals with SCD have a baseline level of anaemia due to their chronic haemolysis. Blood transfusions are not given to correct this baseline anaemia or for acute pain episodes. Instead, transfusions are given to correct acute severe anaemia where the haemoglobin falls significantly below that individual's baseline, and the resulting impairment in oxygen delivery to body tissues would otherwise propagate further sickling of deoxygenated Hb. Examples include red cell aplasia caused by Parvovirus B19 infection, acute splenic sequestration or hyperhaemolysis crises [71]. In an acute setting, transfusion is also used to bridge periods of severe physiologic stress like major surgery or critical illness including acute chest crises. In this setting, blood transfusion with HbS-negative blood reduces the proportion of circulating haemoglobin that is able to sickle, and hence reducing vessel occlusion and haemolysis from abnormal sickle RBCs. Long-term transfusions are instituted as a disease-modifying treatment in specific situations, such as to prevent stroke. The issues that arise as a result of long term transfusion complications include: (i) Allo-immunization, where after receiving a blood transfusion an individual develops antibodies to an antigen on the transfused red cells, which can increase the risk of having haemolytic reactions to blood that they are transfused in future; (ii) Iron overload, although treatment of iron overload is becoming more tolerable with the new oral chelators and, (iii) Risk of transfusion-transmitted infections, especially in countries where only limited screening of donated blood is available [39,72].

9.4. Bone Marrow Transplantation (BMT)

BMT is the only current cure for SCD and is one of the newer methods of treatments available. Results indicate an event-free survival rate of approximately 91% and a mortality rate of less than 5% [51]. BMT carries significant risks, such as the new bone marrow producing leucocytes attacking hosts tissue cells which is known as Graft-versus-host-disease (GVHD) [73]. Tissues affected include skin, liver, gastrointestinal tract and eyes, symptoms include nausea, weight loss and jaundice. The risk of developing GVHD is low when the donor and the recipient are related and matched for HLA type. When the donor and recipient aren't related or there is a mismatch in HLA types, there is greater the likelihood of developing GVHD; strategies for careful immunosuppression after transplant can reduce the risk of GVHD [74]. Other risks from undergoing BMT include strokes, fatal infection, organ damage, and fits. Thus, BMT requires specialist centres with highly experienced teams and advanced technological resources. Due to the current levels of risk, a bone marrow transplant is only usually recommended if the symptoms and complications of SCD are severe enough to warrant the risks of BMT [75].

10. New and Emerging Therapies for Sickle Cell Disease

Researchers are studying several novel and existing medicines for SCD, in order to address different pathophysiological mechanisms. Candidates in the "pipeline" of clinical studies include adhesion blockers, HbS polymerization blockers, antioxidants, regulators of inflammation and activation, and promoters for nitric oxide. Developing a range of mechanistic targets may allow combination therapies to be developed, both to prevent and to treat acute sickle cell complications. For this reason, many phase II and III studies have included patients already established on hydroxycarbamide, to see if combination treatments can provide additional benefit. Examples of some of the key agents under investigation are discussed below.

10.1. Treatments that Reduce HbS Polymerisation

GBT440 (Voxelotor) is an oral small molecule designed to increase the oxygen affinity of HbS, shifting the oxygen dissociation curve of oxy-HbS to the left [76]. It does this by reversibly binding with the N-terminal valine of alpha (α) chain of Haemoglobin, changing its conformational structure and stabilizing the oxygenation form of the molecule. This reduces the concentration of deoxygenated

HbS, which is the form of the molecule that polymerises to give the sickle phenotype. An initial phase I/II study showed Voxelotor to be well tolerated, with predictable pharmacodynamics and pharmacokinetics [76].

10.2. Nutritional Supplements

Omega-3 fatty acids have been purified from fish oil and tested for benefits as antioxidant, antithrombotic, and anti-inflammatory benefit. The clinical trials have used products with different purity, different proportions of types of omega-3 fatty acids, and different dosages. A trial in Georgia showed significantly decreased pain and decreased platelet activation in adults with sickle cell anemia on large daily quantities of fish oil capsules compared to adults on large daily quantities of olive oil capsules as placebo control [31,77,78]. A large trial in Sudan showed school absences were significantly decreased in children with sickle cell anemia taking fish oil compared to those taking placebo [77].

Folic acid is widely prescribed for SCD with the rationale that increased erythropoiesis causes increased risk of folate deficiency. A Cochrane Review evaluated the one double-blinded placebo-controlled clinical trial that was conducted in the 1980's and concluded that the trial presents mixed evidence of benefit in children and no trials were found in adults [79]. Although the Cochrane reviewers recommend further investigation, they also state that no further trials of folic acid in SCD are expected [79].

EvenFlo, an herbal mixture marketed online by Healing Blends, is the only one of several herbal supplements to begin clinical trials. An open-label observational study was published online by the company in 2017 [78] and https://healingblendsglobal.com/2017/02/clinical-study-evenflo/. A randomized controlled trial was recently completed and submitted for peer reviewed publication, still pending at the time of this writing.

A traditional herbal product used to treat SCD in Nigeria, Niprisan, showed promising pre-clinical data although it is likely to have drug interactions from its significant inhibition of cytochrome CYP3A4 activity. Niprisan was awarded "Orphan Drug Status" by the FDA [32,80]. However, financial barriers halted production and Niprisan has not progressed to clinical trials [81].

10.3. Agents that Reduce Cell Adhesion to Activated Microvascular Endothelium: Targeted Selectin Inhibitors (Crizanlizumab, Rivipansel, Heparins and Heparin-Derived Molecules)

Selectins are transmembrane glycoproteins that are important for cell trafficking for the innate immune system, lymphocytes and platelets. Different families of selectins are expressed on endothelial cells, leucocytes and platelets. Leucocyte rolling and tethering by P and E-selectin, expressed on the surface of activated microvascular endothelium may contribute to reduced blood flow velocity and increased sickling and vaso-occlusion. Therefore, targeted P-selectin inhibitors (Crizanlizumab (SEG101, previously SELG1)), pan-selectin inhibitors (Rivipansel/GMI-1070) have undergone phase II trials. Crizanlizumab was evaluated in a double-blind, randomized, placebo-controlled phase II trial which assigned participants aged 16 to 65 years to either low-dose intravenous Crizanlizumab (2.5 mg/kg), high-dose intravenous Crizanlizumab (5.0 mg/kg), or placebo, administered over 30 min, 14 times throughout the course of one year. Results showed that a 43 percent relative risk reduction in annual acute pain episodes (1.63 vs. 2.98) occurred when comparing the high-dose Crizanlizumab and placebo treatment groups ($p = 0.01$). Not only did the therapy decrease the annual acute pain episode rate, but the high dose of Crizanlizumab also delayed the first and second acute pain episodes when compared with placebo (first episode, 4.07 months vs. 1.38 months, $p = 0.001$; second episode, 10.32 months vs. 5.09 months, $p = 0.02$; respectively [31,82].

Heparins are able to bind selectins and it has been posited that this allows heparins to reduce sickle cell adhesion to activated endothelium. A double-blind placebo-controlled randomised trial reported a statistically significant reduction in duration of painful crisis and duration of hospital admission with use of tinzaparin, a low molecular weight heparin, compared with supportive care only, amongst 253 patients with SCD admitted with acute painful crisis. Sevuparin is a novel heparin-derived compound in which the anticoagulant effect has been removed, but which retains the selectin-binding effect of heparins [83,84].

10.4. Agents that Improve Blood Flow through Anticoagulant Effect: Antiplatelet and Anticoagulant Agents

10.4.1. Prasugrel

Prasugrel inhibits ADP-mediated platelet aggregation. Previous research suggested that activated platelets adhere to endothelium during vaso-occlusive episodes and recruit leucocytes. A phase III study of 341 children with SCD did not show a significant reduction in vaso-occlusive events per person-year in children taking Prasugrel compared with those taking placebo. It also did not show a significant reduction in diary-reported pain events [85,86].

10.4.2. Apixaban

Apixaban is an oral direct Factor Xa inhibitor, which therefore prevents the activation of prothrombin to thrombin. A phase III randomised placebo-controlled trial is underway investigating the effectiveness of prophylactic dose Apixaban at reducing mean daily pain scores in adults with SCD [87].

10.5. Agents that Restore Depleted Nitric Oxide within the Microvasculature: Statins, L-Arginine, PDE9

Nitric oxide released from endothelium promotes vessel smooth muscle relaxation, resulting in vasodilatation and improved blood flow. It also suppresses platelet aggregation, as well as reducing expression of cell adhesion molecules on endothelium and reducing release of procoagulant factors. Intravascular haemolysis results in release of free haemoglobin into the patient's plasma [63]. This acts as a nitric oxide scavenger. In addition, arginase released from lysed red cells breaks down arginine, which is a substrate used to make endogenous nitric oxide. Both these events result in depletion of nitric oxide levels. Two drug groups that have been investigated for their effect on improving nitric oxide reserves in SCD are statins and L-arginine. Statins inhibit Rho kinase resulting in endothelial nitric oxide synthase activation [35,88].

10.6. Gene Therapy

Gene therapy is in early studies as a possible cure for sickle cell anaemia. The approach is based on stem cells and gene therapy; instead of using embryonic stem cells, host stem cells are derived by manipulating and reprogramming cells from patient's own blood cells with genetic engineering used to correct the inborn genetic error. Because the cells are provided by the patient, there is no need to find another person to serve as a donor of stem cells and there should be no risk of GVHD. The aim is to transform a patient's blood cells into pluripotent stem cells and replace the defective portion of the gene. These cells will then be coaxed into becoming hematopoietic cells which can specifically regenerate the entire range of red blood cells. At the time of this writing, a handful of people have apparently been cured of SCD in three gene therapy clinical studies with different lentiviral vectors [89].

A number of new sickle cell therapeutic options are on the horizon; the promise of combination therapy is no longer a far-fetched aspiration. This calls for an urgent debate with regards to the correct combinations, the right patient phenotype and access for the majority of patients. It is therefore timely to commission such a review on newborn sickle cell screening not just for European countries which of course face the migration challenge, but also Africa and India [90].

Author Contributions: B.P.D.I. designed the manuscript which was reviewed by L.L.H., W.A., N.K., K.A.A. offering substantial modification and further development of sections. A.P. had written an essay of the role of thrombosis in SCD, some of the concepts were included. K.O.-E. reviewed the manuscript. All authors approved the manuscript.

Acknowledgments: Temiladeoluwa Bademosi who wrote an essay on a related topic in sickle cell disease as a medical student.

References

1. Herrick, J.B. Peculiar Elongated and Sickle-shaped Red Blood Corpuscles in a Case of Severe Anemiaa. *Yale J. Biol. Med.* **2001**, *74*, 543–548.
2. Hoban, M.D.; Orkin, S.H.; Bauer, D.E. Genetic treatment of a molecular disorder: Gene therapy approaches to sickle cell disease. *Blood* **2016**, *127*, 839–848. [CrossRef] [PubMed]
3. Ingram, V.M. Anecdotal, Historical and Critical Commentaries on Genetics Sickle-Cell Anemia Hemoglobin: The Molecular Biology of the First "Molecular Disease"—The Crucial Importance of Serendipity. *Genetics* **2004**, *167*, 1–7. [CrossRef] [PubMed]
4. Ballas, S.K.; Kesen, M.R.; Goldberg, M.F.; Lutty, G.A.; Dampier, C.; Osunkwo, I.; Wang, W.C.; Hoppe, C.; Hagar, W.; Darbari, D.S.; et al. Beyond the Definitions of the Phenotypic Complications of Sickle Cell Disease: An Update on Management. *Sci. World J.* **2012**, *2012*, 949535. [CrossRef]
5. Weatherall, D.J. The inherited diseases of hemoglobin are an emerging global health burden. *Blood* **2010**, *115*, 4331–4336. [CrossRef] [PubMed]
6. American Society of Haematology. Sickle Cell Disease Family Fact Sheet 2015. Available online: http://www.michigan.gov/documents/mdch/Sickle_Cell_Fact_Sheet_465285_7.pdf (accessed on 10 February 2019).
7. Ansong, D.; Akoto, A.O.; Ocloo, D.; Ohene-frempong, K. Sickle Cell Disease: Management Options and Challenges in Developing Countries. *Mediterr. J. Hematol. Infect. Dis.* **2013**, *5*, e2013062. [CrossRef] [PubMed]
8. Piel, F.B.; Steinberg, M.H.; Rees, D.C. Sickle Cell Disease. *N. Engl. J. Med.* **2017**, *376*, 1561–1573. [CrossRef]
9. Steinberg, M.H. Genetic etiologies for phenotypic diversity in sickle cell anemia. *Sci. World J.* **2009**, *9*, 46–67. [CrossRef]
10. De Montalembert, M. Management of children with sickle cell anemia: A collaborative work. *Arch. Pediatr.* **2002**, *9*, 1195–1201. [PubMed]
11. Weatherall, D.J. The challenge of haemoglobinopathies in resource-poor countries. *Br. J. Haematol.* **2011**, *154*, 736–744. [CrossRef]
12. Grosse, S.D.; Odame, I.; Atrash, H.K.; Amendah, D.D.; Piel, F.B.; Williams, T.N. Sickle cell disease in Africa: A neglected cause of early childhood mortality. *Am. J. Prev. Med.* **2011**, *41*, S398–S405. [CrossRef] [PubMed]
13. Piel, F.B.; Patil, A.P.; Howes, R.E.; Nyangiri, O.A.; Gething, P.W.; Dewi, M.; Temperley, W.H.; Williams, T.N.; Weatherall, D.J.; Hay, S.I. Global epidemiology of sickle haemoglobin in neonates: A contemporary geostatistical model-based map and population estimates. *Lancet* **2013**, *381*, 142–151. [CrossRef]
14. Cronin, E.K.; Normand, C.; Henthorn, J.S.; Hickman, M.; Davies, S.C. Costing model for neonatal screening and diagnosis of haemoglobinopathies. *Arch. Dis. Child. Fetal Neonatal Ed.* **1998**, *79*, F161–F167. [CrossRef] [PubMed]
15. Martinez, P.A.; Angastiniotis, M.; Eleftheriou, A.; Gulbis, B.; Pereira, M.D.; Petrova-Benedict, R.; Corrons, J.L. Haemoglobinopathies in Europe: Health & migration policy perspectives. *Orphanet J. Rare. Dis.* **2014**, *9*, 97.
16. Modell, B.; Petrou, M.; Layton, M.; Slater, C.; Ward, R.H.; Rodeck, C.; Varnavides, L.; Nicolaides, K.; Gibbons, S.; Fitches, A.; et al. Audit of prenatal diagnosis for haemoglobin disorders in the United Kingdom: The first 20 years. *BMJ* **1997**, *315*, 779–784. [CrossRef]
17. Cela, E.; Bellón, J.M.; de la Cruz, M.; Beléndez, C.; Berrueco, R.; Ruiz, A.; Elorza, I.; Díaz de Heredia, C.; Cervera, A.; Vallés, G.; et al. National registry of hemoglobinopathies in Spain (REPHem). *Pediatr. Blood Cancer* **2017**, *64*, e26322. [CrossRef] [PubMed]
18. Huntsman, R.G. Hemoglobinopathies: How big a problem? *Can. Med. Assoc. J.* **1978**, *119*, 675. [PubMed]
19. Inusa, B.P.; Colombatti, R. European migration crises: The role of national hemoglobinopathy registries in improving patient access to care. *Pediatr. Blood Cancer* **2017**, *64*, e26515. [CrossRef] [PubMed]
20. Lindenau, J.D.; Wagner, S.C.; Castro, S.M.; Hutz, M.H. The effects of old and recent migration waves in the distribution of HBB* S globin gene haplotypes. *Genet. Mol. Biol.* **2016**, *39*, 515–523. [CrossRef]
21. Dormandy, E.; James, J.; Inusa, B.; Rees, D. How many people have sickle cell disease in the UK? *J. Public Health* **2017**, *40*, e291–e295. [CrossRef]
22. Lobitz, S.; Telfer, P.; Cela, E.; Allaf, B.; Angastiniotis, M.; Backman Johansson, C.; Badens, C.; Bento, C.; Bouva, M.J.; Canatan, D.; et al. Newborn screening for sickle cell disease in Europe: Recommendations from a Pan-European Consensus Conference. *Br. J. Haematol.* **2018**, *183*, 648–660. [CrossRef] [PubMed]

23. Grosse, R.; Lukacs, Z.; Cobos, P.N.; Oyen, F.; Ehmen, C.; Muntau, B.; Timmann, C.; Noack, B. The prevalence of sickle cell disease and its implication for newborn screening in Germany (Hamburg metropolitan area). *Pediatr. Blood Cancer* **2016**, *63*, 168–170. [CrossRef] [PubMed]
24. Colombatti, R.; Martella, M.; Cattaneo, L.; Viola, G.; Cappellari, A.; Bergamo, C.; Azzena, S.; Schiavon, S.; Baraldi, E.; Dalla Barba, B.; et al. Results of a multicenter universal newborn screening program for sickle cell disease in Italy: A call to action. *Pediatr. Blood Cancer* **2019**, *66*, e27657. [CrossRef] [PubMed]
25. Telfer, P.; Coen, P.; Chakravorty, S.; Wilkey, O.; Evans, J.; Newell, H.; Smalling, B.; Amos, R.; Stephens, A.; Rogers, D.; et al. Clinical outcomes in children with sickle cell disease living in England: A neonatal cohort in East London. *haematologica* **2007**, *92*, 905–912. [CrossRef] [PubMed]
26. Quinn, C.T.; Rogers, Z.R.; McCavit, T.L.; Buchanan, G.R. Improved survival of children and adolescents with sickle cell disease. *Blood* **2010**, *115*, 3447–3452. [CrossRef]
27. Makani, J.; Cox, S.E.; Soka, D.; Komba, A.N.; Oruo, J.; Mwamtemi, H.; Magesa, P.; Rwezaula, S.; Meda, E.; Mgaya, J.; et al. Mortality in sickle cell anemia in Africa: A prospective cohort study in Tanzania. *PLoS ONE* **2011**, *6*, e14699. [CrossRef]
28. Chakravorty, S.; Williams, T.N. Sickle cell disease: A neglected chronic disease of increasing global health importance. *Arch. Dis. Child.* **2015**, *100*, 48–53. [CrossRef]
29. Kuznik, A.; Habib, A.G.; Munube, D.; Lamorde, M. Newborn screening and prophylactic interventions for sickle cell disease in 47 countries in sub-Saharan Africa: A cost-effectiveness analysis. *BMC Health Serv. Res.* **2016**, *16*, 304. [CrossRef]
30. Makani, J.; Soka, D.; Rwezaula, S.; Krag, M.; Mghamba, J.; Ramaiya, K.; Cox, S.E.; Grosse, S.D. Health policy for sickle cell disease in Africa: Experience from Tanzania on interventions to reduce under-five mortality. *Trop. Med. Int. Health* **2015**, *20*, 184–187. [CrossRef] [PubMed]
31. Gardner, R.V. Sickle Cell Disease: Advances in Treatment. *Ochsner J.* **2018**, *18*, 377–389. [CrossRef]
32. Manwani, D.; Frenette, P.S. Vaso-occlusion in sickle cell disease: Pathophysiology and novel targeted therapies. *Blood* **2013**, *122*, 3892–3898. [CrossRef] [PubMed]
33. Hebbel, R.P. Ischemia-reperfusion injury in sickle cell anemia: Relationship to acute chest syndrome, endothelial dysfunction, arterial vasculopathy, and inflammatory pain. *Hematol. Oncol. Clin. North Am.* **2014**, *28*, 181–198. [CrossRef]
34. Sebastiani, P.; Nolan, V.G.; Baldwin, C.T.; Abad-Grau, M.M.; Wang, L.; Adewoye, A.H.; McMahon, L.C.; Farrer, L.A.; Taylor, J.G.; Kato, G.J.; et al. A network model to predict the risk of death in sickle cell disease. *Blood* **2007**, *110*, 2727–2735. [CrossRef]
35. Frenette, P.S.; Atweh, G.F. Sickle cell disease: Old discoveries, new concepts, and future promise. *J. Clin. Investig.* **2007**, *117*, 850–858. [CrossRef]
36. Akinsheye, I.; Alsultan, A.; Solovieff, N.; Ngo, D.; Baldwin, C.T.; Sebastiani, P.; Chui, D.H.; Steinberg, M.H. Fetal hemoglobin in sickle cell anemia. *Blood* **2011**, *118*, 19–27. [CrossRef]
37. Bhatnagar, P.; Purvis, S.; Barron-Casella, E.; DeBaun, M.R.; Casella, J.F.; Arking, D.E.; Keefer, J.R. Genome-wide association study identifies genetic variants influencing F-cell levels in sickle-cell patients. *Eur. J. Hum. Genet.* **2011**, *56*, 316. [CrossRef]
38. Watson, J. A study of sickling of young erythrocytes in sickle cell anemia. *Blood* **1948**, *3*, 465–469.
39. Inati, A. Recent advances in improving the management of sickle cell disease. *Blood Rev.* **2009**, *23*, S9–S13. [CrossRef]
40. Bonds, D.R. Three decades of innovation in the management of sickle cell disease: The road to understanding the sickle cell disease clinical phenotype. *Blood Rev.* **2005**, *19*, 99–110. [CrossRef]
41. Watson, R.J.; Burko, H.; Megas, H.; Robinson, M. The hand-foot syndrome in sickle-cell disease in young children. *Pediatrics* **1963**, *31*, 975–982.
42. Piel, F.B.; Tewari, S.; Brousse, V.; Analitis, A.; Font, A.; Menzel, S.; Chakravorty, S.; Thein, S.L.; Inusa, B.; Telfer, P.; et al. Associations between environmental factors and hospital admissions for sickle cell disease. *Haematologica* **2017**, *102*, 666–675. [CrossRef]
43. Brousse, V.; Buffet, P.; Rees, D. The spleen and sickle cell disease: The sick (led) spleen. *Br. J. Haematol.* **2014**, *166*, 165–176. [CrossRef]
44. Minhas, P.S.; KVirdi, J.; Patel, R. Double whammy-acute splenic sequestration crisis in patient with aplastic crisis due to acute parvovirus infection. *J. Commun. Hosp. Int. Med. Perspect.* **2017**, *7*, 194–195. [CrossRef] [PubMed]

45. Tubman, V.N.; Makani, J. Turf wars: Exploring splenomegaly in sickle cell disease in malaria-endemic regions. *Br. J. Haematol.* **2017**, *177*, 938–946. [CrossRef] [PubMed]
46. Booth, C.; Inusa, B.; Obaro, S.K. Infection in sickle cell disease: A review. *Int. J. Infect. Dis.* **2010**, *14*, e2–e12. [CrossRef] [PubMed]
47. Morrissey, B.J.; Bycroft, T.P.; Almossawi, O.; Wilkey, O.B.; Daniels, J.G. Incidence and predictors of bacterial infection in febrile children with sickle cell disease. *Hemoglobin* **2015**, *39*, 316–319. [PubMed]
48. Rezende, P.V.; Viana, M.B.; Murao, M.; Chaves, A.C.; Ribeiro, A.C. Acute splenic sequestration in a cohort of children with sickle cell anemia. *J. Pediatr. (Rio J.)* **2009**, *85*, 163–169. [CrossRef]
49. Araujo, A.N. Acute splenic sequestration in children with sickle cell anemia. *J. Pediatr. (Rio J.)* **2009**, *85*, 373–374. [CrossRef]
50. Habara, A.; Steinberg, M.H. Minireview: Genetic basis of heterogeneity and severity in sickle cell disease. *Exp. Biol. Med.* **2016**, *241*, 689–696. [CrossRef]
51. National Heart Lung and Blood Institute. Evidence-Based Management of Sickle Cell Disease: Expert Panel Report. 2014. Available online: https://www.nhlbi.nih.gov/health-topics/evidence-based-management-sickle-cell-disease (accessed on 10 February 2019).
52. Oteng-Ntim, E.; Meeks, D.; Seed, P.T.; Webster, L.; Howard, J.; Doyle, P.; Chappell, L.C. Adverse maternal and perinatal outcomes in pregnant women with sickle cell disease: Systematic review and meta-analysis. *Blood* **2015**, *125*, 3316–3325. [CrossRef]
53. Anie, K.A.; Green, J. Psychological therapies for sickle cell disease and pain. *Cochrane Database Syst. Rev.* 2015. [CrossRef]
54. Mulder, N.; Nembaware, V.; Adekile, A.; Anie, K.A.; Inusa, B.; Brown, B.; Campbell, A.; Chinenere, F.; Chunda-Liyoka, C.; Derebail, V.K.; et al. Proceedings of a Sickle Cell Disease Ontology workshop—Towards the first comprehensive ontology for sickle cell disease. *Appl. Transl. Genom.* **2016**, *9*, 23–29. [CrossRef]
55. Hsu, L.L.; Green, N.S.; Ivy, E.D.; Neunert, C.E.; Smaldone, A.; Johnson, S.; Castillo, S.; Castillo, A.; Thompson, T.; Hampton, K.; et al. Community health workers as support for sickle cell care. *Am. J. Prev. Med.* **2016**, *51*, S87–S98. [CrossRef]
56. Ohaeri, J.U.; Shokunbi, W.A. Psychosocial burden of sickle cell disease on caregivers in a Nigerian setting. *J. Natl. Med. Assoc.* **2002**, *94*, 1058. [PubMed]
57. Sickle Cell Society. Standards for the Clinical Care of Adults with Sickle Cell Disease in the UK—2018. Available online: https://www.sicklecellsociety.org/sicklecellstandards/ (accessed on 10 Fbruary 2019).
58. Dampier, C.; LeBeau, P.; Rhee, S.; Lieff, S.; Kesler, K.; Ballas, S.; Rogers, Z.; Wang, W.; Comprehensive Sickle Cell Centers (CSCC) Clinical Trial Consortium (CTC) Site Investigators. Health-related quality of life in adults with sickle cell disease (SCD): A report from the comprehensive sickle cell centers clinical trial consortium. *Am. J. Hematol.* **2011**, *86*, 203–205. [CrossRef] [PubMed]
59. Lebensburger, J.D.; Miller, S.T.; Howard, T.H.; Casella, J.F.; Brown, R.C.; Lu, M.; Iyer, R.V.; Sarnaik, S.; Rogers, Z.R.; Wang, W.C.; et al. Influence of severity of anemia on clinical findings in infants with sickle cell anemia: Analyses from the BABY HUG study. *Pediatr. Blood Cancer* **2012**, *59*, 675–678. [CrossRef] [PubMed]
60. Vichinsky, E.P. Comprehensive care in sickle cell disease: Its impact on morbidity and mortality. *Semin. Hematol.* **1991**, *28*, 220–226.
61. Matthews, C.; Walton, E.K.; Inusa, B. Sickle cell disease in childhood. *Stud. BMJ* **2014**, *22*. [CrossRef]
62. Murad, M.H.; Hazem, A.; Prokop, L. Hydroxyurea for Sickle Cell Disease: A Systematic Review of Benefits, Harms, and Barriers of Utilization, 2012 Prepared for the National Heart, Lung, and Blood Institute (NHLBI) Prepared by the Knowledge and Encounter Research Unit. *Mayo Clin.* **2012**, *2012*, 1–116.
63. Ware, R.E. Optimizing hydroxyurea therapy for sickle cell anemia. *ASH Educ. Program Book* **2015**, *2015*, 436–443. [CrossRef]
64. Steinberg, M.H.; Barton, F.; Castro, O.; Pegelow, C.H.; Ballas, S.K.; Kutlar, A.; Orringer, E.; Bellevue, R.; Olivieri, N.; Eckman, J.; et al. Effect of hydroxyurea on mortality and morbidity in adult sickle cell anemia: Risks and benefits up to 9 years of treatment. *JAMA* **2003**, *289*, 1645–1651. [CrossRef] [PubMed]
65. Strouse, J.J.; Lanzkron, S.; Beach, M.C.; Haywood, C.; Park, H.; Witkop, C.; Wilson, R.F.; Bass, E.B.; Segal, J.B. Hydroxyurea for sickle cell disease: A systematic review for efficacy and toxicity in children. *Pediatrics* **2008**, *122*, 1332–1342. [CrossRef] [PubMed]
66. Inusa, B.P.D.; Atoyebi Wale, A.A.; Idhate, T.; Dogara, L.; Ijei, I.; Qin, Y.; Anie, K.; Lawson, J.O.; Hsu, L.

Low-dose hydroxycarbamide therapy may offer similar benefit as maximum tolerated dose for children and young adults with sickle cell disease in low-middle-income settings. *F1000Research* **2018**, *7*, F1000 Faculty Rev-1407. [CrossRef]

67. Qureshi, A.; Kaya, B.; Pancham, S.; Keenan, R.; Anderson, J.; Akanni, M.; Howard, J.; British Society for Haematology. Guidelines for the use of hydroxycarbamide in children and adults with sickle cell disease: A British Society for Haematology Guideline. *Br. J. Haematol.* **2018**, *181*, 460–475. [CrossRef]
68. Hassan, A.; Awwalu, S.; Okpetu, L.; Waziri, A.D. Effect of hydroxyurea on clinical and laboratory parameters of sickle cell anaemia patients in North–West Nigeria. *Egypt J. Haematol.* **2017**, *42*, 70. [CrossRef]
69. Niihara, Y.; Miller, S.T.; Kanter, J.; Lanzkron, S.; Smith, W.R.; Hsu, L.L.; Gordeuk, V.R.; Viswanathan, K.; Sarnaik, S.; Osunkwo, I.; Guillaume, E. A phase 3 trial of L-glutamine in sickle cell disease. *N. Engl. J. Med.* **2018**, *379*, 226–235. [CrossRef]
70. Quinn, C.T. L-glutamine for sickle cell anemia: More questions than answers. *Blood* **2018**, *132*, 689–693. [CrossRef]
71. Danaee, A.; Inusa, B.; Howard, J.; Kesse-Adu, R.; Robinson, S. hyperhaemolysis in patients with haemoglobinopathies: A single centre experience: 229. *Br. J. Haematol.* **2014**, *165*, 96.
72. Adewoyin, A.S.; Obieche, J.C. Hypertransfusion therapy in sickle cell disease in Nigeria. *Adv. Hematol.* **2014**, *2014*, 923593. [CrossRef]
73. Kassim, A.A.; Sharma, D. Hematopoietic stem cell transplantation for sickle cell disease: The changing landscape. *Hematol. Oncol. Stem Cell Ther.* **2017**, *10*, 259–266. [CrossRef]
74. Wiebking, V.; Hütker, S.; Schmid, I.; Immler, S.; Feuchtinger, T.; Albert, M.H. Reduced toxicity, myeloablative HLA-haploidentical hematopoietic stem cell transplantation with post-transplantation cyclophosphamide for sickle cell disease. *Ann. Hematol.* **2017**, *96*, 1373–1377. [CrossRef] [PubMed]
75. Hashmi, S.K.; Srivastava, A.; Rasheed, W.; Adil, S.; Wu, T.; Jagasia, M.; Nassar, A.; Hwang, W.Y.; Hamidieh, A.A.; Greinix, H.T.; et al. Cost and quality issues in establishing hematopoietic cell transplant program in developing countries. *Hematol. Oncol. Stem Cell Ther.* **2017**, *10*, 167–172. [CrossRef]
76. Metcalf, B.; Chuang, C.; Dufu, K.; Patel, M.P.; Silva-Garcia, A.; Johnson, C.; Lu, Q.; Partridge, J.R.; Patskovska, L.; Patskovsky, Y.; et al. Discovery of GBT440, an orally bioavailable R-state stabilizer of sickle cell hemoglobin. *ACS Med. Chem. Lett.* **2017**, *8*, 321–326. [CrossRef] [PubMed]
77. Daak, A.A.; Ghebremeskel, K.; Hassan, Z.; Attallah, B.; Azan, H.H.; Elbashir, M.I.; Crawford, M. Effect of omega-3 (n−3) fatty acid supplementation in patients with sickle cell anemia: Randomized, double-blind, placebo-controlled trial. *Am. J. Clin. Nutr.* **2012**, *97*, 37–44. [CrossRef] [PubMed]
78. Tomer, A.; Kasey, S.; Connor, W.E.; Clark, S.; Harker, L.A.; Eckman, J.R. Reduction of pain episodes and prothrombotic activity in sickle cell disease by dietary n-3 fatty acids. *Thromb. Haemost.* **2001**, *85*, 966–974. [CrossRef]
79. Dixit, R.; Nettem, S.; Madan, S.S.; Soe, H.H.; Abas, A.B.; Vance, L.D.; Stover, P.J. Folate supplementation in people with sickle cell disease. *Cochrane. Database Syst. Rev.* 2018. [CrossRef]
80. Adzu, B.; Masimirembwa, C.; Mustapha, K.B.; Thelingwani, R.; Kirim, R.A.; Gamaniel, K.S. Effect of NIPRISAN® on CYP3A4 activity in vitro. *Eur. J. Drug Metab. Pharmacokinet.* **2015**, *40*, 115–118. [CrossRef]
81. Cordeiro, N.J.; Oniyangi, O. Phytomedicines (medicines derived from plants) for sickle cell disease. *Cochrane Database Syst. Rev.* 2004. [CrossRef]
82. Ataga, K.I.; Kutlar, A.; Kanter, J.; Liles, D.; Cancado, R.; Friedrisch, J.; Guthrie, T.H.; Knight-Madden, J.; Alvarez, O.A.; Gordeuk, V.R.; et al. Crizanlizumab for the prevention of pain crises in sickle cell disease. *N. Engl. J. Med.* **2017**, *376*, 429–439. [CrossRef]
83. Kelley, D.; Jones, L.T.; Wu, J.; Bohm, N. Evaluating the safety and effectiveness of venous thromboembolism prophylaxis in patients with sickle cell disease. *J. Thromb. Thrombolysis* **2017**, *43*, 463–468. [CrossRef]
84. Van Zuuren, E.J.; Fedorowicz, Z. Low-molecular-weight heparins for managing vasoocclusive crises in people with sickle cell disease: A summary of a cochrane systematic review. *Hemoglobin* **2014**, *38*, 221–223. [CrossRef]
85. Heeney, M.M.; Hoppe, C.C.; Abboud, M.R.; Inusa, B.; Kanter, J.; Ogutu, B.; Brown, P.B.; Heath, L.E.; Jakubowski, J.A.; Zhou, C.; et al. A multinational trial of prasugrel for sickle cell vaso-occlusive events. *N. Engl. J. Med.* **2016**, *374*, 625–635. [CrossRef]
86. Hoppe, C.C.; Styles, L.; Heath, L.E.; Zhou, C.; Jakubowski, J.A.; Winters, K.J.; Brown, P.B.; Rees, D.C.;

Heeney, M.M. Design of the DOVE (Determining Effects of Platelet Inhibition on Vaso-Occlusive Events) trial: A global Phase 3 double-blind, randomized, placebo-controlled, multicenter study of the efficacy and safety of prasugrel in pediatric patients with sickle cell anemia utilizing a dose titration strategy. *Pediatr. Blood Cancer* **2016**, *63*, 299–305.

87. Telen, M.J. Beyond hydroxyurea: New and old drugs in the pipeline for sickle cell disease. *Blood* **2016**, *127*, 810–819. [CrossRef] [PubMed]
88. Zhang, D.; Xu, C.; Manwani, D.; Frenette, P.S. Neutrophils, platelets, and inflammatory pathways at the nexus of sickle cell disease pathophysiology. *Blood* **2016**, *127*, 801–809. [CrossRef] [PubMed]
89. Ribeil, J.A.; Hacein-Bey-Abina, S.; Payen, E.; Magnani, A.; Semeraro, M.; Magrin, E.; Caccavelli, L.; Neven, B.; Bourget, P.; El Nemer, W.; et al. Gene therapy in a patient with sickle cell disease. *N. Engl. J. Med.* **2017**, *376*, 848–855. [CrossRef]
90. Inusa, B.P.; Anie, K.A.; Lamont, A.; Dogara, L.G.; Ojo, B.; Ijei, I.; Atoyebi, W.; Gwani, L.; Gani, E.; Hsu, L. Utilising the 'Getting to Outcomes®' Framework in Community Engagement for Development and Implementation of Sickle Cell Disease Newborn Screening in Kaduna State, Nigeria. *Int. J. Neonatal Screen.* **2018**, *4*, 33. [CrossRef]

18

Second Tier Molecular Genetic Testing in Newborn Screening for Pompe Disease: Landscape and Challenges

Laurie D. Smith [1,2], Matthew N. Bainbridge [3,4], Richard B. Parad [5,*] and Arindam Bhattacharjee [2,*]

1 Department of Pediatrics, UNC Hospitals, Chapel Hill, NC 27599, USA; laurie_d_smith@yahoo.com
2 Laboratory Services Division, Baebies, Inc., Durham, NC 27709, USA
3 Codified Genomics, Houston, TX 77004, USA; mbainbridge@rchsd.org
4 Rady Children's Institute for Genomic Medicine, San Diego, CA 92123, USA
5 Department of Pediatric Newborn Medicine, Brigham & Women's Hospital, Harvard Medical School, Boston, MA 02115, USA
* Correspondence: rparad@bwh.harvard.edu (R.B.P.); abhattac2@gmail.com (A.B.);

Abstract: Pompe disease (PD) is screened by a two tier newborn screening (NBS) algorithm, the first tier of which is an enzymatic assay performed on newborn dried blood spots (DBS). As first tier enzymatic screening tests have false positive results, an immediate second tier test on the same sample is critical in resolving newborn health status. Two methodologies have been proposed for second tier testing: (a) measurement of enzymatic activities such as of Creatine/Creatinine over alpha-glucosidase ratio, and (b) DNA sequencing (a molecular genetics approach), such as targeted next generation sequencing. (tNGS). In this review, we discuss the tNGS approach, as well as the challenges in providing second tier screening and follow-up care. While tNGS can predict genotype-phenotype effects when known, these advantages may be diminished when the variants are novel, of unknown significance or not discoverable by current test methodologies. Due to the fact that criticisms of screening algorithms that utilize tNGS are based on perceived complexities, including variant detection and interpretation, we clarify the actual limitations and present the rationale that supports optimizing a molecular genetic testing approach with tNGS. Second tier tNGS can benefit clinical decision-making through the use of the initial NBS DBS punch and rapid turn-around time methodology for tNGS, that includes copy number variant analysis, variant effect prediction, and variant 'cut-off' tools for the reduction of false positive results. The availability of DNA sequence data will contribute to the improved understanding of genotype-phenotype associations and application of treatment. The ultimate goal of second tier testing should enable the earliest possible diagnosis for the earliest initiation of the most effective clinical interventions in infants with PD.

Keywords: newborn screening; lysosomal storage diseases; variant cut-off; next generation sequencing; diagnosis; dried blood spots

---

1. Introduction

Newborn screening (NBS) for Pompe disease (PD), utilizes dried blood spots (DBS) to detect deficient alpha-glucosidase (GAA) activity. As part of currently employed NBS algorithms for PD screening in public health laboratories (PHLs), a first tier biochemical test based on MS/MS or digital microfluidics measures the enzyme activity. The disease is suspected if the enzyme activity is below a previously established cut-off value [1]. However, without two tiered or reflex testing, programs using only first tier biochemical assays would yield poor positive predictive values with high false positive rates or risk high false negative rates due to stringent first tier cut-offs [2]. False-positive results on first tier testing of PD create a high referral burden, often related to the prevalence in the population of non-disease causing pseudodeficiency alleles that lead to low enzyme activity without causing PD. Inclusion of a second tier test, on first tier positive NBS samples provides an opportunity to resolve these false-positives prior to reporting, thus avoiding re-contact, needless referrals and creation of parental anxiety. When GAA activity is below established cutoff values, a second tier test can confirm or disprove the diagnosis of PD. Current algorithms applied by NBS programs may perform repeat sampling and redo the GAA enzyme activity test [3]; or use a second tier test (in-house or as a send-out service) such as DNA sequencing that uses traditional DNA Sanger sequencing technique [4], or the newer targeted next generation sequencing (tNGS) method. Recently, a new second tier test marker—the ratio of creatine/creatinine to alpha-glucosidase activity—has also been proposed [5].

From a clinical standpoint, PD has a wide spectrum of phenotypes ranging from early onset with muscle and cardiac involvement (infantile-onset PD; IOPD) to later juvenile or adult onset (later-onset PD; LOPD). LOPD symptomatology may overlap with other neuromuscular disorders, and timely diagnosis is challenging for both forms of the disease. Most early onset cases are symptomatic in some form at birth. Two NBS algorithms for diagnostic confirmation have been developed by a group of international experts on both NBS and PD, the Pompe Disease Newborn Screening Working Group, based on whether DNA sequencing is performed as part of the screening algorithm [6]. Applying the recommendations of either algorithm can lead to a diagnostic characterization as: (a) classic IOPD, (b) "predicted" LOPD, or (c) no disease/not affected/carrier. In both algorithms, a variety of clinical tests are necessary to confirm the diagnosis and generate a treatment plan, including DNA sequencing, since the *GAA* gene variant analysis is essential for confirming the diagnosis and developing a treatment strategy of PD [6]. A challenge to pursuing DNA sequencing as part of NBS algorithms is that many NBS PHLs and clinical referral centers do not perform or have ready access to sequencing resources on premises. When an NBS laboratory does not provide rapid DNA sequencing results through either send-out services or sequencing on premises, the responsibility of obtaining the *GAA* gene sequencing result that is necessary for diagnosis and treatment initiation falls directly on the referral center. Delays in obtaining DNA sequencing results may lead to poorer outcomes or possible loss to follow-up. Loss to follow-up is a concern given the spectrum of phenotypes, many of which present with a delay in onset of symptoms and loss in benefit opportunity of early treatment. If an infant is found to have any form of disease, follow-up with appropriate treatment is necessary and should start early. Recent reports on IOPD continue to shed light on some of the unique challenges care providers face in diagnosing and managing this genetic disease [2,7]. While delays in PD symptom onset and diagnosis are less common in IOPD (under 3–4 months) compared to LOPD, based on the Pompe Registry data [8], the IOPD cases with cross-reactive immunological material (CRIM), negative statuses almost invariably develop high antibody titers to enzyme replacement therapy (ERT). As high antibody titers to ERT reduce the effectiveness of ERT treatment, CRIM-negative patients require immunomodulation therapy prior to initiation of ERT. If CRIM negative IOPDs are not identified in the newborn period, and if immune modulation therapy and ERT treatment are not initiated within days of birth, 100% ventilator free-survival is unlikely, and death may occur within the first two years of life [2,9]. Several Australian IOPD cases that were not identified by NBS, but identified by clinical examination alone have responded poorly to ERT and developed high antibody titres [7]. CRIM-positive IOPDs can also show high antibody titres, which may be predicted based on genotype [10,11]. Rapid recognition of PD at the molecular genetics level, in conjunction with clinical characterization, can guide treatment strategies that may include ERT for IOPD (with or without immune modulation therapy) and LOPD, and may be critical to ensuring the best patient outcomes while preventing irreversible clinical changes [2,12,13]. Given the clinical workup necessary after NBS to confirm a PD diagnosis and direct therapeutic strategy, and the time sensitive nature of the treatment in some PD cases, it may be imperative to also choose a second tier tNGS test that aligns with clinical algorithms and avoids delayed initiation of beneficial PD treatment. Stepwise serial testing between NBS and referral centers, can lead to obtaining DNA results in weeks, delaying initiation of treatment. The typical confirmatory diagnostic DNA sequencing test takes 3–6 weeks and may require reimbursement authorization, and therefore, is inadequate for the prompt genetic testing required for PD. If rapid DNA sequencing testing is included as part of NBS second tier testing, such delays are avoided. Furthermore, such testing may be more equitable for individuals who have no insurance coverage for post-NBS DNA sequencing test. Such decisions, of course, have cost implications for NBS programs.

We therefore also present the rationale for optimizing second tier molecular genetic testing emphasizing (a) fast turn-around time; (b) inclusion of variant effects such as cross-reactive immunological material (CRIM) status, predicted age of symptom onset and heuristics that impact treatment strategies; (c) incorporation of copy number variation and library preparation methods from DBS as part of a tNGS second tier algorithm; and (d) variant prioritization 'cut-off' tools to reduce the number of false positives and to help with PD phenotype prediction. Challenges in addressing health information privacy, policy, regulation, parental consent, and secondary or incidental findings associated with genetic tests are topics beyond the scope of this review.

2. Current Approach to Second Tier and Follow-Up Testing

The Taiwanese PD NBS algorithm measures GAA, neutral α-glucosidase (NAG), and maltase-glucoamylase (MGA) activities in separate fluorometric assays, using commercially available fluorogenic (4-methylumbelliferone) substrates [2] normalized to protein concentrations. These values discriminate between true GAA deficiency-confirmed positives from false-positives. The percentage of acarbose inhibition as a second tier test, for samples with inconclusive results, further improves the performance of testing in this algorithm.

A second tier test marker for NBS of PD recently reported by Tortorelli et al. [5] describes a reduced false-positive rate through the use of a ratio calculated between the creatine/creatinine (Cre/Crn) ratio as the numerator and the activity of acid α-glucosidase (GAA) as the denominator. This ratio is incorporated alongside a post-analytical tool: Collaborative Laboratory Integrated Reports (CLIR; https://clir.mayo.edu) and routinely used in second tier evaluations to address the issue of false positives due to pseudodeficiency.

Because DBS GAA enzyme activity measured in the first tier NBS cannot predict PD phenotype, additional follow-up evaluation using chest X-ray, electrocardiogram (EKG), creatine kinase (CK) levels, pro-B-type natriuretic peptide (pro-BNP) levels, echocardiogram and genotyping or DNA sequencing (to confirm the presence of two pathogenic variants) is required. Western blot analysis of cultured skin fibroblast lysates has been the gold standard for determining cross-reactive immunologic material (CRIM) status [14], although rapid blood-based assays are also available. Other follow-up tests such as urinary Glc4 levels are also recommended [2,6].

3. The Variant Spectrum of Pompe Disease

PD is an autosomal recessive disorder resulting from two pathogenic variants, including multi-exonic deletions, in the GAA gene. The variant spectrum in the *GAA* gene is highly heterogeneous. To date, over 500 pathogenic (P) or likely pathogenic (LP) variants and numerous benign variants and variants of unknown significance (VUS) in the *GAA* gene have been reported (ClinVar, 2017; Erasmus MC University Medical Center, 2017; Aggregation Databases (ExAC, gnomAD), 2017; Leiden Open Variation Database (LOVD), 2018; The Human Genome Mutation Database (HGMD), 2017). A review of *GAA* variants suggests that missense variants are the most frequent molecular genetic cause of PD (~50%), followed by small deletions [8,15]. Variant hotspots are also known, such as the c.-32-13T>G splice site single nucleotide variant and the exon 18 deletion (c.2481+102_2646+31del). These and other ethnic variants are well described [8,15], but require detection by DNA sequencing methods that can identify both single nucleotide variations (SNVs), as well as copy number variations (CNVs, also known as deletion/duplication events), and these are discussed later.

4. Hybrid Capture tNGS as a Second Tier Method

For NBS programs utilizing second tier DNA sequencing, both tNGS on small panels of genes and exome sequencing are considered (see Section 9). Cost and time efficiency needs, along with specimen requirements and future expansion needs, make DNA hybrid-capture based sequencing protocols for tNGS ideal for PD screening/diagnostic algorithms (see Section 5 below for additional considerations). A reduced time through the pipeline due to a more efficient process means shorter time to results and needed treatment for affected infants. A hybrid-capture based tNGS workflow [16], as outlined in Figure 1, may be performed on 1–2 newborn DBS punches, with end-to-end testing time from sample receipt to initiating reports of ~35 h (Figure 1a). In our experience, this approach used for the NBS second tier testing of PD and other lysosomal storage disorders leads to the return of results in less than a week. Reagents used are typically 'kit-based' and the processing protocol may be optimized specifically as needed. Most send-out DNA sequencing services typically have a turn-around time of several weeks, as well as referral and sample redraw, making this process challenging for the rapidity needed in NBS protocols. In our experience of processing second tier tNGS for several US PHLs, we have been able to report variant information in seven days, and reduce the referral burden in some cases by 70% (reports that did not have any P/LP variant or had exclusively pseudodeficiency variants). These reports, therefore, were capable of providing carrier status, CRIM prediction, and severity of the known reportable variants, which would not otherwise be possible.

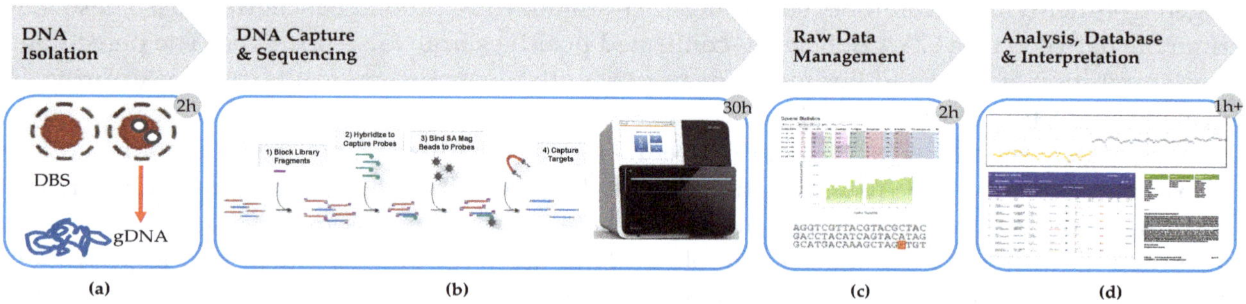

Figure 1. Hybrid Capture-Sequencing tNGS Workflow. Many components of the workflow may be automated: (**a**) DNA Isolation—This step in the workflow may be performed with two 3.2 mm DBS punches, takes 2 h (h) to perform and is an essential requirement of second tier testing as most tNGS protocols call for 2–10 mL of blood; (**b**) DNA hybrid Capture and Sequencing—DNA capture requires library preparation and bait based DNA hybridization-based capture of target regions, which is followed by DNA sequencing (Illumina MiniSeq). (**c**) Raw data management—Involves moving data across secure compliant environments for storage, processing and linking into databases; (**d**) Analysis, database and interpretation—Involves analysis for single nucleotide variants and copy number variant callers, comparative analysis with other database annotations, interpretation and reporting. This overall process takes ~35 h. Adapted from Bhattacharjee et al. [16].

DNA library preparation involves sonication or a kit-based enzymatic DNA fragmentation step (amenable to automation and high throughput) followed by subsequent adaptor ligation/indexing. Indexed DNA fragments are then hybridized to custom DNA enrichment probes in order to target the specific genes on the panel (Figure 1b). Such DNA probes are available from various commercial sources and may be custom designed to target 100–200 genes. Sequencing may be performed on several sequencing platforms. The Illumina MiniSeq platform shown in the example (Figure 1b), takes around 14h to complete a run and can parallel process 20 samples per run. The bioinformatics workflow (raw data management) is processed mostly in parallel and can take an additional 2 h. Custom QC metrics provide insight into sequence quality for each sample as well as coverage gap analysis (Figure 1c). A custom copy number variation (CNV) caller can be used on the same sequence dataset to identify CNVs (Figure 1d, Figure 2a). Strict quality metrics prevent CNV calling on samples with low coverage. An in-house variant database with a well-established analysis platform, such as from Opal™ (Fabric Genomics), can appropriately annotate the data set in real-time and help generate sequencing reports more efficiently. Automated variant scoring allows a reduction in time for data interpretation, and thus drives higher throughput.

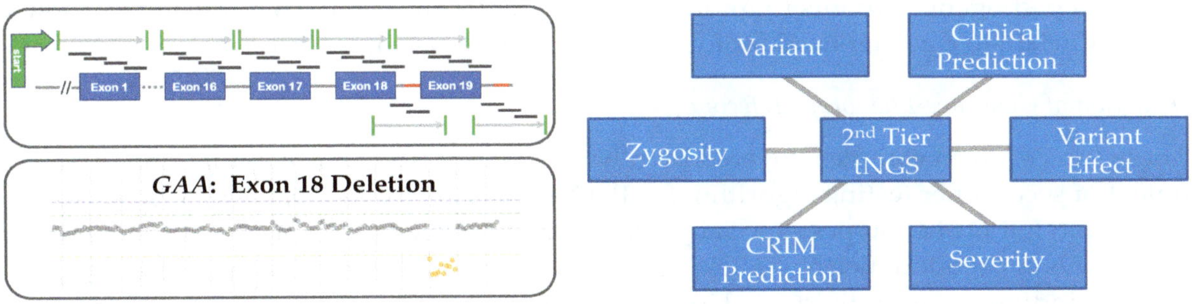

(a) (b)

Figure 2. Second tier Testing features: (**a**) Top panel shows how *GAA* gene structure is targeted for sequencing with overlapping single stranded DNA or RNA probes of 60–200 nucleotides in target exonic regions (blue rectangles), adjoining splice junctions (marked in green), and known hotspots (red). The bottom panel shows the results of a in-house algorithm that integrates detection of copy number variation (CNV) or del/dup events in Pompe disease, such as the *GAA* exon 18 deletion; (**b**) 2nd tier tNGS provides variant (genotype) information for better clinical predictions and management of care. Pseudodeficient alleles, variant effect, and cross-reactive immunologic material (CRIM) prediction can be elucidated from previously observed data [8,14].

5. Ideal PD Second Tier tNGS Testing Features

5.1. Timeliness

The US Federal and State Public Health programs emphasize the importance of timeliness of NBS, setting benchmarks for the efficient collection, transportation, testing, and reporting of results. First and second tier tests are combined to optimize detection of cases at a false positive rate as low as possible and keep overall costs of the combined tests low. Upon referral, necessary diagnostic tests are done. For many diseases that progress slowly, the split in the burden between screening and diagnostic phases may be sufficient. However, this tiered/serial testing and patient recall can cause delays in time-sensitive PD. For most of the LOPD cases that progress slowly, this approach would be sufficient without causing harm. However, for suspected IOPD cases, time to treatment initiation within two weeks is critical. Therefore, timely second tier tNGS reporting in IOPD may be the only option for avoiding diagnostic and treatment delays and avoiding a negative impact on quality of life and potentially on lifespan [7,13]. The treating clinician, in the case of classic IOPD, would need DNA sequencing data in the diagnostic-phase to determine treatment-associated predictive sequence information (CRIM status and phenotype onset predictions) prior to initiating enzyme replacement therapy [2,6]. Although controversial, suspected LOPD patients identified by NBS second tier tNGS may also benefit from follow-up and earlier intervention [2,13,17]. Rapid return of results is a frequent claim by providers of DNA sequencing for diagnostic testing. However, the DNA sequencing turnaround time is generally inadequate for early onset PD (minimum industry standard is three weeks' turnaround). Such inefficiencies make utilization of most commercial resources untenable for the required timeframe of treatment following the diagnostic phase. Second tier tNGS workflow services, if performed end-to-end, may be completed in ~35 h, and reports can be finalized consistently within 5–7 days of receiving the sample. If NBS programs routinely perform tNGS on premises, or use DNA sequencing services that return results within 7 days, then overall reporting and treatment initiation may occur within 10 days, benefiting classic IOPD or CRIM-negative IOPD cases. Starting ERT within this timeframe for CRIM-negative IOPD, and before the immune system has matured, might also enable natural immune tolerance [7]. Omitting the tNGS assay as the second tier PD NBS test and putting the burden on the follow-up referral centers to obtain a molecular diagnostic result, while providing a faster NBS turn-around time may delay treatment initiation. Due to the fact that the optimal effectiveness of ERT in IOPD hinges on the prompt identification of two *GAA* pathogenic variants in-trans [6], a second tier tNGS assay may actually be beneficial by shortening the time to treatment initiation. Identification of one or two pathogenic variants (without *cis* or *trans* determination), combined with a low GAA activity is sufficient to consider need for further confirmatory testing.

5.2. Prediction of Genotype-Phenotype Effects

These topics have been well covered by other reviews [8,15], and therefore only discussed in the context of second tier testing algorithm for PD NBS (Figure 2). In PD, the genotype is generally fully penetrant; IOPD phenotypes especially demonstrate limited heterogeneity. A pseudodeficiency allele is always a pseudodeficiency allele as it causes low measured GAA activity that does not change from individual to individual. However, predicted CRIM status may not exactly correlate as observed in some patients with Western blot analysis of cultured skin fibroblast lysates or for splice variants and may require additional studies [14]. Identification of variants in the *GAA* gene provides valuable information for determining variant-phenotypes, establishing genotype–phenotype correlations, confirming diagnosis or carrier status and counseling about the significance of these findings [6]. Measuring first tier GAA activity, genotyping, and determination of CRIM status from genotype (important for phenotype onset prediction) is necessary to start therapy [14,18].

5.3. Prediction of CRIM Status

In general, for babies with IOPD who have cardiac involvement, treatment with recombinant human GAA (rhGAA) is initiated immediately after confirmation of GAA deficiency and positive CRIM status, either by genotyping prediction or by western blot [2,6]. ERT is started after the cardiac involvement is confirmed, unless immunomodulation therapy to prevent anti-GAA antibodies production is planned. For infants without cardiac involvement, close follow up is needed and ERT treatment is delayed until symptoms appear. As confirmatory biochemical tests and assays are not readily available for PD, and additional testing may delay initiation of therapy, sequence variant identification may be useful to predict CRIM status, thereby directing treatment decisions [14,18]. The presence of two nonsense or frameshift-termination variants is a good predictor of CRIM status, typically resulting in CRIM-negative status, unless the premature stop codon is in the last exon of the gene [14].

5.4. Copy Number Variation (CNV) and False Negative Risk

Due to the fact that CNV events such as those reported in *GAA* exon 18 [8,15] and other heterogeneous CNVs comprise a significant fraction of pathogenic PD variants, a PD NBS second tier tNGS assay must integrate detection of CNV events. While data from targeted small gene panels are scarce, recent reports of PD whole exome sequences provide insight into CNVs. Mori et al. [19] evaluated whole exome sequencing to identify infantile- and late-onset PD (n = 93), concluding that some pathogenic variants may have been missed, since the variant pipeline used did not identify variant hotspots such as the exon 18 deletion (Figure 2a), and c.-32–13 single nucleotide variant. A sensitivity of near 100% can be achieved if issues with custom design, gap filling, improving >20X sequence coverage and deletion duplication coverage are addressed.

5.5. False Positives Resolved by Second Tier tNGS Testing

The variant burden and its effect on an individual is unknown at birth, and phenotype characterized by biochemical activity alone may be imprecise. Low GAA enzyme activity detected by first tier assays may identify pseudodeficiency cases and carriers of a single pathogenic *GAA* variant as a false positive, thus enzyme activity results alone are not definitive and cannot differentiate between true PD and newborns who carry pseudodeficiency alleles or sometimes PD carriers (P/LP variants). Such cases can be distinguished by genetic testing.

5.6. Other Considerations

Occasionally it may be difficult to resolve a false positive with second tier tNGS. Hypothetically, if a sample has a low enzyme activity value on first tier testing and there are no findings on second tier tNGS, the etiology of the low enzyme activity has not been identified and the result can be called negative in screening, or an additional biochemical test can be done. The etiology of discordant results may involve sample mix up or other technical issues. A sample mix up can sometimes be addressed by comparing imputed sex from tNGS data to that reported on accession data. Monitoring of additional DBS enzyme activity values may also indicate false positive risk. For example, if some additional enzyme activity values are all low, it may suggest issues with stability, storage or transportation. As mentioned, new post-analytical tools, such as Collaborative Laboratory Integrated Reports (CLIR; https://clir.mayo.edu) and second tier biochemical testing are becoming available to address these issues [5,17]. A tNGS false negative result when the first tier has low enzyme value is very unlikely given the recessive nature of PD, where the presence of at least two causal variants in trans is expected. We discuss below the post-analysis of tNGS data, including statistical tools to predict and reduce the number of false positives and understand PD phenotypes.

6. Genome Scale Data and Its Impact on PD Screening

We evaluated how information in public genomic databases would inform and impact PD NBS that utilized second tier tNGS. In order to identify potential pathogenic variants for the detection of PD through NBS, we reviewed *GAA* allele frequencies in the gnomAD database. Based on gnomAD and ClinVar, pathogenic and likely pathogenic (P/LP) variants have a total allele frequency of 0.635%. Assuming these alleles segregate independently and are fully penetrant, the probability of inheriting two such alleles is the square of 0.635 or 0.004%. This roughly equates to an expected incidence of 1/24,780 births, which is in the expected range for PD (1/14,000 to 1/100,000). This means that a significant proportion of the variant alleles that cause PD are known and can be automatically identified in a high-throughput fashion.

For the sake of timeliness, it is critical to have a tNGS assay that can identify all genetic variations in a single test. To assemble relevant variants for the diagnosis of PD through NBS, we reviewed alleles in the gnomAD database for potential CRIM status. GnomAD's *GAA* sequences from 141,456 individuals revealed 213 (0.15%) predicted LOF variants (pLOF) at 82 unique sites, of which approximately 50% were frameshift termination and 25% each were splice-site and stop-gain variants. None of these mutations were present in a homozygous state and although an additional mutation may be present in trans; it is more likely that these individuals are presumed carriers. Based on gnomAD data, the carrier frequency of unique pLOF variants is 0.15% (213/141,456) in the population, which is 4-fold less than P/LP variants in gnomAD. Estimates of carriers in general uncovered by NBS is a fraction (0.007–0.013%) of that observed frequency in gnomAD [17]. Although some may be, most PD carriers will not be detected by NBS program based on pLoF or P/LP variant frequencies in gnomAD. While reporting on carrier status is not the aim of most NBS programs (most try to avoid detecting carriers), parents of affected PD patients are obligate carriers. The risk for two carrier parents to have an affected child is 25% with each pregnancy. Thus, the mode and impact of reporting carrier status to parents after detection through a PD tNGS second tier NBS algorithm require careful consideration. Other NBS disorders deal with this issue routinely (e.g., cystic fibrosis carriers via a DNA based second tier, or sickle cell anemia via electrophoresis).

A family history of negative PD screens without carrier information gives families a false sense of security, as reported in the Australian PD cases [7]. A significant fraction of FPs will be due to recurrent carriers or pseudodeficiencies with low enzyme values, and a likely source of anxiety or rightful concern in future newborn births in those families. Thus, a delay in relaying carrier or pseudodeficiency information may have secondary consequences that may need to be considered. Recently, the BabySeq Project (a part of NSIGHT), evaluated newborn diseases using genome scale sequencing in a randomized clinical trial pilot. The cohort studied included both well newborns and those admitted to a neonatal intensive care unit [20,21]. In a cohort of 159 newborns that underwent genome scale NGS based whole exome sequencing (WES), one carrier of a pathogenic *GAA* variant was identified. As part of that study protocol, the in-person genetic counseling was provided to the family.

We also queried 14,821 WES individuals referred for clinical genetic testing to determine a 'hit rate' for *GAA*, generating a list of reportable variants by curating pathogenic and likely pathogenic variants from reputable sources in ClinVar and from manual literature curation. These estimates are useful in understanding PD causal variant frequencies and database quality. This curation resulted in over 100 *GAA* reportable variants. For each case, the exome variant file (variant call format (VCF) file) was scanned through our database and scored as to whether that sample was identified ("hit"). Only one homozygous hit (allele fraction > 90%) was observed for *GAA*. Due to the fact that testing was performed on single samples, it was not possible to know if multiple variants were in cis or trans. Thus, we defined a compound heterozygous hit as having two or more variants in a single gene, in a single sample, from our reportable list of variants. Only two cases had reportable variants in *GAA* and thus the potential "hits" for the referred population was 2/14,821 (0.014%), a value that was consistent with the incidence of PD. These types of analyses have several limitations: (a) no ethnicity control was available, as ethnicity of patients was not known, and therefore impact on actual screening could be variable; (b) consanguinity of patients was not known; (c) patients in the dataset were likely depleted of traditional PD; (d) it was not possible to distinguish the cis and trans configuration of multiple hits in a single individual; (e) this analysis did not take into account novel variants, nor did it take into account copy number variants; (f), variant calls were affected by coverage of the gene/base and particularities of the caller. Thus, while it was not possible to perfectly match the false positive /false negative rate of the caller, this effect was likely small.

7. Variant 'Cut off' for PD

To reduce the burden of interpreting variants of uncertain significance (VUS), we considered a 'cut off' model to filter variants that are too common in population to cause disease. We estimated the maximum credible allele frequency (MCAF), using a statistical framework that was previously reported for a recessive inheritance model by Wiffin et al. [22] Variants that occur more frequently than the MCAF cutoff should not be considered as a causative variant for the disease.

The equation to calculate MCAF is as follows (1):

$$\mathrm{MCAF} = \mathrm{sqrt}(v) \times c \times \mathrm{sqrt}(g) \times 1/\mathrm{sqrt}(p) \tag{1}$$

where c is the maximum allelic contribution, which represents the proportion of cases that are attributable to the gene that is attributable to an individual variant, g is the maximum genetic contribution representing the proportion of all cases that are due to the gene, v is the prevalence and p is the penetrance. This value can be further refined by assuming that the most common causative alleles are known.

For the *GAA* gene, we identified common alleles that were both expertly curated and present in ClinVar. Furthermore, we established a set of trusted ClinVar submissions (multiple sites with no conflicts (GeneDx and Invitae)) and identified all P/LP variants. From this we identified the most common pathogenic variants that contribute to the disease (ClinVar and trusted submitters). We then made the assumption that once the most common variants are accounted for, the maximum allelic contribution of any additional variant is 5%. We use 0.000025 (1/40,000) as the incidence of high-risk PD, 1 as the penetrance and assume all causes of PD are attributable to variants in *GAA*. The calculation for MCAF is then: sqrt(0.000025) × 0.05 × sqrt(1) × 1/sqrt(1) or 0.00025. We then compare this to the maximum MAF in manually curated or trusted submitter (Table 1). This value can then be used to remove likely spurious entries in ClinVar from further consideration. Furthermore, novel variants (VUSes) with MAFs above this cut-off can likely be discarded as likely benign.

Table 1. Maximum Credible Allele Frequency (MCAF): Allelic Contribution, Penetrance, MAF cutoff, pathogenic variants in ClinVar from Trusted submitters and final MAF cutoff.

Prevalence	Max. Allelic Contribution	Penetrance	MCAF (Whiffin et al. [22])	Max. MAF in ClinVar	Final Cut Off
0.000025	0.05	1	0.00025	0.00358	0.00025

8. Follow-Up Infrastructure for Families, Screen Positive Infants and Carrier Status

Some of the most difficult issues generated by NBS for PD will be the follow-up care, for not only the infants who screen positive, but also for the parents and families. As of 2017, the Pompe Disease Newborn Screening Working Group has proposed options for including DNA sequencing as part of the screening algorithm or follow-up [6]. The Pompe Registry, a long-term, multinational observational program (NCT002314000), designed to improve understanding of the natural history and outcomes of patients with PD, started in 2004, and is sponsored and administered by Sanofi Genzyme (Cambridge, MA), the pharmaceutical company that markets PD ERT. The Pompe Registry has *GAA* variants and phenotypes for 1079 patients [8]. Despite the existence of this network, challenges surround the referral of those patients to appropriate care centers, to ensure that up to date care guidelines that reflect the current standards of the PD NBS community are adhered to. Given that current disease modifying treatments for PD may depend on knowing the specific genetic defect, it is critical and ethically required, that all screen positive infants have timely access to genetic testing, as either part of NBS or as referral within the timeframe. Testing should define the specific variants and access to appropriate follow up clinical expertise, so that the appropriate treatment is provided. Future therapies, once approved, such as chaperones, c.-32-splice switching antisense oligonucleotides and AAV-directed gene therapies will need variant information.

Testing parents to determine which parent carries which PD variant is necessary to provide appropriate counseling regarding future reproductive risk for family members. Knowing familial variants for PD can be useful for reproductive planning and the avoidance of recurrence, but is not the primary goal of NBS. Most guidelines recommend against carrier testing of minors and minor siblings, as there is no medical benefit until reaching reproductive age and age of consent [23–25].

Some screen positive infants will have an early-onset form of the disease while others will develop LOPD. Knowing the precise genetic defect in a screen positive IOPD case is critical for the prediction of the long-term clinical outcome of ERT and the development of antibodies against the infused enzyme. An analysis of CRIM status for every IOPD patient within the first two weeks of life is essential. For this reason, sequence analysis of the GAA gene may be justified as a tiered testing step for PD NBS programs or a rapid turnaround confirmatory test for the referral center. Some first tier screen positive newborns may have resolution on a tNGS second tier test, as they may carry pseudodeficiency alleles or a variant burden, that are otherwise low risk. For parents of screen positive infants with identified variant(s), familial testing is relatively simple and may be considered in reproductive planning. Normal GAA enzyme activity, or an above threshold value on a PD NBS, does not confirm a non-carrier status. It is possible that a pathogenic variant may have been missed or that a phenotype may manifest later. The potential therefore exists for misconstruing a negative PD NBS. Further studies must evaluate whether all infants identified with disease or as carriers have received adequate follow-up, including diagnostic confirmation after a positive screen, referral to appropriate clinical care centers and delivery of best practice treatment and management across the lifespan. State NBS programs must have a short-term follow-up plan in place to ensure tracking of screen positive newborns for the receipt of proper referral to appropriate care centers for diagnosis and treatment. Ideally, this short-term follow-up program should have access to resources that include: (a) *GAA* sequencing availability or referral for rapid turnaround DNA sequencing for screen positive infants; (b) the ability to provide cascade genetic testing of both family and extended family members; and (c) the ability to carry out all necessary confirmatory testing. Furthermore, referral sites should be able to appropriately triage infants found to have incidental findings like other overlapping neuromuscular diseases, such as Limb Girdle muscular dystrophy. Since it is recommended that CK levels be determined in all infants in whom 1st and 2nd tier testing is suspicious of PD, there will likely be utility in determining baseline CK levels from DBS at the time of initial enzyme testing. This would be helpful not only for confirming the diagnosis and establishing a baseline level prior to starting treatment, but also allowing for early identification of other neuromuscular disorders if there is persistence of hyperCKemia, despite negative testing for PD. As with all genetic testing, identifying and implementing appropriate educational programs is key. Improving health care provider and parental genetic literacy about genetic disorders is required.

9. Current and Future Utilization of tNGS Testing

PD was added to the U.S. Recommended Universal Screening Panel (RUSP) in 2015. Targeted NGS could reduce the treatment delay for those identified by PD screening by allowing analysis, interpretation, and appropriate reporting of healthcare related information in a timely manner. Already several PHLs in the USA have adopted second tier tNGS in-house or as a service [26,27]. New York and California PHLs have strong DNA sequencing second tier programs including tNGS for PD and other NBS disorders. Several other NBS PHLs use 'send-out second tier tNGS services' for PD. Given developments in genome scale technologies, such as WES or whole genome sequencing (WGS), the utilization of tNGS may be co-opted for needs in second tier testing of PD. Recently, the Utah PHL has started implementing a second tier exome sequencing protocol for genes associated with newborn screening abnormalities [28]. Furthermore, tNGS based testing can avoid constraints or complicating factors associated with biochemical testing, such as the infant's gestational age at birth, transfusion status, age at sample collection, need for repeat sampling (rescreens or redraws), and metabolic and feeding states. The NIH funded NSIGHT consortium (Newborn Sequencing in Genomic Medicine and Public Health) evaluated newborn diseases using genome scale sequencing in randomized clinical trials [21,22,29]. This is an exciting time to be at the forefront of applying genomic information to rapidly identifying and treating genetic disorders such as PD. We envision that population level screening as first tier WES or WGS, or even first tier small gene panel based tNGS testing, is unlikely to be the avenue by which PD may be identified in the near term, due to considerations such as cost and complexity. However, with improvements in technology and a decrease in cost, this may likely be the NBS of the future.

10. Conclusions

In summary, molecular based NGS testing approaches are suitable for NBS of PD, and may be used in algorithms that include either a tandem second tier test or in a contingent fashion. The primary goal of NBS is identifying patients who can be treated to establish significant health gain. Secondary goals, such as shortening the diagnostic odyssey, identifying carriers and providing information for reproductive options are of lesser concern. However, as PD is a spectrum disease simply providing biochemical screen positive information alone delays treatment initiation in those phenotypes with rapid disease progression, which impacts the ultimate outcome. PD has both pseudodeficiencies as well as early-onset and late-onset clinical phenotypes, presenting a special challenge to families and medical follow-up centers. Early genotype information in PD management allows for prompt treatment initiation and the potential for better clinical outcomes, especially in infantile onset disease [2,3,9,12,13]. Considering the recommended diagnostic algorithm [2,6], of which DNA sequencing is a part, the use of second tier tNGS sequencing is only logical, irrespective of whether the PHL yet has sequencing capabilities, since NBS may be the only way to provide molecular genetic information for early determination and treatment of PD in an equitable manner. Several PHLs including New York and California have already introduced DNA sequencing in their PD NBS algorithms. While second tier biochemial tests are capable of PD identification, second tier tNGS test for PD can provide rapid and precise information on highly penetrant recurrent pathogenic variants, distinguish pseudodeficiency alleles with lower biochemical values that are false-positives, provide clues for CRIM status, and identify variants associated with IOPD or LOPD phenotypes. A combination of early detection, close monitoring, and early ERT is likely to be beneficial to LOPD patients, but additional data are needed. Consistent with the original intent of NBS, PD must be considered a time critical condition, for which all PD NBS results including second tier should be provided as early as possible. Given the ever-increasing population-based variation outcome data for PD [30], implementation of tNGS second tier testing of PD from a DBS [16], is both feasible and sufficient in the required time frame for NBS and follow up.

Acknowledgments: We thank Rebecca Kitchener and Viren Amin for the figures, technical details and review of the manuscript.

References

1. Gelb, M.; Lukacs, Z.; Ranieri, E.; Schielen, P. Newborn Screening for Lysosomal Storage Disorders: Methodologies for Measurement of Enzymatic Activities in Dried Blood Spots. *Int. J. Neonatal Screen.* **2018**, *5*, 1. [CrossRef] [PubMed]
2. Chien, Y.-H.; Hwu, W.-L.; Lee, N.-C. Newborn Screening: Taiwanese Experience. *Ann. Transl. Med.* **2019**, *7*, 281. [CrossRef] [PubMed]
3. Yang, C.-F.; Liu, H.-C.; Hsu, T.-R.; Tsai, F.-C.; Chiang, S.-F.; Chiang, C.-C.; Ho, H.-C.; Lai, C.-J.; Yang, T.-F.; Chuang, S.-Y.; et al. A Large-Scale Nationwide Newborn Screening Program for Pompe Disease in Taiwan: Towards Effective Diagnosis and Treatment. *Am. J. Med Genet. Part A* **2013**, *164*, 54–61. [CrossRef]
4. Wasserstein, M.P.; Caggana, M.; Bailey, S.M.; Desnick, R.J.; Edelmann, L.; Estrella, L.; Holzman, I.; Kelly, N.R.; Kornreich, R.; Kupchik, S.G.; et al. The New York Pilot Newborn Screening Program for Lysosomal Storage Diseases: Report of the First 65,000 Infants. *Genet. Med.* **2018**, *21*, 631–640. [CrossRef] [PubMed]
5. Tortorelli, S.; Eckerman, J.S.; Orsini, J.J.; Stevens, C.; Hart, J.; Hall, P.L.; Alexander, J.J.; Gavrilov, D.; Oglesbee, D.; Raymond, K.; et al. Moonlighting Newborn Screening Markers: The Incidental Discovery of a Second-Tier Test for Pompe Disease. *Genet. Med.* **2017**, *20*, 840–846. [CrossRef] [PubMed]
6. Burton, B.K.; Kronn, D.F.; Hwu, W.-L.; Kishnani, P.S. The Initial Evaluation of Patients after Positive Newborn Screening: Recommended Algorithms Leading to a Confirmed Diagnosis of Pompe Disease. *Pediatrics* **2017**, *140*, S14–S23. [CrossRef] [PubMed]
7. Saich, R.; Brown, R.; Collicoat, M.; Jenner, C.; Primmer, J.; Clancy, B.; Holland, T.; Krinks, S. Is Newborn Screening the Ultimate Strategy to Reduce Diagnostic Delays in Pompe Disease? The Parent and Patient Perspective. *Int. J. Neonatal Screen.* **2020**, *6*, 1. [CrossRef]
8. Reuser, A.J.J.; Ploeg, A.T.; Chien, Y.H.; Llerena, J.; Abbott, M.A.; Clemens, P.R.; Kimonis, V.E.; Leslie, N.; Maruti, S.S.; Sanson, B.J.; et al. On Behalf of the Pompe Registry Sit. GAA Variants and Phenotypes among 1079 Patients with Pompe Disease: Data from the Pompe Registry. *Hum. Mutat.* **2019**, *40*, 2146–2164. [CrossRef]
9. Owens, P.; Wong, M.; Bhattacharya, K.; Ellaway, C. Infantile-Onset Pompe Disease: A Case Series Highlighting Early Clinical Features, Spectrum of Disease Severity and Treatment Response. *J. Paediatr. Child Health* **2018**, *54*, 1255–1261. [CrossRef]
10. Desai, A.K.; Li, C.; Rosenberg, A.S.; Kishnani, P.S. Immunological Challenges and Approaches to Immunomodulation in Pompe Disease: A Literature Review. *Ann. Transl. Med.* **2019**, *7*, 285. [CrossRef]
11. Groot, A.D.; Kazi, Z.; Martin, R.; Terry, F.; Desai, A.; Martin, W.; Kishnani, P. HLA- and Genotype-Based Risk Assessment Model to Identify Infantile Onset Pompe Disease Patients at High-Risk of Developing Significant Anti-Drug Antibodies (ADA). *Clin. Immunol.* **2019**, *200*, 66–70. [CrossRef] [PubMed]
12. Yang, C.-F.; Chu, T.-H.; Huang, L.-Y.; Liao, H.-C.; Soong, W.-J.; Niu, D.-M. AB028. Very Early Treatment for Infantile-Onset Pompe Disease Contributes to Better Outcomes: 10-Year Experience in One Institute. *Ann. Transl. Med.* **2017**, *169*, 174–180. [CrossRef]
13. Chien, Y.-H.; Lee, N.-C.; Chen, C.-A.; Tsai, F.-J.; Tsai, W.-H.; Shieh, J.-Y.; Huang, H.-J.; Hsu, W.-C.; Tsai, T.-H.; Hwu, W.-L. Long-Term Prognosis of Patients with Infantile-Onset Pompe Disease Diagnosed by Newborn Screening and Treated since Birth. *J. Pediatr.* **2015**, *166*, 985–991. [CrossRef] [PubMed]
14. Bali, D.; Goldstein, J.; Banugaria, S.; Dai, J.; Mackey, J.; Rehder, C.; Kishnani, P. Predicting Cross Reactive

Immunological Material (CRIM) Status in Pompe Disease Using GAA Mutations: Lessons Learned from 10 Years of Clinical Laboratory Testing Experience. In *American Journal of Medical Genetics Part C: Seminars in Medical Genetics*; John Wiley & Sons: Hoboken, NJ, USA, 2012.

15. Peruzzo, P.; Pavan, E.; Dardis, A. Molecular Genetics of Pompe Disease: A Comprehensive Overview. *Ann. Transl. Med.* **2019**, *7*, 278. [CrossRef]
16. Bhattacharjee, A.; Sokolsky, T.; Wyman, S.K.; Reese, M.G.; Puffenberger, E.; Strauss, K.; Morton, H.; Parad, R.B.; Naylor, E.W. Development of DNA Confirmatory and High-Risk Diagnostic Testing for Newborns Using Targeted Next-Generation DNA Sequencing. *Genet. Med.* **2014**, *17*, 337–347. [CrossRef]
17. Millington, D.; Bali, D. Current State of the Art of Newborn Screening for Lysosomal Storage Disorders. *Int. J. Neonatal Screen.* **2018**, *4*, 24. [CrossRef]
18. Kishnani, P.S.; Goldenberg, P.C.; Dearmey, S.L.; Heller, J.; Benjamin, D.; Young, S.; Bali, D.; Smith, S.A.; Li, J.S.; Mandel, H.; et al. Cross-Reactive Immunologic Material Status Affects Treatment Outcomes in Pompe Disease Infants. *Mol. Genet. Metab.* **2010**, *99*, 26–33. [CrossRef]
19. Mori, M.; Haskell, G.; Kazi, Z.; Zhu, X.; Dearmey, S.M.; Goldstein, J.L.; Bali, D.; Rehder, C.; Cirulli, E.T.; Kishnani, P.S. Sensitivity of Whole Exome Sequencing in Detecting Infantile- and Late-Onset Pompe Disease. *Mol. Genet. Metab.* **2017**, *122*, 189–197. [CrossRef]
20. Holm, I.A.; Agrawal, P.B.; Ceyhan-Birsoy, O.; Christensen, K.D.; Fayer, S.; Frankel, L.A.; Genetti, C.A.; Krier, J.B.; Lamay, R.C.; Levy, H.L.; et al. The BabySeq Project: Implementing Genomic Sequencing in Newborns. *BMC Pediatr.* **2018**, 18. [CrossRef]
21. Ceyhan-Birsoy, O.; Machini, K.; Lebo, M.S.; Yu, T.W.; Agrawal, P.B.; Parad, R.B.; Holm, I.A.; Mcguire, A.; Green, R.C.; Beggs, A.H.; et al. A Curated Gene List for Reporting Results of Newborn Genomic Sequencing. *Genet. Med.* **2017**, *19*, 809–818. [CrossRef]
22. Whiffin, N.; Minikel, E.; Walsh, R.; O'Donnell-Luria, A.H.; Karczewski, K.; Ing, A.Y.; Barton, P.J.R.; Funke, B.; Cook, S.A.; Macarthur, D.; et al. Using High-Resolution Variant Frequencies to Empower Clinical Genome Interpretation. *Genet. Med.* **2017**, *19*, 1151–1158. [CrossRef] [PubMed]
23. Botkin, J.R.; Belmont, J.W.; Berg, J.S.; Berkman, B.E.; Bombard, Y.; Holm, I.A.; Levy, H.P.; Ormond, K.E.; Saal, H.M.; Spinner, N.B.; et al. Points to Consider: Ethical, Legal, and Psychosocial Implications of Genetic Testing in Children and Adolescents. *Am. J. Hum. Genet.* **2015**, *97*, 501. [CrossRef]
24. *Report on the Genetic Testing of Children 2010*; British Society for Human Genetics: Birmingham, UK, 2010.
25. Ethical and Policy Issues in Genetic Testing and Screening of Children. *Pediatrics* **2013**, *131*, 620–622. [CrossRef] [PubMed]
26. Tang, H.; Feuchtbaum, L.; Sciortino, S.; Matteson, J.; Mathur, D.; Bishop, T.; Olney, R.S. The First Year Experience of Newborn Screening for Pompe Disease in California. *Int. J. Neonatal Screen.* **2020**, *6*, 9. [CrossRef]
27. Burton, B.K.; Charrow, J.; Hoganson, G.E.; Fleischer, J.; Grange, D.K.; Braddock, S.R.; Hitchins, L.; Hickey, R.; Christensen, K.M.; Groeppner, D.; et al. Newborn Screening for Pompe Disease in Illinois: Experience with 684,290 Infants. *Int. J. Neonatal Screen.* **2020**, *6*, 4. [CrossRef]
28. Ruiz-Schultz, N.; Oakson, K.; Jones, D.; Rindler, M.; Hart, K.; Rohrwasser, A. Targeted Second-Tier Confirmatory Next Generation Sequencing Newborn Screening Pipeline. In *Poster Abstracts 2019*; Newborn Screening & Genetic Testing Symposium: Chicago, IL, USA, 7–10 April 2019.
29. Milko, L.V.; Odaniel, J.M.; Decristo, D.M.; Crowley, S.B.; Foreman, A.K.M.; Wallace, K.E.; Mollison, L.F.; Strande, N.T.; Girnary, Z.S.; Boshe, L.J.; et al. An Age-Based Framework for Evaluating Genome-Scale Sequencing Results in Newborn Screening. *J. Pediatr.* **2019**, *209*, 68–76. [CrossRef]
30. Bergsma, A.J.; In't Groen, S.L.; van den Dorpel, J.J.; van den Hout, H.J.; van der Beek, N.A.; Schoser, B.; Toscano, A.; Musumeci, O.; Bembi, B.; Dardis, A.; et al. A Genetic Modifier of Symptom Onset in Pompe Disease. *EBioMedicine* **2019**, *43*, 553–561. [CrossRef]

19

It All Depends What You Count—The Importance of Definitions in Evaluation of CF Screening Performance

Natasha Heather [1,2,*] and Dianne Webster [1,2]

1 National Newborn Metabolic Screening programme, LabPlus, Auckland City Hospital, Auckland 1148, New Zealand; diannew@adhb.govt.nz
2 Liggins Institute, University of Auckland, Auckland 1023, New Zealand
* Correspondence: NHeather@adhb.govt.nz

Abstract: Screening metrics are essential to both quality assessment and improvement, but are highly dependent on the way positive tests and cases are counted. In cystic fibrosis (CF) screening, key factors include how mild cases of late-presenting CF and CF screen positive, inconclusive diagnosis (CFSPID) are counted, whether those at prior increased risk of CF are excluded from the screened population, and which aspects of the screening pathway are considered. This paper draws on the New Zealand experience of almost forty years of newborn screening for CF. We demonstrate how different definitions impact the calculation of screening sensitivity. We suggest that, to enable meaningful comparison, CF screening reports should clarify what steps in the screening pathway are included in the assessment, as well as the algorithm used and screening target.

Keywords: newborn screen; target disorder; missed case; sensitivity; cystic fibrosis; CFSPID; immunoreactive trypsin; meconium ileus

---

1. Introduction

Most newborn screening programmes want to know how they are performing. Local metrics, such as transit times for samples or the efficiency of short-term followup of unsuitable samples, are influenced by local conditions and can usefully be compared from time to time within a programme. Global metrics such as those used in public health (e.g., screening sensitivity, specificity, and positive predictive value) are widely used to compare performance between programmes. However, the comparison may not be based on equivalent counting of positive tests and detected and missed cases. This article explores the different definitions used in cystic fibrosis (CF) screening and the effects on screening metrics.

2. Factors to Consider

2.1. Target Disorder

When newborn screening started in the 1960s the understanding of disease was simpler—a baby either had PKU or not. As time went by it was recognized that a milder form existed and the baby had PKU or hyperphenylalaninemia. Then it became clear the borders between these conditions were not sharp, and considerable effort (phenylalanine loads) went into deciding whether a baby with a raised phenylalanine level had hyperphenylalaninemia type one to five (from benign to severe). Finally, the spectrum of disease was recognized, and now it is considered that each person with raised blood phenylalanine has their own disease determined not only by variants in the phenylalanine hydroxylase gene but also by other protein-metabolizing and amino acid-transporting systems.

Similarly, at the time that screening for CF started in the late 1970s [1] it was considered to be a uniformly serious childhood condition. However, since the discovery of the cystic fibrosis transmembrane regulator (CFTR) [2], the CF phenotype has been broadened to include mild and late-presenting disease, such as otherwise healthy males presenting with infertility and older adults with mild respiratory symptoms but found to carry two "pathogenic" CFTR variants [3]. Many CF screening programmes have only been in place for a few years. The recognition of a broadened CF phenotype has created problems in defining the outcome as well as the target of screening.

The biological level at which screening and confirmatory investigations are performed (genetic and/or functional assessment) impacts the number and severity of cases that will be detected [4]. The 2017 CF Foundation consensus guidelines reinforce the importance of a sweat test in establishing a diagnosis of CF [5]. The NewSTEPS case definition acknowledges that a sweat test is the gold standard, but accepts that a diagnosis could also be established by genotyping [6]. Furthermore, most screening programmes would say that a detected case is an infant with a positive newborn screen who went on to be diagnosed with CF. However, some infants have ambiguous genotypes (e.g., one pathogenic variant and another variant of unknown significance) and/or biochemical phenotypes (low but still abnormal sweat chlorides, such as 30–59 mmol/L) and may or may not develop classical CF symptoms later. These infants are now described as CF screen positive, inconclusive diagnosis (CFSPID) [7,8].

This raises the question—what is a diagnosis? When an infant presents with meconium ileus or failure to thrive, the diagnosis is CF. When an infant has a positive screen, confirmatory tests (sweat and pancreatic function) and possibly previously unidentified clinical features can also lead to the early diagnosis of CF. However, infants with CFSPID are apparently healthy, asymptomatic infants who are essentially diagnosed based on their newborn screen, as further tests have been inconclusive. CFSPID sounds like a disease, which creates anxiety and confusion for families [9]. Yet, such infants may go on to either develop symptoms of CF or remain healthy. Screening and sometimes confirmatory investigations provide an indication of the risk of disease [4]. In newborn screening, post-analytical tools, such as the Collaborative Laboratory Integrated Report (CLIR), are being developed to assist with such assessments of risk [10]. It may be that the outcomes of screening could be CF confirmed, CF remains possible, CF unlikely—and results communicated to families in that way.

Screening metrics are used for programme evaluation and to inform quality improvements. Whilst some programmes aim to detect all possible cases, others apply pragmatic boundaries to missed cases such as those presenting in early childhood with severe disease. It is not clear from the literature whether different programmes consider CFSPID as cases of screen-detected CF, and we think it likely that CFSPID is sometimes counted and sometimes not. Whatever approach is taken, the case definition should be clear and consistent, as it impacts screening metrics. In order to inform quality improvements, outcome data must also be available within a reasonable timeframe. The benefit of knowing about a case missed more than a decade prior is arguable given likely changes to the test methodology and algorithms in the intervening period.

2.2. Screened Population

Definitions of population screening vary but generally include a statement about screening only being appropriate for persons not at increased prior risk of having the disorder [11]. The argument for this is that at-risk infants, such as those with a family history of CF, should have genetic and functional diagnostic testing performed regardless of the newborn screen result (with genetic testing taking the particular family CFTR variants into account).

The impact of including at-risk infants in screening metrics varies depending on the screening algorithm used, and hence what is defined as a positive test.

- If the first step of the algorithm is whether family history or meconium ileus is present, and all are reported as positive screens, then all CF cases within this high-risk group will be counted as detected by screening.

- If the first step of the algorithm is to measure immunoreactive trypsin (IRT), then only those with raised IRT will be reported as screen positive, and those who have a family history but do not have raised IRT (as is common in severe disease, especially with meconium ileus detected [12]) will be counted as missed cases.
- If, following a raised IRT, the second step of the algorithm is CFTR variant analysis using a common CFTR variant panel, the screen will also miss those with family histories and a raised IRT but uncommon CFTR variants that are not included in the panel used.

2.3. *Programme Boundaries*

When calculating screening metrics, jurisdictions apply variable boundaries to the screening programme. Many jurisdictions only count missed cases if a normal screen result was issued. As a result, the count of missed cases is limited to those occurring within the laboratory, and due to either screening protocols or error. Whilst this definition may focus on aspects under the control of the screening laboratory, it will result in fewer missed cases and higher reported sensitivity than jurisdictions which apply a broader definition of missed cases.

CF can be missed at all steps of the screening and diagnostic pathway, including where no screening occurred or during the short-term followup [13,14]. Some jurisdictions count missed cases that occur early in the screening pathway because either the test is not offered or the family declines. Others consider the screening pathway to begin with the acceptance of a screening offer, and so would not count cases where families have declined screening because the family has effectively removed itself from the screened population. Cases may also be missed at the level of short-term followup, because the appropriate followup did not occur, or because the diagnostic test was either misinterpreted or incorrectly performed. This is particularly relevant to CF, as both methodological and biological variation can impact measured sweat chloride [15].

2.4. *CF Screening Sensitivity Example*

Newborn screening for CF by the measurement of IRT in dried blood spots was developed in New Zealand [1], and this was the first national programme to adopt CF screening in 1981 [16]. The programme now follows a two-step algorithm whereby samples with raised IRT (top 1%) reflex to analysis for common CFTR variants (F508del, G542X, G551D and in later years R117H). Aside from the addition of R117H, the algorithm remained the same over the period reported. The ethnic composition of New Zealand births has changed over the past decades [17] and was recently described for the period 2010–2017 [18].

Those with at least one CFTR variant are reported as positive CF screening tests. All positive tests within the Auckland region are referred to the multidisciplinary CF team at Starship Children's Hospital, who are also referred likely cases of CF from community and hospital teams within the region. We utilized the Starship Children's Hospital CF clinical database to identify new CF cases and to review CF screening in the Auckland region between 2003 and 2017.

In this time period, 325,000 babies were screened. There were 113 cases of CF diagnosed, of whom 89 were diagnosed as a result of positive newborn screening tests and 24 were clinically detected. Eight CF cases were excluded from further analysis as they had been born abroad and not screened in New Zealand. Of note, seven of these had not been screened for CF and one had a positive screen followed by a sweat test result that was considered to be normal. Table 1 outlines the relevant screening factors for the 16 New Zealand-born CF cases that were diagnosed clinically.

The calculation of screening sensitivity (the number of true positive screens divided by the sum of true positive and false negative screens, expressed as a percentage) varies depending on which clinically diagnosed CF cases are included in the count of missed cases.

- If sensitivity is calculated by counting all missed cases: 89/105 = 84.8%

- If the sensitivity calculation does not include those outside the screened population (i.e., screening declined, family history or meconium ileus) as missed cases: 89/102 = 87.3%
- If the sensitivity calculation only counts missed cases as those which occurred within the laboratory (in-range IRT, no CFTR variants on panel): 89/100 = 89.0%

Table 1. Clinically diagnosed cystic fibrosis, Auckland region 2003–2017.

	No Other Factors	Other Factors	Screening Boundary	Total
No screen			1 declined	1
In-range IRT †	9	1 MI ††		10
CFTR variant not on panel	2	1 FH †††		3
Positive screen			2 normal sweat test	2
Total				16

† IRT = immunoreactive trypsin; †† MI = meconium ileus; ††† FH = family history.

3. Conclusions

While screening metrics are essential for both the quality assessment and improvement of programmes, they are highly dependent on the way positive tests and cases are counted. It is difficult to compare programme metrics unless definitions of the target disorder, the screened population, and the screening programme boundaries are clear and constant over time. This is particularly true for CF, where screening algorithms vary and there is a broad phenotype, as well as infants labelled with CFSPID. We suggest that in order to enable the meaningful comparison of performance data, CF screening reports should clarify what steps in the screening pathway are included in the assessment, as well as the algorithm used and screening target.

Author Contributions: Conceptualization, N.H. and D.W.; writing—original draft preparation, N.H.; writing—review and editing, D.W. All authors have read and agreed to the published version of the manuscript.

Acknowledgments: We acknowledge the ongoing support of the National Screening Unit, Ministry of Health.

References

1. Crossley, J.R.; Elliott, R.B.; Smith, A. Dried-blood spot screening for cystic fibrosis in the newborn. *Lancet* **1979**, *1*, 472–474. [CrossRef]
2. Kerem, B.; Rommens, J.M.; Buchanan, J.A.; Markiewicz, D.; Cox, T.K.; Chakravarti, A.; Buchwald, M.; Tsui, L.C. Identification of the cystic fibrosis gene: Genetic analysis. *Science* **1989**, *245*, 1073–1080. [CrossRef] [PubMed]
3. Gilljam, M. Clinical manifestations of cystic fibrosis among patients with diagnosis in adulthood. *Chest* **2004**, *126*, 1215–1224. [CrossRef] [PubMed]
4. Pollitt, R.J. Different viewpoint: International perspectives on newborn screening. *J. Med. Biochem.* **2015**, *34*, 18–22. [CrossRef] [PubMed]
5. Farrell, P.M.; White, T.B.; Ren, C.L.; Hempstead, S.E.; Accurso, F.; Derichs, N.; Howenstine, M.; McColley, S.A.; Rock, M.; Rosenfeld, M.; et al. Diagnosis of Cystic Fibrosis: Consensus Guidelines from the Cystic Fibrosis Foundation. *J. Pediatr.* **2017**, *181S*, S4–S15.e1. [CrossRef] [PubMed]
6. Sontag, M.K.; Sarkar, D.; Comeau, A.M.; Hassell, K.; Botto, L.D.; Parad, R.; Rose, S.R.; Wintergerst, K.A.; Smith-Whitley, K.; Singh, S.; et al. Case definitions for conditions identified by newborn screening public health surveillance. *Int. J. Neonatal Screen* **2018**, *4*, 16. [CrossRef] [PubMed]
7. Munck, A.; Mayell, S.J.; Winters, V.; Shawcross, A.; Derichs, N.; Parad, R. Cystic Fibrosis Screen Positive, Inconclusive Diagnosis (CFSPID): A new designation and management recommendations for infants with an inconclusive diagnosis following newborn screening. *J. Cyst. Fibros.* **2015**, *14*, 706–713. [CrossRef] [PubMed]
8. Levy, H.; Farrell, M. New challenges in the diagnosis and management of cystic fibrosis. *J. Pediatr.* **2015**, *166*, 1337–1341. [CrossRef] [PubMed]

9. Johnson, F.; Southern, K.W.; Ulph, F. Psychological impact on parents of an inconclusive diagnosis following newborn bloodspot screening for cystic fibrosis: A qualitative study. *Int. J. Neonatal Screen* **2019**, *5*, 23. [CrossRef]
10. Collaborative Laboratory Integrated Reports. Available online: https://clir.mayo.edu (accessed on 25 May 2020).
11. National Health Committee. *Screening to Improve Health in New Zealand*; Ministry of Health: Wellington, New Zealand, 2003.
12. Sontag, M.K.; Corey, M.; Hokanson, J.E.; Marshall, J.A.; Sommer, S.S.; Zerbe, G.O.; Accurso, F.J. Genetic and physiologic correlates of longitudinal immunoreactive trypsinogen decline in infants with cystic fibrosis identified through newborn screening. *J. Pediatr.* **2006**, *149*, 650–657. [CrossRef] [PubMed]
13. Holtzman, C.; Slazyk, W.E.; Cordero, J.F.; Hannon, W.H. Descriptive epidemiology of missed cases of phenylketonuria and congenital hypothyroidism. *Pediatrics* **1986**, *78*, 553–558. [PubMed]
14. Henry, R.L.; Boulton, T.J.; Roddick, L.G. False negative results on newborn screening for cystic fibrosis. *J. Paediatr. Child Health* **1990**, *26*, 150–151. [CrossRef] [PubMed]
15. Collie, J.T.; Massie, R.J.; Jones, O.A.; LeGrys, V.A.; Greaves, R.F. Sixty-five years since the New York heat wave: Advances in sweat testing for cystic fibrosis. *Pediatr. Pulmonol.* **2014**, *49*, 106–117. [CrossRef] [PubMed]
16. Wesley, A.W.; Smith, A.; Elliott, R.B. Experience with neonatal screening for cystic fibrosis in New Zealand using measurement of immunoreactive trypsinogen. *Aust. Paediatr. J.* **1989**, *25*, 151–155. [CrossRef] [PubMed]
17. Albert, B.B.; Cutfield, W.S.; Webster, D.; Carll, J.; Derraik, J.G.B.; Jefferies, C.; Gunn, A.J.; Hofman, P.L. Etiology of increasing incidence of congenital hypothyroidism in New Zealand from 1993–2010. *J. Clin. Endocrinol. Metab.* **2012**, *97*, 3155–3160. [CrossRef] [PubMed]
18. Heather, N.L.; Derraik, J.G.; Webster, D.; Hofman, P.L. The impact of demographic factors on newborn TSH levels and congenital hypothyroidism screening. *Clin. Endocrinol. (Oxf.)* **2019**, *91*, 456–463. [CrossRef] [PubMed]

20

Cost and Cost-Effectiveness Assessments of Newborn Screening for Critical Congenital Heart Disease Using Pulse Oximetry

Scott D. Grosse [1,*], Cora Peterson [2], Rahi Abouk [3], Jill Glidewell [1] and Matthew E. Oster [1,4]

1 Centers for Disease Control and Prevention, National Center on Birth Defects and Developmental Disabilities, 4770 Buford Highway NE, Mail Stop E-87, Atlanta, GA 30341, USA; MGlidewell@cdc.gov (J.G.); OsterM@kidsheart.com (M.E.O.)

2 Centers for Disease Control and Prevention, National Center for Injury Prevention and Control, Atlanta, GA 30341, USA; CPeterson2@cdc.gov

3 Cotsakos College of Business, William Paterson University, Wayne, NJ 07470, USA; AboukR@wpunj.edu

4 Children's Healthcare of Atlanta, Emory University School of Medicine, Atlanta, GA 30341, USA

* Correspondence: sgrosse@cdc.gov;

Abstract: Screening newborns for critical congenital heart disease (CCHD) using pulse oximetry is recommended to allow for the prompt diagnosis and prevention of life-threatening crises. The present review summarizes and critiques six previously published estimates of the costs or cost-effectiveness of CCHD screening from the United Kingdom, United States, and China. Several elements that affect CCHD screening costs were assessed in varying numbers of studies, including screening staff time, instrumentation, and consumables, as well as costs of diagnosis and treatment. A previous US study that used conservative assumptions suggested that CCHD screening is likely to be considered cost-effective from the healthcare sector perspective. Newly available estimates of avoided infant CCHD deaths in several US states that implemented mandatory CCHD screening policies during 2011–2013 suggest a substantially larger reduction in deaths than was projected in the previous US cost-effectiveness analysis. Taking into account these new estimates, we estimate that cost per life-year gained could be as low as USD 12,000. However, that estimate does not take into account future costs of health care and education for surviving children with CCHD nor the costs incurred by health departments to support and monitor CCHD screening policies and programs.

Keywords: neonatal screening; critical congenital heart disease; economic evaluation; cost-effectiveness; health policy

---

1. Introduction

Newborn screening (NBS) can save both lives and healthcare costs, although testing for any given condition may accomplish only one or the other [1]. However, the up-front costs and logistical challenges of instituting screening of all or almost all newborn infants, few of whom will be found to be affected, can deter policy makers from instituting new screening programs or adding conditions to an existing program. The economic balance between the costs and benefits of screening has long been recognized as a desirable attribute of population screening programs [2]. Although some jurisdictions require a prospective economic assessment to inform decisions on the expansion of NBS [3], screening policy decisions have often not required a demonstration of cost-effectiveness in practice [4,5].

Although most NBS is done through centralized laboratory analyses of dried bloodspot specimens collected from newborns, point-of-care NBS for certain conditions is typically performed before discharge from the birthing facility [6]. In particular, screening for various types of critical congenital heart disease (CCHD) (Table 1) can be done using pulse oximetry, a simple, non-invasive test for hypoxemia in which sensors measure blood oxygen saturation through light passing through the skin [7]. Neonatal hypoxemia can have either cardiac or non-cardiac causes. When the US Department of Health and Human Services added CCHD to its Recommended Uniform Screening Panel in 2011, it requested the Centers for Disease Control and Prevention (CDC) to conduct a cost-effectiveness analysis (CEA) of newborn screening for CCHD [8,9]. That information was intended to inform policy decisions by state governments. In 2013, CDC researchers (Peterson et al.) published the first full CEA of CCHD screening in the US setting [10]. Although previous studies had estimated the cost of screening and the cost per case of CCHD detected [11–17], "Calculating the cost to detect a case tells one nothing about the value of detecting and treating the disease in question and, hence, is not informative of the balance of costs and outcomes" [18]. A full CEA includes estimates of the numbers of deaths averted and avoided healthcare costs associated with prompt diagnosis. Peterson et al. reported a point estimate of roughly USD 40,000 in net cost per life-year saved, a figure consistent with commonly used cost-effectiveness thresholds [19]. More recently, a CEA assessed the potential cost-effectiveness of CCHD screening in different localities in China, reporting that screening could be cost-effective in some settings [20].

Table 1. Types of Critical Congenital Heart Disease and Associated International Classification of Disease, 10th Version (ICD-10) Diagnosis Codes.

CCHD Types	ICD-10 Codes
Aortic interruption or atresia or hypoplasia	Q25.4, Q25.2
Coarctation or hypoplasia of the aortic arch	Q25.1
D-transposition of the great arteries	Q20.3
Double-outlet right ventricle	Q20.1
Ebstein anomaly	Q22.5
Hypoplastic left heart syndrome	Q23.4
Pulmonary atresia	Q22.0
Single ventricle	Q20.4
Teratology of Fallot	Q21.3
Total anomalous pulmonary venous connection	Q26.2
Tricuspid stenosis and atresia	Q22.4
Truncus arteriosus	Q20.0

The present review summarizes and critiques previously published estimates of the costs or cost-effectiveness of CCHD screening—two UK studies in four publications [12–14,17], three US studies in four publications [10,21–23], and one study from China [20]. Updated estimates of costs, outcomes, and summary measures of the economic value of CCHD screening in the United States are also presented. The new estimates address future disease-related treatment costs, shortened life expectancy among CCHD survivors, and a higher estimated number of avoided infant deaths due to screening.

2. Review of Previous Estimates

CEA studies of screening programs or policies require as inputs, estimates of the costs of screening, diagnosis, and intervention, numbers of cases detected in a timely manner as a result of screening, differences in health outcomes with and without screening (i.e., effectiveness), and differences in healthcare and other costs for affected individuals between scenarios with and without screening [18,24]. Each of those parameters is context-specific; therefore, it is difficult to use a given study to generalize as to whether screening may be cost-effective in different contexts. For example, a given screening test may have very different costs and outcomes in different settings depending on the characteristics of the population and how screening is implemented in that setting. In addition, the assessment of cost-effectiveness depends on how much decision makers are willing to pay for an intervention or program in relation to the expected health gains. This means that different stakeholders and jurisdictions that consider the same evidence on costs and outcomes may reach different conclusions about economic value. Therefore, instead of asking whether screening is cost-effective, it may be more constructive to ask when and by whom screening might be considered cost-effective [24,25].

The analytic perspective of an economic evaluation must be specified. From the societal or healthcare sector perspectives, cost refers to the opportunity cost of resources used up in providing a service rather than the direct financial outlay or expenditure of money. Many CEAs of clinical interventions take the healthcare sector (or system) perspective, in which only formal healthcare sector costs are considered [26,27]. A societal perspective analysis should also include informal healthcare costs, such as the time and expenses incurred by patients and families, non-health sector costs such as educational expenditures, and productivity losses resulting from death or premature mortality [28]. Spillover effects of illness or disability on the health of family members and on the time use and economic productivity of family caregivers are also germane for societal-perspective cost-effectiveness analyses [29]. The societal perspective is particularly appropriate for the analysis of public health policies and programs, and such analyses should include the costs of public health activities in support of clinical interventions.

2.1. Cost of Critical Congenital Heart Disease (CCHD) Screening and Follow-Up

The one element common to all previous economic evaluations of CCHD screening is inclusion of the directly estimated cost of screening, which is readily measurable for CCHD screening. Most studies employed a micro-costing approach with separate estimates for staff time, instrumentation, and consumables (Table 2). An exception is a cost-effectiveness study from China that did not report detailed screening costs [20]. The micro-costing estimates from other studies are summarized below separately for labor (Section 2.1.1) and instruments and consumables (Section 2.1.2). In addition to the direct costs of pulse oximetry screening, the incremental cost of CCHD screening includes the costs incurred by the healthcare system for the follow-up and management of patients who screen positive. That includes clinical examinations and diagnostic tests attributable to screening. It also includes the differences in treatment costs that result from early diagnosis. Estimates for those cost components are summarized in Sections 2.1.3 and 2.1.4.

Table 2. Summary of data assumptions of micro-costing studies of critical congenital heart disease screening.

Study	Country and Jurisdiction	Screening Time (Minutes)	Screening Staff Type and Labor Cost per Infant	Type of Probes, and Equipment/Supply Cost per Infant	Total Screening Cost per Infant
Knowles et al. [13,14]	United Kingdom	2.0	Senior house officer £1.54 $2.20 (USD)	Reusable £1.28 $1.83 (USD)	£2.82 (2000–2001 prices) $4.03 (USD)
Roberts et al. [12]	United Kingdom	6.9	Midwives Not reported	Reusable Not reported	£6.24 (2009 prices) $8.80 (USD)
Peterson et al. [21]	United States New Jersey	9.1	Registered nurses $7.36	Mixed types $6.83	$14.19 (2011 prices)
Kochilas et al. [22]	United States Minnesota	5.5	Nursing staff $3.32	Reusable $1.82	$5.10 (2012 prices)
Reeder et al. [23]	United States Utah (two hospitals)	8.4	Medical assistants and nurses $2.60	Disposable $21.92	$24.52 (2014 prices)
		9.8	Nursing assistants $2.35	Reusable $0.25	$2.60 (2014 prices)

Note: all currency conversions were calculated using the purchasing power parity exchange rate for the year of the original cost estimate. Source: https://data.oecd.org/conversion/purchasing-power-parities-ppp.htm.

In principle, the full spectrum of a screening program or policy also includes the costs of a public health program in coordinating the implementation of screening, reporting of screening results, short and long-term follow-up of screen-positive patients, and the surveillance or tracking of short and long-term outcomes. However, no estimates of public health costs associated with CCHD screening have been published to date.

2.1.1. Labor Cost

The cost of staff time per screen is the product of the average number of minutes per screen and the average wage or labor cost per minute (see Table 2). Empirical screening time estimates can be obtained by either asking nursing staff to estimate their own time or by conducting direct observation, i.e., time-and-motion studies. Three time-and-motion studies conducted in birthing hospitals in three US states using the same data collection methods all calculated that nursing staff took on average 9–10 min per newborn to complete a CCHD screen, including preparation and paperwork [21,23,30]. A similar UK study estimated an average time of 7 min per newborn, but preparation time was minimized because parental consent had been obtained before birth [12]. In contrast, studies based on clinical opinion have assumed that screening takes 2–5 min per newborn [11,13,14,31]. Self-reports by nursing staff in two US hospital-based studies reported average screening times of 3.5–5.5 min per newborn [22,32], although that does not include time spent explaining results to families or documenting screening results [22].

The per-minute cost of staff time for CCHD screening is a function of both the pay scale in a given population and the pay grade of the staff who perform the screening, which can vary by clinical setting and time period. Most programs use registered nurses or midwife staff in a newborn unit. Cost estimates from older studies that used research assistants or physicians to conduct screening do not reflect current hospital procedures. Another source of variability in estimates, at least in US studies, is differences in how labor costs were calculated. Some US studies have considered only hourly wages [22], whereas others included total hourly compensation, including taxes and fringe benefits [21,23]. The most recent UK study cited an official database for unit staff costs [12]. An earlier UK study included an adjustment for administrative overhead as well as benefits [14]. Hourly labor costs differ by occupation and geographic labor market; labor cost per minute was roughly three times higher in a US study conducted in New Jersey [21] than in one conducted in Utah [23] using similar methods (Table 2).

2.1.2. Instruments and Consumables

The equipment cost of CCHD screening consists of the amortized costs of the pulse oximeter machine and reusable probes or sensors and the consumable cost of disposable probes or probe tips and straps. The variety of probe types used for screening creates great heterogeneity in cost estimates. Variable cost per newborn is very low when a reusable probe is used for screening compared to the use of a disposable probe, although there are maintenance costs with reusable probes. A US study conducted by Peterson et al. in a statewide sample of hospitals in New Jersey estimated that the equipment cost per infant screened was $0.49 using fully disposable probes, $1.74 using reusable probes with disposable tips, and $13.62 using disposable probes (2014 USD) [21]. A subsequent US study conducted in two facilities in Utah suggested that the total equipment cost per newborn was $21.92 using disposable probes and $0.25 using reusable probes (2014 USD) [23] (Table 2). British economic evaluations have assumed the use of the less expensive reusable probes [12,14,17].

2.1.3. Diagnostic Work-Up

If a newborn does not pass CCHD screening, the newborn is referred for a diagnostic work-up to determine the cause of hypoxemia, whether cardiac or non-cardiac. The diagnostic process may include a clinical evaluation, laboratory and/or imaging tests (including echocardiography), and possibly transportation to another hospital for further evaluation and management. The diagnostic work-up for non-cardiac causes is variable, and no published studies of CCHD screening to date have included estimates of clinical examination to identify potential non-cardiac causes of hypoxemia. Previous UK studies of CCHD screening costs assumed that newborns who do not pass CCHD screening would receive a 30 min diagnostic echocardiographic assessment by a pediatric cardiologist at a cost of roughly £115 pounds per child (2009 GBP) [12,17]. No cost was assigned in that study for transportation.

Peterson et al. estimated costs of echocardiography based on administrative data from a private insurance claims database, with the analysis restricted to inpatient services during infancy. The cost estimate was a truncated arithmetic mean after excluding the top and bottom 1% of observations [10]. Based on data from Florida, indicating that roughly 43% of infants with CCHD were transferred to another hospital during the birth hospitalization [33], it was assumed that 43% of infants who screened positive would require ambulance transport for transfer to a hospital with echocardiography. The cost of ambulance transport was derived using the same methods as the cost of echocardiography [10]. The additional cost of diagnostic echocardiography and transport was estimated to add $0.25 per newborn screened (2011 USD).

2.1.4. Treatment

The potential reduction in treatment costs associated with timely CCHD diagnosis is challenging to estimate, and only one study to date attempted to do so. In an analysis using linked Florida birth defects surveillance and hospital discharge data from 1998 to 2007, Peterson et al. estimated attributable hospitalization costs in the first year of life for infants with CCHD (n = 3603) [33]. Unadjusted costs were higher for infants with CCHD detected prior to discharge from the birth hospitalization than those detected later because severely affected infants are more likely to be detected sooner and to incur more costly treatment. In a statistical analysis that adjusted for CCHD type, maternal race/ethnicity, and other variables, late CCHD detection was found to be associated with 52% more admissions, 18% more hospitalized days, and 35% higher inpatient costs during infancy relative to the early detection of CCHD [33].

The CEA by Peterson et al. projected the avoided cost of hospitalization for infants with screening-detected CCHD in two steps. First, the difference in number of hospitalized days between infants with timely and late detected CCHD was derived from a previous analysis of Florida data [10,33]. Second, average hospital costs per day among infants with selected CCHD conditions were estimated, assuming that the cost per day was the same for early-detected and late-detected cases [10]. The underlying CEA model assumed that with screening, 77.5% of infants with CCHD would be detected prior to discharge, with an average hospital cost during infancy of $156,501 compared to $181,775 for those not detected, a difference of $24,677 per timely-detected CCHD case (2011 USD). Comparing screening and no-screening scenarios, the hospitalization cost was calculated to be $19,111 per infant with CCHD under screening, taking into account false negatives. That amount was equal to $7.48 per newborn infant (2011 USD) [10].

2.2. *Screening Cost per Case Detected*

Besides the direct cost of performing screening, it is straightforward to calculate the number of additional cases of CCHD detected in a timely manner due to screening. However, this number must be assessed in a given population, because the numbers of new CCHD diagnoses that can be made through the follow-up of screening using pulse oximetry is dependent on the use and accuracy of prenatal screening and postnatal clinical detection in that population. In particular, an increased frequency of prenatal diagnosis of CCHD results in fewer additional diagnoses of CCHD following CCHD screening using pulse oximetry [34]. The frequency of delayed CCHD diagnoses in the United States was shown to have decreased over time [35], although no decrease in post-discharge CCHD diagnoses was found in a study from the United Kingdom [36].

Multiple studies have estimated the screening cost per CCHD case detected, with widely varying estimates. For example, UK estimates range from roughly £5000 (2001 GBP) [13] to £24,000 (2009 GBP) per CCHD case detected [12] and US estimates range from approximately $21,000 (2011 USD) per case with timely diagnosis [10] to $46,000 (2012 USD) per case detected [22]. Different assumptions about two cost elements—the cost per newborn screened and the averted costs of care resulting from timely diagnosis—account for much of this variation. In particular, some estimates are of gross screening costs and others are net screening costs, after subtracting the avoided cost of treatment. For example, Kochilas et al. reported a relatively high cost per case detected ($46,000), despite assuming a low screening cost [22]. In contrast, Peterson et al. assumed a higher cost of CCHD screening and reported that screening would cost approximately $21,000 per case with timely diagnosis [10]. The Peterson et al. estimate reflected the *net* cost of screening, after subtracting the estimated savings in hospitalization costs during infancy resulting from timely diagnosis, which offset more than half of the screening cost. The gross cost per case detected in that study was roughly $46,000.

As noted in Section 2.1.3, the choice of reusable or disposable pulse oximeter probes can have an even larger impact on estimated costs of CCHD screening. Peterson et al. assumed average equipment and labor costs of $6.86 and $6.62 per infant, respectively (2011 USD) [10]. The equipment cost was derived from a sample of seven New Jersey hospitals, only one of which used fully reusable probes. If it had been assumed that all hospitals used fully reusable probes, the average equipment cost would have been much lower [21], and the average cost per newborn screened would have been roughly half as great.

2.3. Health Gains

It is challenging to estimate health gains from CCHD screening, which encompass avoided early deaths and improved health outcomes among survivors. Cost-effectiveness guidelines call for both types of health outcomes to be expressed in summary measures of health such as the quality-adjusted life-year (QALY) that take into account changes in life expectancy and morbidity [26–28]. However, evidence of improved health among survivors following timely diagnosis is lacking. In addition, it is challenging to find conceptually and empirically appropriate estimates of utility weights for pediatric conditions that can be used to project QALY gains [37–39]. Consequently, it is common for CEAs of interventions that primarily affect survival to calculate the cost per life-year saved, since it makes little practical difference in ranking the cost-effectiveness ratios for such interventions [40].

Two CEA studies published estimates of numbers of deaths avoided through CCHD screening. First, Peterson et al. conservatively assumed that CCHD screening, if applied to four million US births each year, would avoid 20 infant deaths [10]. This estimate was based on a national estimate of 28 annual deaths associated with delayed diagnosis of CCHD in the absence of universal screening. The estimate of 28 deaths was derived by multiplying four million births by an avoidable mortality rate among infants with late-detected CCHD of 1.8% and a frequency of 38.8 infants with late-detected CCHD per 100,000 births, both calculated from a study of linked births and deaths in Florida prior to the introduction of screening [33]; the overall preventable death rate among infants with CCHD was 0.4%. To calculate the number of life-years saved as a denominator for a cost-effectiveness ratio, Peterson et al. took the estimated number of infant deaths averted by screening and multiplied this by 30.7 years, which was the life expectancy at birth of the US population discounted to the present with a 3.0% discount rate per year [10]. In other words, the investigators assumed that surviving infants would have a normal life expectancy.

Tobe et al. estimated infant deaths from CCHD for three scenarios in three Chinese cities [20]. The base scenario assumed that infant mortality would be the same as in the 1950s (standard practice in CEAs is to use recent estimates as the baseline to compare with an intervention). The authors also assumed that "that infant mortality would reduce to approximately 25% if infants received timely diagnosis and treatment", but did not state the assumed mortality rates with and without screening. The ratio of assumed averted deaths to CCHD cases was 0.225 in Beijing, 0.112 in Shandong, and 0.046 in Gansu. They assumed that access to timely diagnosis and treatment varied across regions (e.g., apparently one-half as high in Shandong as in Beijing), but did not make those assumptions explicit. Tobe et al. also reported outcomes in terms of disability-adjusted life-year (DALY) estimates, a measure analogous to the QALY, but did not explain how the DALY estimates were generated [20].

It should be noted that the "disability" weights used to calculate DALYs refer to "any short-term or long-term loss of health" and hence assess morbidity rather than disability [41].

2.4. Cost-Effectiveness Ratios

It is standard practice for CEAs to report incremental cost-effectiveness ratios (ICERs) for interventions that are found to be both more costly (net positive cost) and to improve health outcomes relative to next most cost-effective strategy analyzed. To calculate the numerator of the ICER, analysts are supposed to subtract any cost offset associated with improved health from the cost of the intervention. The denominator is the difference in the number of health outcomes attained, most commonly in the form of discounted life-years or health-adjusted life-years gained relative to the alternative. In some countries, policy makers set threshold values or ranges for ICERs below which interventions are presumed to be considered cost-effective. For example, thresholds for approval of the coverage of new medications have been estimated at roughly £30,000 (GBP) per QALY in the United Kingdom, CAN$50,000 in Canada, and AUS$42,000 in Australia [42].

Peterson et al. projected that the point estimate of the net cost of screening was just over $40,000 per life-year saved in 2011 US dollars [10]. It is increasingly recommended that CEAs include probabilistic sensitivity analyses in which estimates for multiple parameters are allowed to vary simultaneously within ranges using probability distributions and simulation modeling techniques [43]. Peterson et al. also reported that a probabilistic analysis projected a one in three chance that CCHD screening would be cost-saving (i.e., negative net costs), and a roughly four in four probability that CCHD screening would cost less than $100,000 per life-year gained. It should be noted that there is no official threshold or standard for cost-effectiveness in the United States, although a private organization, the Institute for Clinical and Economic Review, has used a range of $100,000 to $150,000 per QALY to establish a "value price" for new therapies [44]. It should also be recognized, though, that because utility weights are usually less than 1.0 and decrease with advancing age, the number of QALYs gained is necessarily less than the number of life-years saved. Consequently, the cost per QALY gained is larger than the cost per life-year gained, often by at least 15–20%, which can affect the interpretation of ICERs relative to benchmark values [24].

CEAs are recommended to report sensitivity analyses that show the dependence of results on uncertainty in estimates or assumptions of model parameters [26–28]. Peterson et al. reported that the three variables with the greatest influence on the cost-effectiveness of CCHD screening were the reduction in hospitalization costs during infancy from early detection, the baseline proportion of late-detected CCHD cases, and the hospital cost of CCHD screening [10]. Variables that had the least influence on the results were the cost of echocardiography, cost and probability of transport for echocardiography and subsequent treatment, the mortality rate among infants with CCHD detected by screening, and the rate of false positives.

It should be noted that the assumption of 18% higher hospitalization costs with the late detection of CCHD assumed a fixed cost per hospital day. However, patients in critical care incur much higher costs per hospital day, and infants with late-detected CCHD are more likely to be in critical care units. The observed difference in hospitalization costs in infancy associated with late detection was twice as large as the difference in hospital days, 35% vs. 18% [33]. Therefore, the CEA was conservative; if the study had assumed 35% lower hospitalization costs in infancy with early detection, the cost-effectiveness ratio could have been close to zero.

Many CEAs reported in low- and middle-income countries use a threshold of three times per capita gross domestic product (GDP) per DALY, which was endorsed in the early 2000s by a World Health Organization report. Using that approach in China, with GDP per capita calculated by province, Tobe et al. concluded, "the intervention was highly cost-effective in Beijing (Int$7833/DALY); cost-effective in Shandong (Int$27,780/DALY); and not cost-effective in Gansu (Int$167,407)" [20]. However, those are average cost-effectiveness ratios rather than ICERs. The authors' Table 1 indicates ICERs for CCHD screening of Int$15,020, Int$51,636, and Int$307,952, respectively. If the same arbitrary cost-effectiveness threshold had been applied to the ICERs, CCHD screening would not have been considered cost-effective in either Shandong or Gansu. In addition, it should be noted that the three times GDP per capita cost-effectiveness threshold value has been challenged as lacking validity [45].

3. Revised Cost-Effectiveness Estimates

3.1. New Estimates of Averted Infant Deaths

Newly published estimates of the impact of CCHD screening policies in the United States suggest that the actual reduction in CCHD deaths associated with universal screening may be much higher than previous economic evaluations anticipated. A statistical analysis of the association of US state CCHD screening policies that had been adopted by 1 June 2013 with the numbers of early infant (24 h to <6 months of age) deaths coded for CCHD or other/unspecified congenital heart defects (CHDs) through the end of 2013 found that the implementation of CCHD screening mandates was associated with a one-third lower frequency of recognized infant deaths with CCHD as the listed cause (see Supplement) [46]. The reduction in CCHD deaths was not entirely attributable to screening using pulse oximetry, since screening mandates could also have led to a greater clinical awareness and the earlier detection of CCHD using other methods. This reduction in CCHD-associated deaths was roughly six times greater than was assumed in the US CEA of CCHD screening by Peterson et al. based on the frequency of delayed CCHD diagnoses that could be avoided through screening [10]. Adjusting the Peterson et al. model to include 110 deaths averted annually (as opposed to the 20 deaths averted annually assumed in the Peterson et al. original study), the estimated cost per life-year gained becomes approximately $10,000 (2011 USD) (compared to the original reported estimate of approximately $40,000 per life-year gained).

3.2. Shortened Life Expectancy among Survivors

One factor unaddressed by Peterson et al. and other economic evaluations of CCHD screening is shortened life expectancy among individuals with CCHD. In other words, previous economic evaluations have implicitly or explicitly assumed that children with CCHD who survive infancy have the same life expectancy as unaffected children. However, all-cause mortality is higher among children with CHDs than for the general population, even after infancy [47]. For example, it has been widely reported that children and adolescents with CHDs have higher rates of cancer, even after excluding individuals with chromosomal disorders [48]. Survival with a CHD varies widely by condition or type of defect, country, ethnic group, and time period. Dramatic reductions over time in infant and early childhood mortality among cohorts of infants born with a CHD have been widely reported [49–52].

Few studies have reported survival probabilities for patients with CHDs relative to life-table survival probabilities for the general population. A population-based surveillance study conducted in metropolitan Atlanta, Georgia (USA), involving birth cohorts from 1979 to 2005, found that the average infant survival probability for infants with CCHD who had no non-cardiac defects or chromosomal syndromes was 75.2%, but increased from 67.2% during the first 15 years to 82.5% during the more recent 12 years [52]. One implication of the reductions in infant deaths associated with CCHD is a smaller number of deaths that could be potentially averted through screening. The average survival probability from 12 months to 25 years of age was 89.3%, which compares with a 99.3% survival probability for the general US population in the 2009 national life table [53]. A Danish study modeled post-surgery survival to age 25 among children born during 1990–2002 as 85% for all CHDs and from 64% to 87% for specific CCHD types, but the 10-year survival probability for the subsequent birth cohort was substantially greater, 93% vs. 87% overall [54].

It would be reasonable to project that life expectancy among individuals with CCHD who survive infancy could be 10–20% lower than in the general population. That would reduce discounted life-years by three to six years relative to population norms. Adjusting the US CEA model of CCHD screening reported by Peterson et al. to include 110 deaths averted annually and 20% fewer years lived yields an estimated cost per life-year saved of approximately $12,000 (2011 USD).

3.3. CHD-Related Future Medical Costs

It is generally recommended that CEAs include the present value of expected future medical costs for survivors whose deaths are avoided or postponed as a result of a healthcare intervention, although only one-half of CEAs published during 2008–2013 included estimates of future related medical costs [55]. Since infants with complex medical conditions incur substantial medical costs, including future medical costs can make life-saving interventions for such children appear less cost-effective. It is common for CEAs of newborn screening tests to not include future medical costs [40].

No estimates of lifetime medical costs for children with CHDs in general or for the subset with CCHD defects are currently available, with or without adjustment for co-occurring conditions. A US study that used linked birth defects surveillance and administrative data from California dating from the late 1980s estimated lifetime costs for four infants born with one of four specific CCHD conditions: truncus arteriosus, transposition of the great arteries/double-outlet right ventricle, tetralogy of Fallot, and single ventricle [56]. At the time of the study, infant survival was assumed to be low, with <50% of infants with truncus arteriosus or single ventricle reaching one year of age. A CDC publication recalculated the cost estimates with a 3% discount rate; lifetime medical costs per infant varied by condition from $86,000 to $260,000 (1992 USD) [57].

Given dramatic changes in survival and medical technologies, cost estimates from three decades in the past are not currently informative [58]. An analysis of 2005 US private insurance claims data reported that children with severe CHDs (roughly equivalent to CCHD) had mean expenditures during the first three years of life of roughly $210,000 in excess of children without CHDs [58]. The most recent estimates of hospitalization costs associated with birth defects estimated an aggregate burden almost twice as high in 2013 as in 2004 [59]. In 2013, the mean cost for a single inpatient stay with a CCHD diagnosis was $79,011, and aggregate hospital costs for CCHD patients of all ages generated a figure of $2.3 billion [59].

Despite the absence of recent estimates of lifetime costs for infants born with CCHD, it is possible to conduct sensitivity analyses. One potential proxy is the lifetime medical cost for infants born with spina bifida, which was recently estimated as $513,500 (2014 USD) [60]. In the analysis of California data from the late 1980s, medical costs for children born with spina bifida were similar to those born with single ventricle or tetralogy of Fallot and lower than those with truncus arteriosus [56,57]. However, annual medical costs for spina bifida remain elevated across the lifespan [60], whereas costs associated with care for severe CHDs drop off sharply after infancy. Roughly two-thirds of all hospital costs associated with CHD diagnoses are associated with admissions in the first 12 months of life [61]. Therefore, the lifetime medical cost for spina bifida might be an upper-bound estimate of the lifetime medical cost associated with CCHD.

Adjusting the US CEA model of CCHD screening reported by Peterson et al. to include 110 deaths averted annually, 20% fewer years lived, and $450,000 in post-infancy CCHD-attributable discounted future lifetime medical costs (as opposed to $0 included in the original study), yields an estimated cost per life-year saved of approximately $31,000 (2011 USD). That sensitivity analysis yields a conservative estimate of net benefit (i.e., the cost-effectiveness ratio is likely overestimated) since the actual incremental medical cost associated with CCHD is likely less than the proxy estimate that was used. In any case, the estimated cost is still lower than the originally reported estimate of approximately $40,000 per life-year gained.

4. Discussion

To date, all economic analyses of CCHD screening have followed the healthcare sector perspective, as is conventional for clinical interventions. All have included employee compensation costs to employers to estimate the cost of staff time. However, hospitals that have implemented CCHD screening have reported to be able to do so using existing nursing staff and do not incur additional staff costs [21]. From the hospital perspective, the cost of staff time might not need to be included [10]. From a societal perspective, the inclusion of staff time makes sense if nursing time used for CCHD screening could have otherwise been used for other tasks. If nursing time could not be reallocated, the time spent doing the screening would not represent an incremental cost. If that is the case, existing cost estimates could overestimate the incremental cost of CCHD screening.

Economic analyses of CCHD screening as a public policy should also include the costs of public health activities in support of CCHD screening and follow-up, but little is known about those costs. Jurisdictions implementing CCHD screening policies and programs often take varying approaches to the organization and surveillance of CCHD screening [62]. For that reason, it may not be possible to generalize the costs of the public health role in supporting and monitoring CCHD screening.

Notable variations exist in methods and results among the two previously published CEAs of CCHD screening [10,20] and several costing studies included in this review. The level of evidence for some cost elements, notably the cost of CCHD screening based on combined screening time, labor cost, instrumentation, and consumables cost, is reasonably established in some clinical settings. These cost elements still merit reconsideration or reinvestigation for future economic evaluations, for each is dependent on existing conditions in a given clinical setting. Estimates of effectiveness are also variable. Survival among infants with CCHD can vary greatly depending on location and treatment availability, which limits the generalizability of results across settings within countries, as well as across countries.

Other formal healthcare costs associated with CCHD screening are less well established. Some matter more than others, as indicated by their potential magnitude per infant screened. For example, the cost of the diagnostic work-up of screen-positive newborns is not well established, but given the very small numbers of infants who screen positive, this cost element contributes very little to the total cost of screening; perhaps 2% of the total cost [10]. It is likely that the assumption in the Peterson et al. study that 43% of newborns who do not pass CCHD screening require transport to another hospital is a substantial overestimate, but since such transportation contributed only marginally to the estimated total cost of screening in that study, modifying that assumption would have little effect on the results. In contrast, the cost of avoided hospitalizations associated with late-detected CCHD is highly influential [10]. However, that cost estimate in Peterson et al. was based on just one study in one US state conducted prior to the implementation of universal CCHD screening [33]. Furthermore, the Peterson et al. study assumed a high rate of sensitivity of CCHD screening.

Some healthcare costs have been neglected in economic evaluations of CCHD screening. One is the cost and benefits of diagnosing and treating non-CCHD cases among newborns referred following screening. The implicit assumption has been that the costs of diagnostic work-up relative to the size of the newborn population are low, similar to that of CCHD diagnosis. However, the potential health benefits of detecting and treating non-cardiac conditions, such as neonatal sepsis, deserve further attention. Non-health costs have been neglected in published cost-effectiveness analyses of CCHD screening to date. For example, no published information exists on the time costs incurred by family members caring for individuals with CCHD, nor the loss of economic productivity. Although there is evidence of the increased use of special education services among surviving children with CCHD [63,64], the associated costs have not been calculated. Furthermore, it is unknown whether early detection might influence long-term academic outcomes among those children.

Three parameters can substantially affect the overall CEA results and remain underinvestigated: estimates of averted infant CCHD deaths, shortened life expectancy among children with CCHD who survive infancy, and future CCHD-associated medical costs. Previous CEAs have relied on indirect estimates of averted deaths based on estimates of numbers of infant deaths with CCHD, the frequency of delayed diagnosis, and the assumed relative reduction with timely diagnosis; they have excluded the other two parameters. For example, Peterson et al. calculated an expected number of averted deaths based on infant mortality differentials by timing of diagnosis derived before the advent of universal screening [10]. Newly available estimates of the relative reduction in deaths associated with CCHD screening mandates based on a retrospective analysis of CCHD deaths in US states with universal screening policies offer evidence of a greater number of deaths averted [46] than had been projected by Peterson et al. [10] Using the direct estimates of averted deaths associated with mandatory CCHD screening policies from Abouk et al. [46] yields cost-effectiveness ratios more favorable for universal screening policies.

A comparative analysis of life expectancy among CCHD survivors relative to the general population can contribute evidence to improve future economic evaluations of CCHD screening. Where previous CEAs have assumed a normal life expectancy for individuals that through CCHD screening detection avoided CCHD-associated death, accounting for a shorter than average life expectancy will increase the net cost of screening by increasing the cost per life-year gained. Finally, previous CEAs have not accounted for CCHD-related expenditures associated with averted CCHD death in infancy. Accounting for such costs will also presumably increase the net cost of CCHD screening.

In conclusion, uncertainty remains regarding several parameters that are important to the analysis of the cost-effectiveness of CCHD screening. Nonetheless, the ability of universal CCHD screening to detect many newborns with CCHD who would otherwise have remained undiagnosed at the time of discharge—and at risk of severe morbidity and mortality—has been demonstrated [65–67].

Acknowledgments: No funding was received for the preparation or publication of the study.

Author Contributions: Scott D. Grosse and Cora Peterson conceived the review and the new, updated results. Scott D. Grosse conducted the review and wrote most of the paper. Rahi Abouk produced the new estimates of avoided deaths and contributed to the new cost-effectiveness estimates. Jill Glidewell and Matthew E. Oster provided substantive input and clinical expertise in the interpretation of the findings. All authors contributed to the final version of the paper.

References

1. Centers for Disease Control and Prevention. CDC Grand Rounds: Newborn screening and improved outcomes. *Morb. Mortal. Wkly. Rep.* **2012**, *61*, 390–393.
2. Wilson, J.M.; Jungner, Y.G. Principles and practice of mass screening for disease. *Bol. Oficina Sanit. Panam.* **1968**, *65*, 281–393. [PubMed]
3. Grosse, S.D.; Thompson, J.D.; Ding, Y.; Glass, M. The use of economic evaluation to inform newborn screening policy decisions: The Washington state experience. *Milbank Q.* **2016**, *94*, 366–391. [CrossRef] [PubMed]
4. Fischer, K.E.; Grosse, S.D.; Rogowski, W.H. The role of health technology assessment in coverage decisions on newborn screening. *Int. J. Technol. Assess. Health Care* **2011**, *27*, 313–321. [CrossRef] [PubMed]
5. Grosse, S.D. Cost effectiveness as a criterion for newborn screening policy decisions. In *Ethics and Newborn Genetic Screening: New Technologies, New Challenges*; Baily, M.A., Murray, T.H., Eds.; Johns Hopkins University Press: Baltimore, MD, USA, 2009; pp. 58–88.
6. Grosse, S.D.; Riehle-Colarusso, T.; Gaffney, M.; Mason, C.A.; Shapira, S.K.; Sontag, M.K.; Braun, K.V.N.; Iskander, J. CDC Grand Rounds: Newborn screening for hearing loss and critical congenital heart disease. *Morb. Mortal. Wkly. Rep.* **2017**, *66*, 888–890. [CrossRef] [PubMed]
7. Ewer, A.K. Review of pulse oximetry screening for critical congenital heart defects in newborn infants. *Curr. Opin. Cardiol.* **2013**, *28*, 92–96. [CrossRef] [PubMed]
8. Sebelius, K. Letter to the Secretary's Advisory Council on Hereditary Diseases of Newborns and Children. Available online: http://www.hrsa.gov/advisorycommittees/mchbadvisory/heritabledisorders/recommendations/correspondence/cyanoticheartsecre09212011.pdf (accessed on 20 July 2016).
9. Martin, G.R.; Beekman, R.H., III; Mikula, E.B.; Fasules, J.; Garg, L.F.; Kemper, A.R.; Morrow, W.R.; Pearson, G.D.; Mahle, W.T. Implementing recommended screening for critical congenital heart disease. *Pediatrics* **2013**, *132*, e185–e192. [CrossRef] [PubMed]
10. Peterson, C.; Grosse, S.D.; Oster, M.E.; Olney, R.S.; Cassell, C.H. Cost-effectiveness of routine screening for critical congenital heart disease in US newborns. *Pediatrics* **2013**, *132*, e595–e603. [CrossRef] [PubMed]

11. De-Wahl Granelli, A.; Wennergren, M.; Sandberg, K.; Mellander, M.; Bejlum, C.; Inganas, L.; Eriksson, M.; Segerdahl, N.; Agren, A.; Ekman-Joelsson, B.M.; et al. Impact of pulse oximetry screening on the detection of duct dependent congenital heart disease: A Swedish prospective screening study in 39,821 newborns. *BMJ* **2009**, *338*, a3037. [CrossRef] [PubMed]
12. Roberts, T.E.; Barton, P.M.; Auguste, P.E.; Middleton, L.J.; Furmston, A.T.; Ewer, A.K. Pulse oximetry as a screening test for congenital heart defects in newborn infants: A cost-effectiveness analysis. *Arch. Dis. Child.* **2012**, *97*, 221–226. [CrossRef] [PubMed]
13. Griebsch, I.; Knowles, R.L.; Brown, J.; Bull, C.; Wren, C.; Dezateux, C.A. Comparing the clinical and economic effects of clinical examination, pulse oximetry, and echocardiography in newborn screening for congenital heart defects: A probabilistic cost-effectiveness model and value of information analysis. *Int. J. Technol. Assess. Health Care* **2007**, *23*, 192–204. [CrossRef] [PubMed]
14. Knowles, R.; Griebsch, I.; Dezateux, C.; Brown, J.; Bull, C.; Wren, C. Newborn screening for congenital heart defects: A systematic review and cost-effectiveness analysis. *Health Technol. Assess.* **2005**, *9*, 1–152. [CrossRef] [PubMed]
15. Ewer, A.K.; Furmston, A.T.; Middleton, L.J.; Deeks, J.J.; Daniels, J.P.; Pattison, H.M.; Powell, R.; Roberts, T.E.; Barton, P.; Auguste, P.; et al. Pulse oximetry as a screening test for congenital heart defects in newborn infants: A test accuracy study with evaluation of acceptability and cost-effectiveness. *Health Technol. Assess.* **2012**, *16*, 1–184. [CrossRef] [PubMed]
16. Mahle, W.T.; Newburger, J.W.; Matherne, G.P.; Smith, F.C.; Hoke, T.R.; Koppel, R.; Gidding, S.S.; Beekman, R.H., III; Grosse, S.D. Role of pulse oximetry in examining newborns for congenital heart disease: A scientific statement from the American Heart Association and American Academy of Pediatrics. *Circulation* **2009**, *120*, 447–458. [CrossRef] [PubMed]
17. Ewer, A.K.; Middleton, L.J.; Furmston, A.T.; Bhoyar, A.; Daniels, J.P.; Thangaratinam, S.; Deeks, J.J.; Khan, K.S.; PulseOx Study Group. Pulse oximetry screening for congenital heart defects in newborn infants (PulseOx): A test accuracy study. *Lancet* **2011**, *378*, 785–794. [CrossRef]
18. Grosse, S.D. Showing value in newborn screening: Challenges in quantifying the effectiveness and cost-effectiveness of early detection of phenylketonuria and cystic fibrosis. *Healthcare* **2015**, *3*, 1133–1157. [CrossRef] [PubMed]
19. Grosse, S.D. Assessing cost-effectiveness in healthcare: History of the $50,000 per QALY threshold. *Expert Rev. Pharmacoecon. Outcomes Res.* **2008**, *8*, 165–178. [CrossRef] [PubMed]
20. Tobe, R.G.; Martin, G.R.; Li, F.; Mori, R. Should postnatal oximetry screening be implemented nationwide in China? A cost-effectiveness analysis in three regions with different socioeconomic status. *Int. J. Cardiol.* **2016**, *204*, 45–47. [CrossRef] [PubMed]
21. Peterson, C.; Grosse, S.D.; Glidewell, J.; Garg, L.F.; Van Naarden Braun, K.; Knapp, M.M.; Beres, L.M.; Hinton, C.F.; Olney, R.S.; Cassell, C.H. A public health economic assessment of hospitals' cost to screen newborns for critical congenital heart disease. *Public Health Rep.* **2014**, *129*, 86–93. [CrossRef] [PubMed]
22. Kochilas, L.K.; Lohr, J.L.; Bruhn, E.; Borman-Shoap, E.; Gams, B.L.; Pylipow, M.; Saarinen, A.; Gaviglio, A.; Thompson, T.R. Implementation of critical congenital heart disease screening in Minnesota. *Pediatrics* **2013**, *132*, e587–e594. [CrossRef] [PubMed]
23. Reeder, M.R.; Kim, J.; Nance, A.; Krikov, S.; Feldkamp, M.L.; Randall, H.; Botto, L.D. Evaluating cost and resource use associated with pulse oximetry screening for critical congenital heart disease: Empiric estimates and sources of variation. *Birth Defects Res. A Clin. Mol. Teratol.* **2015**, *103*, 962–971. [CrossRef] [PubMed]
24. Grosse, S.D. When is genomic testing cost-effective? Testing for Lynch Syndrome in patients with newly-diagnosed colorectal cancer and their relatives. *Healthcare* **2015**, *3*, 860–878. [CrossRef] [PubMed]
25. Hatz, M.H.; Schremser, K.; Rogowski, W.H. Is individualized medicine more cost-effective? A systematic review. *Pharmacoeconomics* **2014**, *32*, 443–455. [CrossRef] [PubMed]
26. Drummond, M.E.; O'Brien, B.; Stoddart, G.L.; Torrance, G.W. *Methods for the Economic Evaluation of Health Care Programmes*, 2nd ed.; Oxford University Press: Oxford, UK, 1997.
27. Gold, M.R.; Siegel, J.E.; Russell, L.B.; Weinstein, M.C. *Cost-Effectiveness in Health and Medicine*; Oxford University Press: New York, NY, USA, 1996.
28. Sanders, G.D.; Neumann, P.J.; Basu, A.; Brock, D.W.; Feeny, D.; Krahn, M.; Kuntz, K.M.; Meltzer, D.O.; Owens, D.K.; Prosser, L.A.; et al. Recommendations for conduct, methodological practices, and reporting of

cost-effectiveness analyses: Second Panel on Cost-Effectiveness in Health and Medicine. *JAMA* **2016**, *316*, 1093–1103. [CrossRef] [PubMed]

29. Tilford, J.M.; Payakachat, N. Progress in measuring family spillover effects for economic evaluations. *Expert Rev. Pharmacoecon. Outcomes Res.* **2015**, *15*, 195–198. [CrossRef] [PubMed]
30. Centers for Disease Control and Prevention. Assessment of current practices and feasibility of routine screening for critical congenital heart defects—Georgia, 2012. *Morb. Mortal. Wkly. Rep.* **2013**, *62*, 288–291.
31. Walsh, W. Evaluation of pulse oximetry screening in Middle Tennessee: Cases for consideration before universal screening. *J. Perinatol.* **2011**, *31*, 125–129. [CrossRef] [PubMed]
32. Bradshaw, E.A.; Cuzzi, S.; Kiernan, S.C.; Nagel, N.; Becker, J.A.; Martin, G.R. Feasibility of implementing pulse oximetry screening for congenital heart disease in a community hospital. *J. Perinatol.* **2012**, *32*, 710–715. [CrossRef] [PubMed]
33. Peterson, C.; Dawson, A.; Grosse, S.D.; Riehle-Colarusso, T.; Olney, R.S.; Tanner, J.P.; Kirby, R.S.; Correia, J.A.; Watkins, S.M.; Cassell, C.H. Hospitalizations, costs, and mortality among infants with critical congenital heart disease: How important is timely detection? *Birth Defects Res. A Clin. Mol. Teratol.* **2013**, *97*, 664–672. [CrossRef] [PubMed]
34. Ailes, E.C.; Gilboa, S.M.; Honein, M.A.; Oster, M.E. Estimated number of infants detected and missed by critical congenital heart defect screening. *Pediatrics* **2015**, *135*, 1000–1008. [CrossRef] [PubMed]
35. Chang, R.K.; Gurvitz, M.; Rodriguez, S. Missed diagnosis of critical congenital heart disease. *Arch. Pediatr. Adolesc. Med.* **2008**, *162*, 969–974. [CrossRef] [PubMed]
36. Wren, C.; Reinhardt, Z.; Khawaja, K. Twenty-year trends in diagnosis of life-threatening neonatal cardiovascular malformations. *Arch Dis. Child. Fetal Neonatal Ed.* **2008**, *93*, F33–F35. [CrossRef] [PubMed]
37. Grosse, S.D.; Prosser, L.A.; Asakawa, K.; Feeny, D. QALY weights for neurosensory impairments in pediatric economic evaluations: Case studies and a critique. *Expert Rev. Pharmacoecon. Outcomes Res.* **2010**, *10*, 293–308. [CrossRef] [PubMed]
38. Ungar, W.J. Challenges in health state valuation in paediatric economic evaluation: Are QALYs contraindicated? *Pharmacoeconomics* **2011**, *29*, 641–652. [CrossRef] [PubMed]
39. Grosse, S.D. Economic evaluations of newborn screening interventions. In *Economic Evaluation in Child Health*; Ungar, W.J., Ed.; Oxford University Press: New York, NY, USA, 2009; pp. 113–132.
40. Ding, Y.; Thompson, J.D.; Kobrynski, L.; Ojodu, J.; Zarbalian, G.; Grosse, S.D. Cost-Effectiveness/Cost-Benefit Analysis of Newborn Screening for Severe Combined Immune Deficiency in Washington State. *J. Pediatr.* **2016**, *172*, 127–135. [CrossRef] [PubMed]
41. Salomon, J.A.; Vos, T.; Hogan, D.R.; Gagnon, M.; Naghavi, M.; Mokdad, A.; Begum, N.; Shah, R.; Karyana, M.; Kosen, S.; et al. Common values in assessing health outcomes from disease and injury: Disability weights measurement study for the Global Burden of Disease Study 2010. *Lancet* **2012**, *380*, 2129–2143. [CrossRef]
42. Griffiths, E.A.; Hendrich, J.K.; Stoddart, S.D.; Walsh, S.C. Acceptance of health technology assessment submissions with incremental cost-effectiveness ratios above the cost-effectiveness threshold. *Clinicoecon. Outcomes Res.* **2015**, *7*, 463–476. [CrossRef] [PubMed]
43. Briggs, A.H.; Weinstein, M.C.; Fenwick, E.A.; Karnon, J.; Sculpher, M.J.; Paltiel, A.D.; Ispor-Smdm Modeling Good Research Practices Task Force. Model parameter estimation and uncertainty analysis: A report of the ISPOR-SMDM Modeling Good Research Practices Task Force Working Group-6. *Med. Decis. Mak.* **2012**, *32*, 722–732. [CrossRef] [PubMed]
44. Neumann, P.J.; Cohen, J.T. ICER's revised value assessment framework for 2017-2019: A critique. *Pharmacoeconomics* **2017**, *35*, 977–980. [CrossRef] [PubMed]
45. Marseille, E.; Larson, B.; Kazi, D.S.; Kahn, J.G.; Rosen, S. Thresholds for the cost-effectiveness of interventions: Alternative approaches. *Bull. World Health Organ.* **2015**, *93*, 118–124. [CrossRef] [PubMed]
46. Abouk, R.; Grosse, S.D.; Ailes, E.C.; Oster, M.E. Association of US state implementation of newborn screening policies for critical congenital heart disease with early infant cardiac deaths. *JAMA* **2017**, *318*, 2111–2118. [CrossRef] [PubMed]
47. Best, K.E.; Rankin, J. Long-term survival of individuals born with congenital heart disease: A systematic review and meta-analysis. *J. Am. Heart Assoc.* **2016**, *5*, e002846. [CrossRef] [PubMed]
48. Botto, L.D.; Flood, T.; Little, J.; Fluchel, M.N.; Krikov, S.; Feldkamp, M.L.; Wu, Y.; Goedken, R.; Puzhankara, S.; Romitti, P.A. Cancer risk in children and adolescents with birth defects: A population-based cohort study. *PLoS ONE* **2013** *8*, e69077. [CrossRef] [PubMed]

49. Khairy, P.; Ionescu-Ittu, R.; Mackie, A.S.; Abrahamowicz, M.; Pilote, L.; Marelli, A.J. Changing mortality in congenital heart disease. *J. Am. Coll. Cardiol.* **2010**, *56*, 1149–1157. [CrossRef] [PubMed]
50. Nembhard, W.N.; Salemi, J.L.; Ethen, M.K.; Fixler, D.E.; Dimaggio, A.; Canfield, M.A. Racial/Ethnic disparities in risk of early childhood mortality among children with congenital heart defects. *Pediatrics* **2011**, *127*, e1128–e1138. [CrossRef] [PubMed]
51. Wang, Y.; Liu, G.; Druschel, C.M.; Kirby, R.S. Maternal race/ethnicity and survival experience of children with congenital heart disease. *J. Pediatr.* **2013**, *163*, 1437–1442. [CrossRef] [PubMed]
52. Oster, M.E.; Lee, K.A.; Honein, M.A.; Riehle-Colarusso, T.; Shin, M.; Correa, A. Temporal trends in survival among infants with critical congenital heart defects. *Pediatrics* **2013**, *131*, e1502–e1508. [CrossRef] [PubMed]
53. Arias, E. United States Life Tables, 2009. In *National Vital Statistics Reports*; Centers for Disease Control and Prevention, National Center for Health Statistics, National Vital Statistics System: Atlanta, GA, USA, 2014; Volume 62, pp. 1–63.
54. Larsen, S.H.; Olsen, M.; Emmertsen, K.; Hjortdal, V.E. Interventional treatment of patients with congenital heart disease: Nationwide Danish experience over 39 years. *J. Am. Coll. Cardiol.* **2017**, *69*, 2725–2732. [CrossRef] [PubMed]
55. Gros, B.; Soto Alvarez, J.; Angel Casado, M. Incorporation of future costs in health economic analysis publications: Current situation and recommendations for the future. *Expert Rev. Pharmacoecon. Outcomes Res.* **2015**, *15*, 465–469. [CrossRef] [PubMed]
56. Waitzman, N.J.; Romano, P.S.; Scheffler, R.M. *The Cost of Birth Defects*; University Press of America: Lanham, MD, USA, 1996.
57. Centers for Disease Control and Prevention. Economic costs of birth defects and cerebral palsy—United States, 1992. *Morb. Mortal. Wkly. Rep.* **1995**, *44*, 694–699.
58. Boulet, S.; Grosse, S.; Riehle-Colarusso, T.; Correa-Villasenor, A. Health care costs of congenital heart defects. In *Congenital Heart Defects: From Origin to Treatment*; Wyszynski, D., Graham, T., Correa-Villasenor, A., Eds.; Oxford University Press: New York, NY, USA, 2010; pp. 493–501.
59. Arth, A.C.; Tinker, S.C.; Simeone, R.M.; Ailes, E.C.; Cragan, J.D.; Grosse, S.D. Inpatient hospitalization costs associated with birth defects among persons of all ages—United States, 2013. *Morb. Mortal. Wkly. Rep.* **2017**, *66*, 41–46. [CrossRef] [PubMed]
60. Grosse, S.D.; Berry, R.J.; Tilford, J.M.; Kucik, J.E.; Waitzman, N.J. Retrospective assessment of cost savings from prevention: Folic acid fortification and spina bifida in the US. *Am. J. Prev. Med.* **2016**, *50*, S74–S80. [CrossRef] [PubMed]
61. Simeone, R.M.; Oster, M.E.; Hobbs, C.A.; Robbins, J.M.; Collins, R.T.; Honein, M.A. Population-based study of hospital costs for hospitalizations of infants, children, and adults with a congenital heart defect, Arkansas 2006 to 2011. *Birth Defects Res. A Clin. Mol. Teratol.* **2015**, *103*, 814–820. [CrossRef] [PubMed]
62. Glidewell, J.; Olney, R.S.; Hinton, C.; Pawelski, J.; Sontag, M.; Wood, T.; Kucik, J.E.; Daskalov, R.; Hudson, J. State legislation, regulations, and hospital guidelines for newborn screening for critical congenital heart defects—United States, 2011–2014. *Morb. Mortal. Wkly. Rep.* **2015**, *64*, 625–630.
63. Oster, M.E.; Watkins, S.; Hill, K.D.; Knight, J.H.; Meyer, R.E. Academic outcomes in children with congenital heart defects: A population-based cohort study. *Circ. Cardiovasc. Qual. Outcomes* **2017**, *10*, e003074. [CrossRef] [PubMed]
64. Riehle-Colarusso, T.; Autry, A.; Razzaghi, H.; Boyle, C.A.; Mahle, W.T.; Van Naarden Braun, K.; Correa, A. Congenital heart defects and receipt of special education services. *Pediatrics* **2015**, *136*, 496–504. [CrossRef] [PubMed]
65. Ismail, A.Q.; Cawsey, M.; Ewer, A.K. Newborn pulse oximetry screening in practice. *Arch. Dis. Child. Educ. Pract. Ed.* **2016**, *102*, 155–161. [CrossRef] [PubMed]
66. Oster, M.E.; Aucott, S.W.; Glidewell, J.; Hackell, J.; Kochilas, L.; Martin, G.R.; Phillippi, J.; Pinto, N.M.; Saarinen, A.; Sontag, M.; et al. Lessons learned from newborn screening for critical congenital heart defects. *Pediatrics* **2016**, *137*, e20154573. [CrossRef] [PubMed]
67. Narayen, I.C.; Blom, N.A.; Ewer, A.K.; Vento, M.; Manzoni, P.; te Pas, A.B. Aspects of pulse oximetry screening for critical congenital heart defects: When, how and why? *Arch. Dis. Child. Fetal Neonatal Ed.* **2016**, *101*, F162–F167. [CrossRef] [PubMed]
68. Martin, J.A.; Hamilton, B.E.; Osterman, M.J. Births in the United States, 2015. *NCHS Data Brief* **2016**, 1–8.

21

Expanding Newborn Screening for Pompe Disease in the United States: The NewSTEPs New Disorders Implementation Project, a Resource for New Disorder Implementation

Kshea Hale [1,*], Yvonne Kellar-Guenther [2], Sarah McKasson [3], Sikha Singh [1] and Jelili Ojodu [1]

[1] Association of Public Health Laboratories, Silver Spring, MD 20910, USA; sikha.singh@aphl.org (S.S.); jelili.ojodu@aphl.org (J.O.)

[2] Center for Public Health Innovation, Littleton, CO 80120, USA; ykellar-guenther@ciinternational.com

[3] Colorado School of Public Health, Department of Epidemiology, University of Colorado, Anschutz Medical Campus, Aurora, CO 80045, USA; sarah.mckasson@cuanschutz.edu

* Correspondence: kshea.hale@aphl.org;

Abstract: Public health programs in the United States screen more than four million babies each year for at least 30 genetic disorders. The Health and Human Services (HHS) Advisory Committee on Heritable Disorders in Newborns and Children (ACHDNC) recommends the disorders for state newborn screening (NBS) programs to screen. ACHDNC updated the Recommended Uniform Screening Panel (RUSP) to include Pompe disease in March 2015. To support the expansion of screening for Pompe disease, the Association of Public Health Laboratories (APHL) proposed the Newborn Screening Technical assistance and Evaluation Program (NewSTEPs) New Disorders Implementation Project, funded by the HHS' Health Resources and Services Administration (HRSA) Maternal and Child Health Bureau (MCHB). Through this project, APHL provided financial support to 15 state NBS programs to enable full implementation of screening for Pompe disease. As of 27 April 2020, nine of the 15 programs had fully implemented Pompe disease newborn screening and six programs are currently pursuing implementation. This article will discuss how states advanced to statewide implementation of screening for Pompe disease, the challenges associated with implementing screening for this condition, the lessons learned during the project, and recommendations for implementing screening for Pompe disease.

Keywords: newborn screening; Pompe disease; new disorders implementation

---

1. Introduction

Public health programs in the United States screen more than four million babies each year for at least 30 genetic disorders. Through the newborn screening (NBS) program, states identify newborns at risk for certain metabolic, endocrine, hemoglobin, neuromuscular, and other inherited conditions. To guide this process, the Health and Human Services (HHS) Advisory Committee on Heritable Disorders in Newborns and Children (ACHDNC) recommends the disorders for state NBS programs to screen [1]. Each disorder is selected through a vigorous evidence review process. Once approved, these disorders are included on the Recommended Uniform Screening Panel (RUSP).

There are 35 core disorders on the RUSP, as of April 2020 [2]. ACHDNC updated the RUSP to include Pompe disease in March 2015.

Pompe disease is a multi-systemic lysosomal storage disorder (LSD) caused by a deficiency in the acid alpha glucosidase (GAA) enzyme. This enzyme helps lysosomes breakdown glycogen, a complex sugar, in the body. Without this enzyme, glycogen accumulates in the cells, causing them to lose their ability to function properly. If left untreated, babies born with the most severe form of Pompe disease die within their first year of life [3]. In the United States, Pompe disease affects approximately one in 40,000 births. Implementing NBS for Pompe disease allows babies with the disorder to be identified and linked to care, often before symptoms arise. As of April 2020, 23 states in the US screen for Pompe disease, nine of which received direct funding and technical assistance from the Association of Public Health Laboratories (APHL) to implement screening for Pompe disease.

To implement universal screening for Pompe disease, there are many factors for state NBS programs to consider. This includes determining the cost to screen for the disorder, gaining legislative and funding approval to screen, securing fee increases if necessary, selecting a technology and methodology to screen, expanding laboratory space and capacity, acquiring the appropriate equipment, hiring laboratory and follow-up staff, and developing and implementing education initiatives for the public and for clinical providers. While these factors are important for the addition of all new disorders to state screening panels, Pompe disease introduced unique considerations for the newborn screening system. States screening for this disorder must consider establishing algorithms for the detection of infantile Pompe disease in distinction from late onset Pompe disease, defining the duration of short term follow up and late onset Pompe disease and defining the role of NBS in long term follow up (LTFU) for individuals identified with the disorder.

2. Methods

APHL was awarded a cooperative agreement from the HHS' Health Resources and Services Administration (HRSA) Maternal and Child Health Bureau (MCHB) to expand the ability of state NBS programs to screen for Pompe disease. Through the New Disorders Implementation Project, the APHL Newborn Screening Technical assistance and Evaluation Program (NewSTEPs) provided financial support over the course of three years to 15 state NBS programs to enable and accelerate full implementation of newborn screening for Pompe disease [4].

APHL also selected and funded three additional states to serve as Peer Network Resources Centers (PNRCs) during the course of the New Disorders Implementation Project. The PNRCs served as content area experts providing technical assistance and training regarding laboratory techniques, follow-up procedures, and educational processes related to Pompe disease, as well as for other new disorders screening as needed. Each state NBS program and PNRC applied to participate in the project through a competitive request for proposals (RFP) and a subsequent evaluation process. In the RFP, NewSTEPs proposed a four-phase model to stratify the NBS implementation process, as seen in Figure 1 [5]. In their RFP response, each state program indicated where they were in the implementation of screening for Pompe disease, which other new disorders they were seeking support for, what they hoped to accomplish with this funding opportunity, and how they would use the funding.

The 15 participating state NBS programs provided a combination of monthly and annual progress reports where they described activities and progress toward full implementation and also participated in monthly calls with NewSTEPs staff to track and describe their activities and indicate their successes, challenges, needs, lessons learned, and recommendations.

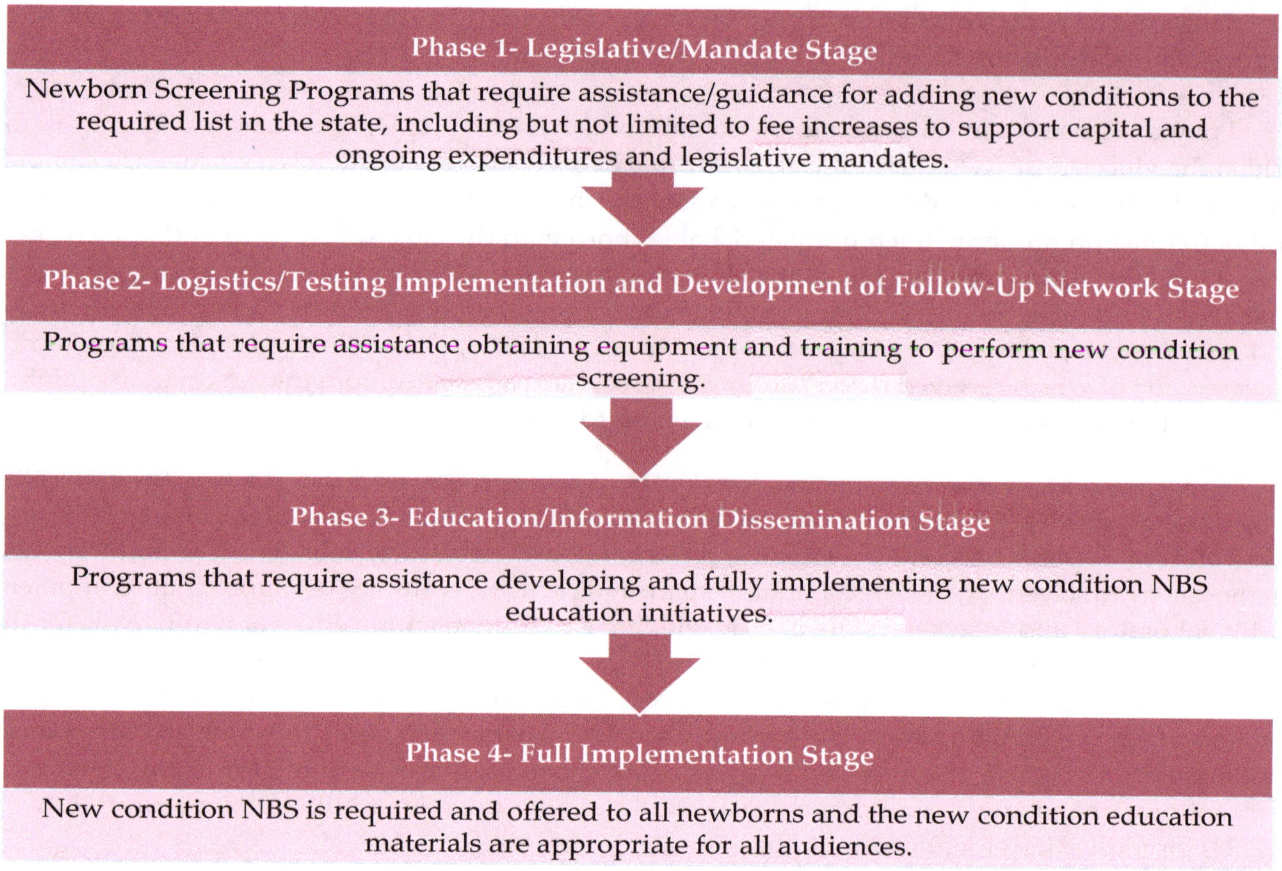

Figure 1. Phases of Implementation for New Disorders Newborn Screening.

3. Results

Of the 15 funded state newborn screening programs, nine were also funded to implement screening for Mucopolysaccharidosis type I (MPS I) and X-linked adrenoleukodystrophy (X-ALD) simultaneously with Pompe disease and six were funded to implement MPS I simultaneously with Pompe disease.

Additionally, the 15 funded programs set varied project goals and objectives to move them toward full implementation of screening for Pompe disease during the funding period. A summary of these goals are found in Table 1.

Table 1. Goals being pursued by the 15 Association of Public Health Laboratories (APHL) funded states for Pompe disease newborn screening implementation.

Project Goals for Pompe Disease Implementation	Number of States (% of Total, $n = 15$)
Full implementation of population screening	5 (33%)
Implementation of education or follow-up activities	4 (27%)
Validation activities and pilot screening	6 (40%)

3.1. Progress toward Pompe Disease NBS Implementation

Upon initiation of the funded project, two of the 15 state NBS programs were working on Phase 1 (Figure 1) to obtain approval and secure fee increases from their NBS Advisory Committee, Board of Health Commissioner, and/or State Budget Authority to screen for Pompe disease.

Upon initiation of the funding project, nine state NBS programs reported that they were working on Phase 2 (Figure 1) toward ensuring infrastructure and staffing readiness for Pompe disease newborn screening. Activities during this time included identifying screening methodologies, acquiring equipment, developing algorithms and protocols for screening, determining cut-off values for analysis, establishing contracts with medical specialists and treatment centers, developing long-term follow-up programs, pursuing assay validation, and integrating Pompe disease reporting features into their Laboratory Information Management Systems (LIMS).

Upon initiation of funding, three state NBS programs reported that they would be working toward Phase 2 (Figure 1) in securing infrastructure and staffing readiness simultaneously with Phase 3 (Figure 1) in developing educational materials for providers, families, and the general public as well as implementing educational and outreach activities.

Upon initiation of funding, only one state NBS program reported that they would be engaging in Phase 1, Phase 2, and Phase 3 (Figure 1) simultaneously.

In their applications, 10 state NBS programs anticipated that they would have implemented Pompe disease screening at the end of the project period, one program anticipated that they would have entered Phase 3 (Figure 1), and two programs anticipated that they would have entered Phase 2 (Figure 1) at the conclusion of the funding period.

3.2. *How States Advanced to Statewide Implementation of Screening for Pompe Disease*

Participating state NBS programs utilized funding from the NewSTEPs New Disorder Implementation Project to purchase equipment and supplies, develop and translate educational materials, develop a statewide outreach program, host a community engagement event, hire laboratory and follow-up personnel, purchase software for sequence analysis, travel to professional meetings or to PNRCs for training, configure LSDs workflow in Laboratory Information Management Systems (LIMS), and develop a long-term follow-up program (Table 2).

Table 2. Utilization of funding by states to implement screening for Pompe disease.

Project Expenses	Number of States (n = 15)
Equipment and supplies	2
Staffing	1
Educational activities	0
Travel	0
Other expenses	0
Equipment, supplies, and travel	2
Equipment, supplies, and educational activities	1
Staffing, travel, educational activities, and other expenses	2
Equipment, supplies, staffing, educational activities, and other expenses	2
Equipment, supplies, staffing, travel, educational activities, and other expenses	3
Equipment, supplies, travel, educational activities, and other expenses	1
Equipment, supplies, staffing, and other expenses	1

Each program engaged at least one PNRC for technical assistance during the project. The PNRCs provided states with LSD standard operating procedures and algorithms, sample panels for validation, technical assistance around LSD test validation, LSD cost data, comparison analysis, second-tier testing guidance for Pompe disease, DNA sequence analyses for Pompe disease, and Pompe disease related educational materials for primary care providers and parents. The PNRCs also retested abnormal LSDs for state programs. One PNRC hosted an annual Tandem Mass Spectrometry, DNA Sequencing, and a Follow-up hands-on workshop. Another program prepared Pompe disease follow-up flow diagrams. State NBS programs also visited PNRCs for direct one-on-one-training to learn laboratory and follow up best practices and to observe processes.

As of 27 April, 2020, nine of the 15 programs that participated in the project had fully implemented Pompe disease newborn screening, offering the screening universally to all newborns in the following states: California, Michigan, Minnesota, Nebraska, New Jersey, Ohio, Tennessee, Virginia, and Washington. The other six programs are currently pursuing screening implementation for Pompe disease.

Programs participating in the NewSTEPs New Disorders Implementation project to implement Pompe Disease Newborn Screening also achieved the following milestones during the course of the funding period: created and deployed an online education module for providers and parents, educated 500 health care professional across the state regarding Pompe disease, implemented second-tier testing for Pompe disease, developed a follow-up quality improvement plan, and hosted a successful deliberative community engagement event.

It is important to note that while the activities for the 15 state newborn screening programs highlighted here are specific to their pursuit of Pompe disease newborn screening, additional disorders (MPS I and x-ALD) were also pursued by a number of these programs. There are several aspects of the newborn screening multiplexing of the screening assay, development of educational materials, and training of implementation activities described above that are generalizable to these other disorders, including laboratory and follow-up staff, establishment of reporting algorithms, among others.

4. Challenges

The participating state NBS programs faced several challenges implementing screening for Pompe disease. As noted above, while many barriers and challenges in implementing newborn screening are generalizable to multiple disorders, the challenges presented below are articulated by the 15 newborn screening programs pursuing Pompe disease newborn screening during the course of the NewSTEPs New Disorders Implementation Project. These challenges are as follows (Table 3):

Table 3. Challenges reported by participating state newborn screening programs when implementing Pompe Disease Newborn Screening during the course of the NewSTEPs New Disorder Implementation Project.

Challenge	Reason Provided
Hiring	Lengthy in-state human resources approval processes Lack of qualified applicants to perform enzyme activity detection and/or genetic testing Lack of qualified applicants to analyze results and perform risk assessments for the various stages of Pompe disease onset
Retention of Staff	Availability of more lucrative positions elsewhere Staff retirements coupled with lack of backfilling these vacancies
Procurement Delays	Complicated and time-consuming state procurement processes Delays by the state procurement office in establishing contracts with vendors to purchase reagents and lease instrumentation to perform the assay for Pompe disease
Instrumentation Challenges	New instrumentation did not perform as expected
Infrastructure Challenges	Delays in the construction of adequate laboratory space to house instrumentation required for the addition of Pompe disease newborn screening
Information Technology	Delays by vendors to complete upgrades to Laboratory Information Management Systems (LIMS) to accommodate results reporting and messaging for newly added disorder (Pompe disease) to the workflow Time and expense involved in gathering system requirements and working with Information Technology (IT) developers and informatics support to modify LIMS and vendor specific software
Clinical Follow-up	The pediatric community and other healthcare providers who would be responsible for caring for babies with an abnormal result have limited knowledge regarding Pompe disease

5. Lessons Learned

When implementing screening for Pompe disease the participating state newborn screening programs recommended allowing for sufficient time to accomplish procurement of instrumentation required for first tier detection of GAA enzyme activity. Multiple methodologies exist to perform a Pompe disease newborn screening assay, including the use of digital microfluidics or tandem mass spectrometry, and programs recommended building in sufficient time to identify the methodology to use [6]. In addition, delays should be anticipated when performing building and space modifications to accommodate Pompe disease newborn screening into the existing workflow. In order to address these delays associated with introducing Pompe disease newborn screening, while maintaining existing quality practices, adequate staffing should be available.

Before implementing full population screening for Pompe disease, the participating states noted that NBS programs should determine second-tier needs, address special populations since these infants can potentially influence the determination of cut-off values for assay analysis and may require repeat screening, and ensure LIMS integration is complete. The introduction of Pompe disease newborn screening can increase the workload for all staff involved in the testing and reporting process, therefore affecting communication with providers.

6. Recommendations

At the end of the NewSTEPs New Disorder Implementation Project, the participating state NBS programs provided recommendations for implementing newborn screening for Pompe disease. The recommendations included participating in APHL NewSTEPs committees and in-person meetings to collaborate and connect with other programs and NBS stakeholders, creating standardized educational materials and long-term follow-up strategies that can be modified for state-specific use, and ensuring that all state stakeholders including pediatric subspecialties and parent representatives are involved in discussing all plans for implementation. Other recommendations include adding second-tier screening to reduce false positives and monitoring screening outcomes and refining cut-off reporting algorithms. Prior to implementing second-tier screening or refining cut-offs, states' programs screening for Pompe disease using tandem mass spectrometry or digital microfluidics reported higher than expected false positive and referral rates, increasing the patient load at NBS follow-up coordinating and genetic centers. Implementing second-tier testing and refining cut-offs reduced false positive and referral rates. Participating state NBS programs also recommended developing long-term follow-up guidelines for cases of Late Onset Pompe Disease (LOPD).

7. Conclusions

The ACHDNC updated the RUSP to include Pompe disease in March 2015. To support the expansion of newborn screening across the United States for Pompe disease, APHL proposed the NewSTEPs New Disorders Implementation Project, funded by HRSA. Through this project, 15 state NBS programs received direct funding through a competitive RFP process to implement screening for Pompe disease and all states had access to technical assistance and training via PNRCs. To provide further support to state NBS programs with the implementation of Pompe disease, APHL hosted national meetings to provide a platform for state programs to share their experiences implementing screening, hosted disease-specific webinars, and convened a NewSTEPs New Disorders Workgroup to serve as educational experts. As a result of the project, all states had access to information and resources regarding Pompe disease screening implementation.

To ensure that all states have the capacity to screen for Pompe disease and newborns living with this disorder are identified and linked to care, APHL will continue to provide support through technical assistance, training, webinars, quality improvement initiatives, and national meetings.

Author Contributions: Conceptualization, S.S., Y.K.-G., and J.O.; methodology, K.H. and Y.K.-G.; data curation, K.H.; writing—original draft preparation, K.H. and S.S.; writing—review and editing, K.H., S.S., Y.K.-G., J.O., and S.M.; visualization, K.H. and S.M.; supervision, S.S.; project administration, K.H.; funding acquisition, J.O. All authors have read and agreed to the published version of the manuscript.

Acknowledgments: The information in this article is based on participation from NBS programs in the following states/territories: California, Florida, Georgia, Iowa, Michigan, Minnesota, Missouri, Nebraska, New Jersey, New York, North Carolina, Ohio, South Carolina, Tennessee, Utah, Virginia, Washington, and Wisconsin.

References

1. Health Resources and Services Administration. Advisory Committee on Heritable Disorders in Newborns and Children. Available online: https://www.hrsa.gov/advisory-committees/heritable-disorders/index.html (accessed on 7 May 2020).
2. Health Resources and Services Administration. Recommended Uniform Screening Panel. Available online: https://www.hrsa.gov/advisory-committees/heritable-disorders/rusp/index.html (accessed on 7 May 2020).
3. National Institutes of Health; U.S. National Library of Medicine. Pompe Disease. Available online: https://ghr.nlm.nih.gov/condition/pompe-disease (accessed on 26 November 2019).
4. Ojodu, J.; Singh, S.; Kellar-Guenther, Y.; Yusuf, C.; Jones, E.; Wood, T.; Baker, M.; Sontag, M.K. NewSTEPs: The Establishment of a National Newborn Screening Technical Assistance Resource Center. *Int. J. Neonatal Screen.* **2018**, *4*, 1. [CrossRef]
5. APHL. Request for Proposals (RFP): Support for Newborn Screening Implementation of New RUSP Disorders. Available online: https://www.aphl.org/rfp/Documents/2017_RFP_Y02%20_New_Disorders_Project_Aug%202017.pdf (accessed on 7 May 2020).
6. Millington, D.S.; Bali, D.S. Current State of the Art of Newborn Screening for Lysosomal Storage Disorders. *Int. J. Neonatal Screen.* **2018**, *4*, 24. [CrossRef]

22

Newborn Screening for SCD in the USA and Canada

Nura El-Haj and Carolyn C. Hoppe *

Department of Hematology-Oncology, UCSF Benioff Children's Hospital Oakland, Oakland, CA 94609, USA; nelhaj@mail.cho.org
* Correspondence: choppe@mail.cho.org;

Abstract: Sickle cell disease (SCD) encompasses a group of inherited red cell disorders characterized by an abnormal hemoglobin, Hb S. The most common forms of SCD in the United States and Canada are identified through universal newborn screening (NBS) programs. Now carried out in all fifty U.S. states and 8 Canadian provinces, NBS for SCD represents one of the major public health advances in North America. The current status of NBS programs for hemoglobinopathies and the screening techniques employed in many regions worldwide reflect in large part the U.S. and Canadian experiences. Although the structure, screening algorithms and laboratory procedures, as well as reporting and follow up, vary between NBS programs, the overall workflow is similar. The current review summarized the historical background, current approaches, and methods used to screen newborns for SCD in the United States and Canada.

Keywords: hemoglobinopathies; newborn screening; methods; review

---

1. Introduction

Sickle cell disease (SCD) refers to a clinically heterogeneous group of disorders characterized by a structurally abnormal hemoglobin, hemoglobin S (Hb S), inherited in either a homozygous fashion (Hb SS) or in combination with other Hb variants (e.g., Hb SC, Hb SD, Hb S/O-Arab) or a beta thalassemia mutation (Hb S/beta thalassemia).

Under hypoxic conditions, Hb S polymerizes causing red blood cells to become rigid and deformable [1]. These sickled red blood cells adhere to the vascular endothelium, as well as circulating blood cells, leading to vaso-occlusion and impaired tissue oxygenation [2]. Repeated sickling also damages the red blood cell membrane, resulting in a chronic hemolytic anemia.

Elevated levels of fetal hemoglobin (Hb F) normally present at birth prevent Hb S polymerization and hemolysis and protect affected newborns from complications. As Hb F becomes replaced by Hb S in the first few months of life infants with sickle cell disease (SCD) become at risk for life-threatening complications associated with sickling and hemolysis. These complications, including infection and acute splenic sequestration, are associated with increased morbidity and mortality in the first five years of life [3].

In the USA and Canada, the rationale for newborn hemoglobinopathy screening is based on the benefit provided by penicillin prophylaxis against life-threatening pneumococcal infection in infants with SCD [4]. Since implementation of universal NBS for SCD in the United States, mortality has decreased by 50% in affected children ages 1 to 4 years, and the overall life expectancy has increased from a median of 14.3 years to between 42 and 53 years in males, and between 46 to 58.5 years in females [5]. Additional benefits of NBS include prompt clinical intervention for infection or splenic sequestration episodes, and early education of caretakers about the signs and symptoms of illness in infancy and early childhood [6]. Early parent education on assessment of spleen size reduced mortality due to splenic sequestration by nearly 10-fold in an observational study [7]. Moreover, in a 7-year follow up study, NBS was found to be most effective in reducing mortality when coupled with comprehensive medical care and parent education [5,8].In addition to the public health impact on affected infants, NBS carries the added benefit of identifying at-risk couples, providing the opportunity for genetic counseling regarding options for future pregnancies.

2. Epidemiology

SCD affects over 300,000 newborns per year worldwide [9]. Although hemoglobin disorders are most prevalent in sub-Saharan Africa, throughout Asia, the Middle East, and around the Mediterranean, population migration from these regions has changed the demographic landscape in North America, where the carrier rates for SCD and other hemoglobin disorders have increased in recent years [10]. Contemporary national data regarding the overall prevalence of sickle cell disease in the United States is lacking. However, data derived from the U.S. Census and NBS programs estimates a sickle cell carrier frequency of 8–10% in African-Americans and 0.6% in Hispanics, respectively, and an overall disease prevalence of 100,000 Americans [11].

Using national birth cohort data spanning the 20-year period from 1991–2010, Therrell et al. reported an overall annual birth prevalence of 1:1941 across the USA [12]. Although the absolute number of affected births is lower in Canada, annual birth prevalence rates of SCD in provinces with large multi-ethnic populations, such as Ontario and Quebec, are similar to those in the USA [13]

In Canada, an estimated 3000 to 5000 individuals are living with SCD, the majority of whom reside in Ontario and Quebec. As in the USA, the estimated annual birth incidence of SCD varies geographically with reported estimates of 1:17,721 births in British Columbia, 1:5650 births in Ontario and 1:1852 births in Quebec with the highest rates of 1:2800 births observed in populations of African, Middle Eastern, and Mediterranean descent [14].

3. History of NBS for SCD

The evolution of NBS for SCD, from the initial discovery of a laboratory test to detect sickle hemoglobin to the development of a complex state-based public health program, has been previously described in detail [15]. An overview of the landmark events leading to NBS for SCD is shown in Figure 1. In the USA, population screening for SCD began in the late 1960's in response to mounting political pressure by African American advocacy groups. Only a few states performed testing for SCD in newborns and only on a selective basis.

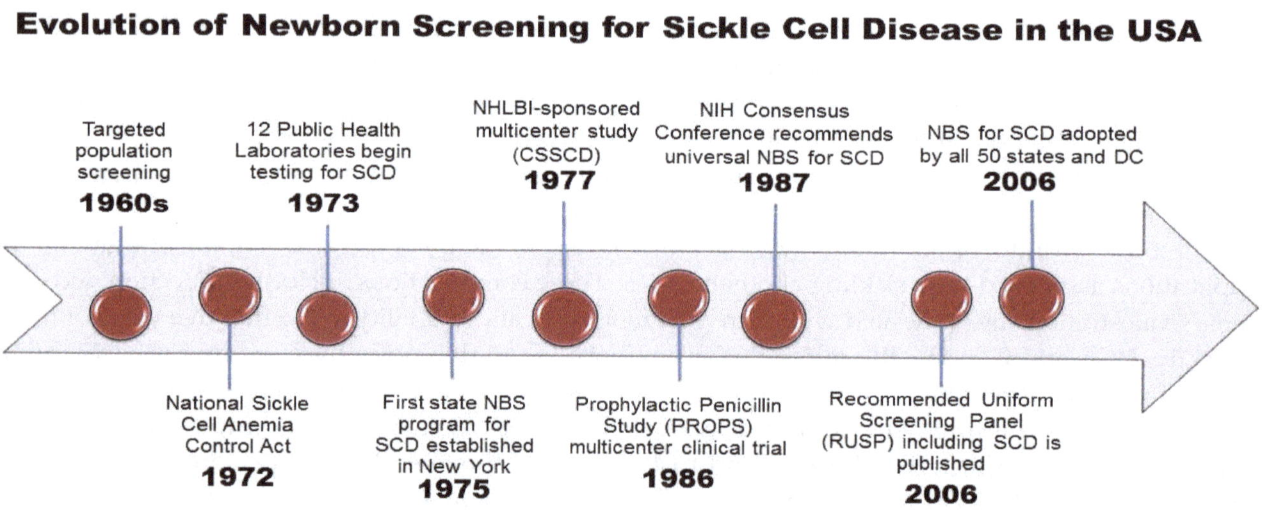

Figure 1. SCD includes Hb SS, Hb S/beta thalassemia and Hb SC genotypes. Abbreviations: ACMG, American College of Medical Genetics; CSSCD, Cooperative Study of Sickle Cell Disease; HHS, Health and Human Services; HRSA, Health Resources and Services Administration; NBS, newborn screening; NHLBI, National Heart, Lung and Blood Institute; NIH, National Institutes of Health; RUSP, Recommended Uniform Screening Panel.

With increasing recognition of SCD as a significant public health issue, Congress passed the National Sickle Cell Anemia Control Act in 1972, which gave authority to establish education, screening, testing, counseling, research, and treatment programs [16]. At the same time, dried blood spots were introduced as an effective method to collect and test blood samples from newborns [17]. By 1973, 12 state public health laboratories had adopted some form of sickle cell screening program and the first statewide NBS program for SCD was established in New York in 1975 [18].

As the first federal program to support a genetic disease, The National Sickle Cell Disease Program funded over 250 general screening programs, 41 sickle cell centers and clinics, as well as 69 research grants and contracts with numerous locally supported screening, education, and counseling clinics [19]. A centralized Hemoglobinopathy Reference Laboratory was also created at the U.S. Centers for Disease Control (CDC) serving as a national resource to assist states in testing for SCD and other hemoglobinopathies, and to provide external proficiency testing and continuing education [20]. After the CDC Hemoglobinopathy Reference Laboratory's closure in 1993, screening and confirmation for all hemoglobin disorders was left to the individual state programs and the proficiency testing program was subsequently transitioned to the Laboratory Quality Assurance Program.

Despite national recognition and federal funding for NBS, states outside of New York, were slow to follow in implementing universal NBS [15,21]. By 1983 only 3 states, New York, Colorado, Texas, had added hemoglobinopathies to the screening panel. The landmark Prophylactic Penicillin Study (PROPS) multicenter clinical trial demonstrating the lifesaving benefit of penicillin prophylaxis against pneumococcal infection in infants and young children with SCD, provided the impetus and justification for universal NBS in the USA [4]. Following publication of this study, the National Institutes of Health convened a consensus conference that resulted in unanimous support for universal NBS for SCD, as mandated by state law [22]. Regionally-centered laboratory services were also recommended in order to improve efficiency and minimize potential errors.

Automated dried blood spot (DBS) punching facilitated expanded screening by significantly reducing the sample preparation time and effort. U.S. and Canadian programs were the first to apply computerized data management to NBS in the 1980s. In 1993, the Agency for Health Care Policy and Research (AHCPR) concluded that NBS for SCD combined with comprehensive health care could significantly reduce infant morbidity and mortality rates, and the agency recommended universal screening rather than targeted screening based on race [23].

By 1999, all but nine states in the USA had implemented universal NBS for SCD. However, there was still no national process to ensure uniformity among states in quality of testing, interpretation of results, or collection of outcome data. In response, the Health Resources and Services Administration commissioned the American College of Medical Genetics to gather expert opinion for a consensus document outlining a core panel of conditions, minimum standards, policies, and procedures for NBS programs nationally [24]. Three SCD genotypes (SS, S/beta thalassemia, and SC) were included in the recommended core panel of state-mandated screening conditions. All other hemoglobinopathies were listed as recommended secondary targets for optional screening. By 2006, all 50 states, the District of Columbia, and many U.S. territories had adopted universal NBS for SCD [15].

Although all NBS programs in the US currently screen for the most common forms of SCD (HbSS, Hb SC, and Hb S/β thalassemia), there is wide variability across states with respect to screening, reporting, and referral of other hemoglobinopathies identified in the course of screening for the core panel conditions. Some states screen for a number of secondary conditions, such as Hb SD, that are concomitantly detected by the screening test methods. A few states have expanded the core screening panel to include clinically relevant non-sickling hemoglobin disorders, such as beta thalassemia and Hb H disease, but most states consider these as secondary screening targets and will refer newborns with a screening test showing a Hb F-only pattern or elevated Bart's hemoglobin for definitive molecular testing [25]. Hemoglobin H disease, an alpha thalassemia disorder prevalent in Southeast Asian, Middle Eastern, and Mediterranean populations, has been given consideration for inclusion as a core condition on the Recommended Uniform Screening Panel (RUSP) RUSP, but lacks sufficient evidence to meet selection criteria [26]

All states require newborn screening, and with the exception of two NBS programs, state statutes that govern screening do not require parental consent. Another 13 states require that parents be informed about NBS prior to testing. All states, except one, allow parents to refuse NBS on religious or personal grounds [27].

Unlike the U.S. where NBS for SCD has been a consideration since 1975, with complete coverage by 2006, screening in Canada was only formalized in one program in 2006, with others slowly coming on board. Targeted screening for SCD began in Quebec in 1988 [13]. The Committee for Development of Newborn Screening for Sickle Cell Disease in Ontario followed in 1989 by launching initiatives and lobbying for universal NBS in Canada. Universal NBS was first implemented in 2006 in Ontario, followed by British Columbia and Yukon in 2009. In 2013, Quebec piloted a universal screening program based on the results from the earlier targeted screening program in Montreal and ultimately implemented a province-wide universal NBS in 2016 [28]. Universal SCD screening is now carried out in 7 Canadian provinces (British Columbia, Ontario, Quebec, New Brunswick, Nova Scotia, Yukon, and Prince Edward Island). Inclusion of SCD on the core NBS panel in Alberta is under consideration pending available funds and service capacity [28].

With no national NBS policy in either the USA or Canada, individual NBS programs screen for a variable number of conditions beyond the recommended core panel, and employ different methods and procedures to carry out screening. Government funding and political support for NBS also vary by region in both countries. Similar to the state governed NBS programs in the USA, universal NBS is under provincial jurisdiction in Canada. Whereas NBS for a recommended core panel of conditions, including SCD, is mandated by individual states in the USA, NBS is considered standard of care in Canada [29]. Moreover, there is no formal province-wide mechanism to document consent, and health care providers are responsible for giving sufficient information to allow parents to make informed decisions, and for documenting parental consent or refusal in the infant's medical record and/or a signed form indicating parent refusal [27].

4. Components of Newborn Screening for SCD

Although logistical aspects, testing methods, and referral policies vary across NBS programs in the United States and Canada, the overarching system for NBS is the same and is comprised of six parts: (1) Education, (2) Screening, (3) Short-Term Follow-Up (STFU), (4) Diagnosis, (5) Management, and (6) Evaluation and Long-Term Follow-Up (LTFU) [30]. NBS programs in both countries follow a similar workflow using newborn DBS specimens, which are tested in specialized screening laboratories and linked to clinical follow-up programs for confirmatory testing and referral to subspecialty comprehensive care [29]. In keeping with national guidelines, state NBS programs in the United States have developed policy and procedure manuals following uniform standards for the performance and documentation of all NBS testing [31].

5. Screening

5.1. Specimen Collection

NBS programs in the United States and Canada have incorporated SCD into the existing laboratory algorithms, and initial screening is now performed in conjunction with testing for other selected congenital disorders. Both countries perform screening using blood spots collected by heel-prick between 24 to 72 h of age, or prior to discharge from the hospital or birthing facility. The timing of collection for repeat blood specimens varies by state. Almost one-third of states require collection of a second sample at age 1–2 weeks [32]. For infants transfused prior to newborn screening, a repeat specimen is recommended between 90 to 120 days after transfusion, unless DNA testing is part of the NBS protocol.

5.2. Specimen Submission

Dried blood spot specimens are sent to a laboratory that is designated by the state or territory within 24–72 h after collection to avoid hemoglobin degradation from prolonged storage and exposure to heat and humidity [33]. Quality checks are performed and the data from the DBS card are entered into a database. Testing is performed within 72 h, typically on the same day the specimen is received in the laboratory.

5.3. Testing Methods

Current methodologies recommended by The Agency for Health Care Policy and Research (AHCPR) for initial and second-tier screening include isoelectric focusing (IEF), high performance liquid chromatography (HPLC), and capillary electrophoresis, which are more sensitive and specific than alkaline and acid gel electrophoresis [34]. Less common screening techniques that are continuing to evolve include tandem mass spectrometry (MS/MS) and various molecular methods [35].

Most NBS programs still use a two-tiered approach, wherein the initial test is followed by a complementary method, such as IEF, HPLC, CE, or dual citrate and cellulose acetate electrophoresis [20]. Alternatively, some NBS laboratories use a modified protocol to improve resolution of the initial test method as the second-tier method. Most NBS laboratories in the US and Canada use HPLC and/or IEF to screen for SCD.

As of 2015, an equal number of NBS laboratories participating in the CDC newborn screen quality assurance proficiency testing program used either HPLC or IEF as the primary screening method [20]. Although HPLC and IEF are highly sensitive and specific, results and interpretation can be confounded by extreme prematurity, previous blood transfusion, or degradation of hemoglobin on the DBS [31].

The increasing availability of automated, reliable, and relatively inexpensive molecular technologies has expanded the use of DNA-based methods for confirmation or definitive diagnosis of NBS results. Molecular techniques can be used either as a second-tier screening method or as a confirmatory test. DNA analysis is performed for second-tier testing in three states (New York, Texas, and Washington). In California, DNA testing on a second specimen is included as part of the screening protocol. In Canada, molecular testing may be requested for NBS results indicating a presumptive β-thalassemia or other genetic variants. Samples are referred to a centralized specialty laboratory for testing at no cost [36].

6. Short Term Follow up

6.1. Primary Screening Results Reporting

As with the provision of NBS laboratory services, follow up and education are also defined by individual NBS programs in both the USA and Canada. Short-term follow up begins with communication of the presumptive positive screening results to the submitting hospital, physician of record, and/or designated NBS follow-up program.

In Canada, all screen-positive test results are reported to the primary care provider, as well as to the provincial Regional Treatment Centers responsible for tracking all presumptive positive cases [36]. The primary care provider (PCP) is given recommendations for the necessary follow up, including initiation of penicillin prophylaxis and is responsible for arranging confirmatory testing on a second liquid blood sample "recall specimen."

A few state NBS programs have incorporated a web-based screening information system allowing follow-up staff at regional coordinating centers and health care providers to directly access the NBS results [37]. This system has been shown to facilitate tracking of positive results and timely enrollment of infants into a comprehensive treatment program.

6.2. *Confirmatory Testing*

All abnormal or unusual screening results require follow-up of the presumptive screen-positive result through a confirmatory testing protocol to verify the screening result. Policies and practices for confirmatory testing of hemoglobinopathies vary by state. Even in cases where molecular testing on the initial NBS specimen has confirmed the likelihood of a disorder, additional testing is necessary to verify the specimen identification, determine the type of SCD, and to prove or disprove an initial result indicating a presumptive hemoglobinopathy of potential clinical significance. A screening result report of "Other" or "Unknown" hemoglobin variant(s) (often abbreviated as "Hb V") usually indicates the presence of a hemoglobin variant for which the proper comparison to a validated control has not been made. In Canada, confirmatory testing of SCD follows a similar pathway, performed on a liquid blood sample, in contracted reference laboratories, using similar laboratory techniques, either HPLC and/or IEF.

In both the US and Canada, abnormal screening results are reported to a dedicated follow-up agency, sickle cell treatment center or provider to ensure that the newborn and the family have access to appropriate follow-up care. Each US state and Canadian province is responsible for directing its follow-up program state involving NBS program staff, primary care providers, hematologists, and genetic counselors [38]

In the USA, the processes and algorithms for notification and follow-up of newborns with confirmed SCD often place the primary care physician as the initial "medical home," which ideally includes specialists with expertise in SCD, as well as families and community-based organizations working in partnership to obtain the comprehensive services needed. Many states have long-standing contracts with academic SCD and thalassemia centers to provide follow-up services [39]. However, the extent of the comprehensive services provided by the "medical home" is variable and often limited by a lack of resources, competing priorities or incomplete understanding of child health quality measures and care [39].

7. Long-term Follow-up

Long term follow-up is part of the quality assurance component of the NBS system, specifically the evaluation of the effectiveness of the NBS follow-up program in ensuring access to treatment and preventive care throughout the lifespan [40]. In both Canada and the US, treatment and follow-up services are delivered through programs that are either government sponsored, private or public-private collaborations [29]. Currently, all states are required to follow established standards for laboratory practices [41]. All laboratories that perform testing for state NBS programs voluntarily participate in the CDC's Newborn Screening Quality Assurance Program (NSQAP) to verify the accuracy of the screening tests performed.

However, many state programs fall short in tracking the long-term data from comprehensive care centers and specialists, and in evaluating the outcomes. The absence of standard case definitions across states has also been identified as a barrier to aggregate data for comparative analyses. To address this challenge, a HRSA-funded data repository, the Newborn Screening Technical assistance and Evaluation Program (NewSTEPs), was created to facilitate data collection using a uniform nomenclature [42]. These case definitions have been piloted, but not yet validated. State NBS programs are encouraged to utilize the case definitions and to enter case data into the repository [42].

The Health Resources and Services Administration (HRSA)-sponsored Registry and Surveillance System for Hemoglobinopathies (RuSH) is another example of a data resource for evaluating the quality of NBS follow-up by linking multiple data sources across seven states for population-level surveillance of newborns and individuals with SCD [43].

8. Challenges of NBS for SCD

Newborn screening has improved the prognosis for individuals with SCD through early intervention measures, such as penicillin prophylaxis and immunization and early education. However, there remain ongoing challenges with regards to the timely follow-up and implementation of comprehensive care [44]. Wide variation in reporting of screening results by states has led to delays in early intervention [38]. Other states have reported gaps in compliance with early medical intervention, parental education, and the provision of comprehensive health services.

As state NBS programs have different systems for capturing data, the use of different case definitions to evaluate the burden and birth prevalence of SCD has been challenging. Federally-sponsored capacity building for long term follow-up data capture is now a focus across many states, using resources to support coordinated data collection and tracking of cohorts of individuals with SCD to evaluate the long term outcomes [45]. While systems linking state NBS programs using common data definitions are in development, there is currently no mechanism linking NBS systems with clinical data systems, nor is there a standardized approach to assess the impact of NBS on health outcomes in children.

Patient registries using medical record linkage with NBS programs are being explored to facilitate the transfer and exchange of information between the NBS program and clinical providers [46]. Health information technology (e.g., electronic medical record exchanges and interoperability standards) provides a tool for consistent data collection, current care practices, and identifying gaps. The costs associated with building this capacity for long term follow-up remains a major challenge. Moreover, the decline in reimbursement for services from public insurance programs has further limited the ability to provide adequate clinical care and education to affected patients [23].

Only a few NBS programs have established activities focused on policy development and system change [47]. Despite the recently published NHLBI evidence-based clinical standards of care for SCD, the available preventative and therapeutic interventions are not reaching the affected individuals [48]. A framework for widespread application of the NHLBI guidelines, using implementation science methods, has been proposed to close the "quality gap" [47].

9. Conclusion

The history of NBS for SCD in the USA and Canada spans many years beginning with the recognition of SCD as a significant public health issue, and the identification of hemoglobinopathies from the same dried blood spot used to screen for other congenital disorders. Many of the screening tests that have become part of routine screening worldwide were initially developed in the U.S. and Canadian laboratories, including hemoglobinopathy testing. In both countries, the components of NBS include a screening process incorporating specimen collection, submission, and a two-tiered testing approach using complementary methods to identify a hemoglobinopathy. However, NBS programs in both countries use different methods of testing and reporting results to public health programs, hospitals, and individual providers, with wide variation in the content and format. Although the implementation of NBS for SCD has led to improved outcomes in children, few studies have evaluated the long-term health outcomes in the growing population of adults with SCD. Efforts to standardize nomenclature and collection of outcomes data through the development of linked registries are a first step in achieving the long-term follow-up goal to ensure appropriate delivery of health care to individuals with SCD identified by the NBS.

Author Contributions: For research articles with several authors, a short paragraph specifying their individual contributions must be provided. The following statements should be used "Conceptualization, N.E.-H. and C.C.H.; Data Curation, N.E.-H.; Writing-Original Draft Preparation, N.E.-H.; Writing-Review & Editing, N.E.-H. and C.C.H.; Supervision, C.C.H.

References

1. Brittenham, G.M.; Schechter, A.N.; Noguchi, C.T. Hemoglobin S polymerization: Primary determinant of the hemolytic and clinical severity of the sickling syndromes. *Blood* **1985**, *65*, 183–189. [PubMed]
2. Frenette, P.S. Sickle cell vaso-occlusion: Multistep and multicellular paradigm. *Curr. Opin. Hematol.* **2002**, *9*, 101–106. [CrossRef] [PubMed]
3. Gill, F.M.; Sleeper, L.A.; Weiner, S.J.; Brown, A.K.; Bellevue, R.; Grover, R.; Pegelow, C.H.; Vichinsky, E. Clinical events in the first decade in a cohort of infants with sickle cell disease. Cooperative Study of Sickle Cell Disease. *Blood* **1995**, *86*, 776–783. [PubMed]
4. Gaston, M.H.; Verter, J.I.; Woods, G.; Pegelow, C.; Kelleher, J.; Presbury, G.; Zarkowsky, H.; Vichinsky, E.; Iyer, R.; Lobel, J.S.; et al. Prophylaxis with oral penicillin in children with sickle cell anemia. A randomized trial. *N. Engl. J. Med.* **1986**, *314*, 1593–1599. [CrossRef] [PubMed]
5. Vichinsky, E.; Hurst, D.; Earles, A.; Kleman, K.; Lubin, B. Newborn screening for sickle cell disease: Effect on mortality. *Pediatrics* **1988**, *81*, 749–755. [PubMed]
6. Frempong, T.; Pearson, H.A. Newborn screening coupled with comprehensive follow-up reduced early mortality of sickle cell disease in Connecticut. *Connect. Med.* **2007**, *71*, 9–12.
7. Emond, A.M.; Collis, R.; Darvill, D.; Higgs, D.R.; Maude, G.H.; Serjeant, G.R. Acute splenic sequestration in homozygous sickle cell disease: Natural history and management. *J. Pediatr.* **1985**, *107*, 201–206. [CrossRef]
8. Vichinsky, E.P. Comprehensive care in sickle cell disease: Its impact on morbidity and mortality. *Semin. Hematol.* **1991**, *28*, 220–226. [PubMed]
9. Piel, F.B. The Present and future global burden of the inherited disorders of hemoglobin. *Hematol. Oncol. Clin. North. Am.* **2016**, *30*, 327–341. [CrossRef] [PubMed]
10. Piel, F.B.; Tatem, A.J.; Huang, Z.; Gupta, S.; Williams, T.N.; Weatherall, D.J. Global migration and the changing distribution of sickle haemoglobin: A quantitative study of temporal trends between 1960 and 2000. *Lancet Glob. Health* **2014**, *2*, e80–e89. [CrossRef]
11. Hassell, K.L. Population estimates of sickle cell disease in the U.S. *Am. J. Prev. Med.* **2010**, *38* (Suppl. 4), S512–S521. [CrossRef] [PubMed]
12. Therrell, B.L., Jr.; Lloyd-Puryear, M.A.; Eckman, J.R.; Mann, M.Y. Newborn screening for sickle cell diseases in the United States: A review of data spanning 2 decades. *Semin. Perinatol.* **2015**, *39*, 238–251. [CrossRef] [PubMed]
13. Robitaille, N.; Delvin, E.E.; Hume, H.A. Newborn screening for sickle cell disease: A 1988-2003 Quebec experience. *Paediatr. Child Health* **2006**, *11*, 223–227. [CrossRef] [PubMed]
14. Davies, C.; Potter, B.K.; Khangura, M.; Hawken, S.; Hawken, J. Epidemiology and health system impact of hemoglobinopathy: Results from Newborn Screening Ontario. 2015 Canadian Newborn and Child Screening Symposium, Ottawa, ON, Canada, 30 April–1 May 2015.
15. Benson, J.M.; Therrell, B.L., Jr. History and current status of newborn screening for hemoglobinopathies. *Semin. Perinatol.* **2010**, *34*, 134–144. [CrossRef] [PubMed]
16. *National Sickle Cell Anemia Control Act*; US Congress: Washington, DC, USA, 1972; Volume 86, p. 136.
17. Garrick, M.D.; Dembure, P.; Guthrie, R. Sickle-cell anemia and other hemoglobinopathies. Procedures and strategy for screening employing spots of blood on filter paper as specimens. *N. Engl. J. Med.* **1973**, *288*, 1265–1268. [CrossRef] [PubMed]
18. Grover, R.; Shahidi, S.; Fisher, B.; Goldberg, D.; Wethers, D. Current sickle cell screening program for newborns in New York City, 1979–1980. *Am. J. Public Health* **1983**, *73*, 249–252. [CrossRef] [PubMed]
19. Schmidt, R.M. Hemoglobinopathy screening: Approaches to diagnosis, education and counseling. *Am. J. Public Health* **1974**, *64*, 799–804. [CrossRef] [PubMed]
20. Laboratories, A.O.P.H. *Hemoglobinopathies: Current Practices for Screening, Confirmation and Follow up*; Centers for Disease Control: Atlanta, GA, USA, 2015.
21. Selekman, J. Update: New guidelines for the treatment of infants with sickle cell disease. Agency for Health Care Policy and Research. *Pediatr. Nurs.* **1993**, *19*, 600–605. [PubMed]
22. Consensus conference. Newborn screening for sickle cell disease and other hemoglobinopathies. *JAMA* **1987**, *258*, 1205–1209. [CrossRef]
23. Smith, J.A.; Kinney, T.R. Sickle cell disease: Screening and management in newborns and infants. Agency for Health Care Policy and Research. *Am. Fam. Phys.* **1993**, *48*, 95–102.

24. Newborn screening: Toward a uniform screening panel and system-executive summary. *Pediatrics* **2006**, *117*, S296–S307. [CrossRef] [PubMed]
25. Calonge, N.; Green, N.S.; Rinaldo, P.; Lloyd-Puryear, M.; Dougherty, D.; Boyle, C.; Watson, M.; Trotter, T.; Terry, S.F.; Howell, R.R.; et al. Committee report: Method for evaluating conditions nominated for population-based screening of newborns and children. *Genet. Med.* **2010**, *12*, 153–159. [CrossRef] [PubMed]
26. Knapp, A.A.; Metterville, D.R.; Kemper, A.R.; Perrin, J.M. *Newborn Screening for Hemoglobin H Disease: A Summary of the Evidence and Advisory Committee Decision*; Health Resources and Services Administration: Rockville, MD, USA, 2010.
27. Hiller, E.H.; Landenburger, G.; Natowicz, M.R. Public participation in medical policy-making and the status of consumer autonomy: The example of newborn-screening programs in the United States. *Am. J. Public Health* **1997**, *87*, 1280–1288. [CrossRef] [PubMed]
28. *Newborn Blood Spot Screening for Galactosemia, Tyrosinemia Type 1, Homocystinuria, Sickle Cell Anemia, Sickle Cell/Beta-Thallassemia, Sickle Cell/Hemoglobin C Disease and Severe Combined Immunodeficiency: Costs and Cost Analysis*; 2016-03; Institute of Health Economics: Edmonton, AB, Canada, 2016.
29. Therrell, B.L.; Adams, J. Newborn screening in North America. *J. Inherit. Metab. Dis.* **2007**, *30*, 447–465. [CrossRef] [PubMed]
30. Therrell, B.L.; Hannon, W.H. National evaluation of US newborn screening system components. *Ment. Retard. Dev. Disabil. Res. Rev.* **2006**, *12*, 236–245. [CrossRef] [PubMed]
31. Campbell, M.; Henthorn, J.S.; Davies, S.C. Evaluation of cation-exchange HPLC compared with isoelectric focusing for neonatal hemoglobinopathy screening. *Clin. Chem.* **1999**, *45*, 969–975. [PubMed]
32. CLSI Document NBS01-A6. *Blood Collection on Filter Paper for Newborn Screening Programs*, 6th ed.; Approved Standard; CLSI: Wayne, PA, USA, 2013.
33. Adam, B.W.; Haynes, C.A.; Chafin, D.L.; De Jesus, V.R. Stabilities of intact hemoglobin molecules and hemoglobin peptides in dried blood samples. *Clin. Chim. Acta* **2014**, *429*, 59–60. [CrossRef] [PubMed]
34. Huisman, T.H. Separation of hemoglobins and hemoglobin chains by high-performance liquid chromatography. *J. Chromatogr.* **1987**, *418*, 277–304. [CrossRef]
35. Boemer, F.; Ketelslegers, O.; Minon, J.M.; Bours, V.; Schoos, R. Newborn screening for sickle cell disease using tandem mass spectrometry. *Clin. Chem.* **2008**, *54*, 2036–2041. [CrossRef] [PubMed]
36. Newborn Screening Ontario. Regional Treatment Centres. Available online: https://www.newbornscreening.on.ca/en/health-care-providers/regional-treatment-centres (accessed on 28 September 2018).
37. Feuchtbaum, L.; Dowray, S.; Lorey, F. The context and approach for the California newborn screening short- and long-term follow-up data system: Preliminary findings. *Genet. Med.* **2010**, *12* (Suppl. 12), S242–S250. [CrossRef]
38. Kavanagh, P.L.; Wang, C.J.; Therrell, B.L.; Sprinz, P.G.; Bauchner, H. Communication of positive newborn screening results for sickle cell disease and sickle cell trait: Variation across states. *Am. J. Med. Genet. Part C Semin. Med. Genet.* **2008**, *148C*, 15–22. [CrossRef] [PubMed]
39. Hinton, C.F.; Feuchtbaum, L.; Kus, C.A.; Kemper, A.R.; Berry, S.A.; Levy-Fisch, J.; Luedtke, J.; Kaye, C.; Boyle, C.A. What questions should newborn screening long-term follow-up be able to answer? A statement of the US Secretary for Health and Human Services' Advisory Committee on Heritable Disorders in Newborns and Children. *Genet. Med.* **2011**, *13*, 861–865. [CrossRef] [PubMed]
40. Kemper, A.R.; Boyle, C.A.; Aceves, J.; Dougherty, D.; Figge, J.; Fisch, J.L.; Hinman, A.R.; Greene, C.L.; Kus, C.A.; Miller, J.; et al. Long-term follow-up after diagnosis resulting from newborn screening: Statement of the US Secretary of Health and Human Services' Advisory Committee on Heritable Disorders and Genetic Diseases in Newborns and Children. *Genet. Med. Off. J. Am. Coll. Med. Genet.* **2008**, *10*, 259–261. [CrossRef] [PubMed]
41. Centers for Disease. Prevention, Good laboratory practices for biochemical genetic testing and newborn screening for inherited metabolic disorders. *MMWR. Recomm. Rep. Morb. Mortal. Wkly. Rep. Recomm. Rep.* **2012**, *61*, 1–44.
42. Sontag, M.K.; Sarkar, D.; Comeau, A.M.; Hassell, K.; Botto, L.D.; Parad, R.; Rose, S.R.; Wintergerst, K.A.; Smith-Whitley, K.; Singh, S.; et al. Case definitions for conditions identified by newborn screening public health surveillance. *Int. J. Neonatal Screen.* **2018**, *4*, 16. [CrossRef] [PubMed]

43. Paulukonis, S.T.; Harris, W.T.; Coates, T.D.; Neumayr, L.; Treadwell, M.; Vichinsky, E.; Feuchtbaum, L.B. Population based surveillance in sickle cell disease: Methods, findings and implications from the California registry and surveillance system in hemoglobinopathies project (RuSH). *Pediatr. Blood Cancer* **2014**, *61*, 2271–2276. [CrossRef] [PubMed]
44. Sox, H.C. Resolving the tension between population health and individual health care. *JAMA* **2013**, *310*, 1933–1934. [CrossRef] [PubMed]
45. Wharton, M.; Chorba, T.L.; Vogt, R.L.; Morse, D.L.; Buehler, J.W. *Case Definitions for Public Health Surveillance*; U.S. Department of Health and Human Services: Atlanta, GA, USA, 1990; pp. 1–43.
46. Wang, Y.; Caggana, M.; Sango-Jordan, M.; Sun, M.; Druschel, C.M. Long-term follow-up of children with confirmed newborn screening disorders using record linkage. *Genet. Med.* **2011**, *13*, 881–886. [CrossRef] [PubMed]
47. DiMartino, L.D.; Baumann, A.A.; Hsu, L.L.; Kanter, J.; Gordeuk, V.R.; Glassberg, J.; Treadwell, M.J.; Melvin, C.L.; Telfair, J.; Klesges, L.M.; et al. The sickle cell disease implementation consortium: Translating evidence-based guidelines into practice for sickle cell disease. *Am. J. Hematol.* **2018**. [CrossRef] [PubMed]
48. Hassell, T.; Hennis, A. Chronic Disease Challenges in the Caribbean. *Glob. Heart* **2016**, *11*, 437–438. [CrossRef] [PubMed]

Permissions

All chapters in this book were first published by MDPI; hereby published with permission under the Creative Commons Attribution License or equivalent. Every chapter published in this book has been scrutinized by our experts. Their significance has been extensively debated. The topics covered herein carry significant findings which will fuel the growth of the discipline. They may even be implemented as practical applications or may be referred to as a beginning point for another development.

The contributors of this book come from diverse backgrounds, making this book a truly international effort. This book will bring forth new frontiers with its revolutionizing research information and detailed analysis of the nascent developments around the world.

We would like to thank all the contributing authors for lending their expertise to make the book truly unique. They have played a crucial role in the development of this book. Without their invaluable contributions this book wouldn't have been possible. They have made vital efforts to compile up to date information on the varied aspects of this subject to make this book a valuable addition to the collection of many professionals and students.

This book was conceptualized with the vision of imparting up-to-date information and advanced data in this field. To ensure the same, a matchless editorial board was set up. Every individual on the board went through rigorous rounds of assessment to prove their worth. After which they invested a large part of their time researching and compiling the most relevant data for our readers.

The editorial board has been involved in producing this book since its inception. They have spent rigorous hours researching and exploring the diverse topics which have resulted in the successful publishing of this book. They have passed on their knowledge of decades through this book. To expedite this challenging task, the publisher supported the team at every step. A small team of assistant editors was also appointed to further simplify the editing procedure and attain best results for the readers.

Apart from the editorial board, the designing team has also invested a significant amount of their time in understanding the subject and creating the most relevant covers. They scrutinized every image to scout for the most suitable representation of the subject and create an appropriate cover for the book.

The publishing team has been an ardent support to the editorial, designing and production team. Their endless efforts to recruit the best for this project, has resulted in the accomplishment of this book. They are a veteran in the field of academics and their pool of knowledge is as vast as their experience in printing. Their expertise and guidance has proved useful at every step. Their uncompromising quality standards have made this book an exceptional effort. Their encouragement from time to time has been an inspiration for everyone.

The publisher and the editorial board hope that this book will prove to be a valuable piece of knowledge for researchers, students, practitioners and scholars across the globe.

List of Contributors

Julia C. van Campen, Elizabeth S. A. Sollars, Rebecca C. Thomas, Clare M. Bartlett, Antonio Milano, Matthew D. Parker, Jennifer Dawe, Peter R. Winship, Gerrard Peck, Darren Grafham, Richard J. Kirk and Ann Dalton
Sheffield Diagnostic Genetics Service (SDGS), Sheffield Children's NHS Foundation Trust, Western Bank, Sheffield S10 2TH, UK

James R. Bonham
Division of Pharmacy, Diagnostics and Genetics, Sheffield Children's NHS Foundation Trust, Western Bank, Sheffield S10 2TH, UK

Anne C. Goodeve
Sheffield Diagnostic Genetics Service (SDGS), Sheffield Children's NHS Foundation Trust, Western Bank, Sheffield S10 2TH, UK
Department of Infection, Immunity & Cardiovascular Disease, Faculty of Medicine, Dentistry & Health, University of Sheffield Medical School, Beech Hill Road, Sheffield S10 2RX, UK

Ilona C. Narayen and Arjan B. te Pas
Department of Paediatrics, Division of Neonatology, Leiden University Medical Center, 2300 RC Leiden, The Netherlands

Nico A. Blom
Division of Paediatric Cardiology, Leiden University Medical Center, 2333 ZA Leiden, The Netherlands

John S. Kim and Christopher M. Rausch
Department of Pediatrics, Heart Institute, Children's Hospital Colorado, University of Colorado School of Medicine, Aurora, CO 80045, USA

Merlin W. Ariefdjohan
Department of Epidemiology, Colorado School of Public Health, University of Colorado Anschutz Medical Campus, Aurora, CO 80045, USA

Marci K. Sontag
Department of Epidemiology, Colorado School of Public Health, University of Colorado Anschutz Medical Campus, Aurora, CO 80045, USA
Center for Public Health Innovation at CI International, Littleton, CO 80120, USA

Ana C. Silva-Pinto
Policy of Integral Attention to People with Sickle Cell Disease (PIAPSCD), Technical Advisory Council for Sickle Cell Disease (TAC-SCD), CGSH/DAET/SAS, Ministry of Health, Asa Norte Brasília 70719-040, Brazil
Regional Blood Center of Ribeirão Preto, HC-FMRP, University of Sao Paulo (USP), Campus Universitário, Ribeirão Preto 14049-900, Brazil

Maria Cândida Alencar de Queiroz
Regional Blood Center of Ribeirão Preto, HC-FMRP, University of Sao Paulo (USP), Campus Universitário, Ribeirão Preto 14049-900, Brazil

Paula Juliana Antoniazzo Zamaro
National Newborn Screening Program Policy (NNSPP)/CGSH/SAS, Ministry of Health, Asa Norte Brasília 70719-040, Brazil

Miranete Arruda
Policy of Integral Attention to People with Sickle Cell Disease (PIAPSCD), Technical Advisory Council for Sickle Cell Disease (TAC-SCD), CGSH/DAET/SAS, Ministry of Health, Asa Norte Brasília 70719-040, Brazil
State Health Secretariat, State of Pernambuco, Recife 50751-530, Brazil

Helena Pimentel dos Santos
Policy of Integral Attention to People with Sickle Cell Disease (PIAPSCD), Technical Advisory Council for Sickle Cell Disease (TAC-SCD), CGSH/DAET/SAS, Ministry of Health, Asa Norte Brasília 70719-040, Brazil
Newborn Screening Program, APAE-Salvador, Salvador 41830-141, Brazil

Joan M. Keutzer
Sanofi Genzyme, Cambridge, MA 02142, USA

Barbara K. Burton and Joel Charrow
Department of Pediatrics, Feinberg School of Medicine of Northwestern University, Chicago, IL 60611, USA
Department of Pediatrics, Ann and Robert H. Lurie Children's Hospital of Chicago, Chicago, IL 60611, USA

Lauren Hitchins and Rachel Hickey
Department of Pediatrics, Ann and Robert H. Lurie Children's Hospital of Chicago, Chicago, IL 60611, USA

George E. Hoganson
Department of Pediatrics, University of Illinois College of Medicine, Chicago, IL 60612, USA

Julie Fleischer and Daniel Groepper
Department of Pediatrics, Southern Illinois University School of Medicine, Springfield, IL 62701, USA

Dorothy K. Grange
Department of Pediatrics, Washington University School of Medicine and St. Louis Children's Hospital, St. Louis, MO 63110, USA

Stephen R. Braddock and Katherine M. Christensen
Department of Pediatrics, Saint Louis University, St. Louis, MO 63104, USA

Heather Shryock and Pamela Smith
Office of Health Promotion, Illinois Department of Public Health, Springfield, IL 62761, USA

Rong Shao and Khaja Basheeruddin
Newborn Screening Laboratory, Illinois Department of Public Health, Chicago, IL 60603, USA

Yvonne Daniel, Cathy Coppinger and Joan Henthorn
Public Health England, NHS Sickle Cell and Thalassemia Screening Programme, London SE16LH, UK

Jacques Elion
Laboratoire d'Excellence GR-Ex, UMR_S1134, Inserm, Université Paris Diderot, Sorbonne Paris Cité, Institut National de la Transfusion Sanguine, 75015 Paris, France

Bichr Allaf
NBS Laboratory for Haemoglobinopathies, Hôpital Universitaire Robert-Debré, 75019 Paris, France

Catherine Badens
Département de génétique médicale, Aix-Marseille Université, Hôpital de la Timone, 13385 Marseille, France

Marelle J. Bouva
National Institute for Public Health and the Environment, Centre for Health Protection, 3720 Bilthoven, The Netherlands

Ian Brincat
Pediatric Medicine Laboratory, Department of Pathology, Mater Dei Hospital, Triq Tal-Qroqq, MSD2090 Msida, Malta

Elena Cela
Department of Pediatric Oncology/Hematology, Hospital Universitario General Gregorio Marañón, Facultad de Medicina, Universidad Complutense Madrid, 28007 Madrid, Spain

Mariane de Montalembert
Department of Pediatrics, Reference Center for Sickle Cell Disease, AP-HP Hôpital Universitaire Necker-Enfants Malades, 75743 Paris, France

Béatrice Gulbis
Department of Clinical Chemistry, Cliniques Universitaires de Bruxelles, Hôpital Erasme—ULB, 1070 Bruxelles, Belgium

Olivier Ketelslegers
Laboratoire—Biologie Clinique, Centre Hospitalier Régional de la Citadelle, 4000 Liège, Belgium

Corrina McMahon
Our Lady's Children's Hospital, Crumlin, D12V004 Dublin, Ireland

Allison Streetly
School of Population Health and Environmental Sciences, Faculty of Life Sciences & Medicine, King's College London, London WC2R2LS, UK
Division of Healthcare Public Health, Health Protection and Medical Directorate, Public Health England, London SE18UG, UK

Raffaella Colombatti
Department of Child and Maternal Health, Clinic of Pediatric Hematology/Oncology, Azienda Ospedaliera-Università di Padova, 35129 Padova, Italy

Stephan Lobitz
Department of Pediatric Oncology/Hematology, Kinderkrankenhaus Amsterdamer Straße, 50735 Cologne, Germany

Elena Cubells, Antonio Nuñez-Ramiro and Isabel Izquierdo
Division of Neonatology, Hospital Universitario y Politécnico La Fe, 46026 Valencia, Spain

Begoña Torres
Instituto de Investigación Sanitaria La Fe, 46026 Valencia, Spain

Manuel Sánchez-Luna
Division of Neonatology, Hospital Universitario Gregorio Marañón, 28007 Madrid, Spain

Máximo Vento
Division of Neonatology, Hospital Universitario y Politécnico La Fe, 46026 Valencia, Spain
Instituto de Investigación Sanitaria La Fe, 46026 Valencia, Spain

Raymond Y. Wang
Division of Metabolic Disorders, CHOC Children's Specialists, Orange, CA 92868, USA
Department of Pediatrics, University of California-Irvine School of Medicine, Orange, CA 92868, USA

Claudia Frömmel
MVZ Alexianer Labor GmbH, Groβe Hamburger Str. 5–11, 10115 Berlin, Germany
Newborn Screening Laboratory, Charité-Universitätsmedizin Berlin, Augustenburger Platz 1, 13353 Berlin, Germany

Rachael E. Armstrong and Kevin W. Southern
Department of Women's and Children's Health, University of Liverpool, Liverpool L12 2AP, UK

Lucy Frith
Institute of Population Health, University of Liverpool, Liverpool L69 3GL, UK

Fiona M. Ulph
Division of Psychology & Mental Health, School of Health Sciences, Faculty of Biology, Medicine and Health, University of Manchester, Manchester Academic Health Science Centre, Manchester M13 9PL, UK

Can Ficicioglu, Rebecca C. Ahrens-Nicklas, Sanmati R. Cuddapah, Brenda S. DiBoscio, Caitlin Menello and Nicole Luongo
Division of Human Genetics/Metabolism, Children's Hospital of Philadelphia, Perelman School of Medicine at the University of Pennsylvania, Philadelphia, PA 19104, USA

Joshua Barch, Nadene Henderson and Damara Ortiz
Department of Pediatrics, Division of Medical Genetics, UPMC Children's Hospital of Pittsburgh, Pittsburgh, PA 15224, USA

James C. DiPerna
PerkinElmer, Mass Spectroscopy Unit, Pittsburgh, PA 15275, USA

Patricia L. Gordon
Division of Human Genetics, Penn State Heath Children's Hospital, Penn State University College of Medicine, Hershey, PA 17033, USA

Mary Heeley and Anthony Heeley
East Anglian Biochemical Genetic Unit, Peterborough, UK

Rui Xiao
Department of Pediatrics, Division of Biostatistics, Children's Hospital of Philadelphia, Philadelphia, PA 19104, USA
Department of Biostatistics, Epidemiology & Informatics, Perelman School of Medicine at the University of Pennsylvania, Philadelphia, PA 19104, USA

Pierre Naubourg, Marven El Osta and Patrick Ducoroy
Biomaneo, 22B boulevard Winston Churchill, F-21000 Dijon, France

David Rageot
CLIPP, Clinical Innovation Proteomic Platform, Université de Bourgogne Franche Comté, F-21000 Dijon, France

Olivier Grunewald, Gilles Renom and Jean-Marc Périni
Newborn Screening Laboratory, Biology and Pathology Center, Lille University Medical Centre, F-59000 Lille, France

Jürg Barben
Division of Paediatric Pulmonology & CF Centre, Children's Hospital of Eastern Switzerland, 9006 St. Gallen, Switzerland

Jane Chudleigh
School of Health Sciences, City, University of London, London EC1V 0HB, UK

Georges Travert
University of Caen Normandy (UNICAEN), 14032 Caen, France
Caen University Hospital, 14040 Caen, France

Anne Bergougnoux
Molecular Genetics Laboratory, CHU Montpellier, EA7402 University of Montpellier, 34093 Montpellier CEDEX 5, France

Maureen Lopez and Emmanuelle Girodon
Molecular Genetics Laboratory, Cochin Hospital, APHP. Centre, University of Paris, 75014 Paris, France

Baba P. D. Inusa
Paediatric Haematology, Evelina London Children's Hospital, Guy's and St Thomas NHS Trust, London SE1 7EH, UK

Lewis L. Hsu
Pediatric Hematology-Oncology, University of Illinois at Chicago, Chicago, IL 60612, USA

Neeraj Kohli
Haematology, Guy's and St Thomas NHS Trust, London SE1 7EH, UK

Anissa Patel
Holborn Medical Centre, GP, London WC1N 3NA, UK

Kilali Ominu-Evbota
Paediatrics Department, Basildon and Thurrock University Hospitals, NHS Foundation Trust, Basildon SS16 5NL, UK

Kofi A. Anie
Haematology and Sickle Cell Centre, London NorthWest University Healthcare NHS Trust, London NW10 7NS, UK

Wale Atoyebi
Department of Clinical Haematology, Cancer and Haematology Centre, Oxford University Hospitals NHS Foundation Trust, Churchill Hospital, Oxford OX3 9DU, UK

Laurie D. Smith
Department of Pediatrics, UNC Hospitals, Chapel Hill, NC 27599, USA
Laboratory Services Division, Baebies, Inc., Durham, NC 27709, USA

Arindam Bhattacharjee
Laboratory Services Division, Baebies, Inc., Durham, NC 27709, USA

Matthew N. Bainbridge
Codified Genomics, Houston, TX 77004, USA
Rady Children's Institute for Genomic Medicine, San Diego, CA 92123, USA

Richard B. Parad
Department of Pediatric Newborn Medicine, Brigham &Women's Hospital, Harvard Medical School, Boston, MA 02115, USA

Natasha Heather and Dianne Webster
National Newborn Metabolic Screening programme, LabPlus, Auckland City Hospital, Auckland 1148, New Zealand
Liggins Institute, University of Auckland, Auckland 1023, New Zealand

Scott D. Grosse and Jill Glidewell
Centers for Disease Control and Prevention, National Center on Birth Defects and Developmental Disabilities, 4770 Buford Highway NE, Mail Stop E-87, Atlanta, GA 30341, USA

Cora Peterson
Centers for Disease Control and Prevention, National Center for Injury Prevention and Control, Atlanta, GA 30341, USA

Rahi Abouk
Cotsakos College of Business, William Paterson University, Wayne, NJ 07470, USA

Matthew E. Oster
Centers for Disease Control and Prevention, National Center on Birth Defects and Developmental Disabilities, 4770 Buford Highway NE, Mail Stop E-87, Atlanta, GA 30341, USA
Children's Healthcare of Atlanta, Emory University School of Medicine, Atlanta, GA 30341, USA

Kshea Hale, Sikha Singh and Jelili Ojodu
Association of Public Health Laboratories, Silver Spring, MD 20910, USA

Yvonne Kellar-Guenther
Center for Public Health Innovation, Littleton, CO 80120, USA

Sarah McKasson
Colorado School of Public Health, Department of Epidemiology, University of Colorado, Anschutz Medical Campus, Aurora, CO 80045, USA

Nura El-Haj and Carolyn C. Hoppe
Department of Hematology-Oncology, UCSF Benioff Children's Hospital Oakland, Oakland, CA 94609, USA

Index

www.ingramcontent.com/pod-product-compliance
Lightning Source LLC
LaVergne TN
LVHW060549210926
848485LV00005B/1284